HEALTH PSYCHOLOGY

Now in its third edition, *Health Psychology* offers the perfect introduction to this rapidly developing field. Clearly explaining the psychological processes that shape health-related behaviours, and affect core functions such as the immune and cardiovascular systems, it shows how these relationships provide the foundation for psychological interventions which can change cognition, perception and behaviour, thereby improving health.

Divided into five parts, the book looks at the biological bases of health and illness, stress and health, coping resources, motivation and behaviour, and applied health psychology. The third edition has been revised to highlight:

- Current research on the biological processes that underpin stress and illness.
- How stress can be best managed at individual, organisational and community levels.
- The ways people's beliefs and attitudes shape motivation and behaviour.
- How health promotion can effectively change beliefs and attitudes to promote health behaviour change.
- The implications of current health psychology research for services.
- How health psychology research can improve healthcare practice.
- Looking at the roles of practitioner health psychologists.

The book is supported by useful in-text features including boxes that highlight key issues, activity boxes and essay questions to engage readers in applying what they have learned from research, and suggestions for further reading to encourage further study.

With its clear structure and ability to eloquently link theory to real-world application, this is the perfect primer for both undergraduates studying health psychology for the first time, and those embarking on postgraduate study in this exciting field.

Charles Abraham is an applied Health Psychologist specialising in translational health research, a registered practising Health Psychologist in the UK and a Professor of Psychology at Deakin University, Melbourne, Australia.

Mark Conner is Professor of Applied Social Psychology at the School of Psychology, University of Leeds, UK.

Fiona Jones is formerly a Visiting Senior Research Fellow in the School of Psychology, University of Leeds, UK.

Daryl O'Connor is Professor of Psychology at the School of Psychology, University of Leeds, UK.

HEALTH PSYCHOLOGY

Third Edition

Charles Abraham,
Mark Conner,
Fiona Jones and
Daryl O'Connor

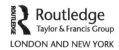

Routledge
Taylor & Francis Group

LONDON AND NEW YORK

Cover Image: Getty Images © Abstract Aerial Art

Third edition published 2024
by Routledge
4 Park Square, Milton Park, Abingdon, Oxon, OX14 4RN

and by Routledge
605 Third Avenue, New York, NY 10158

Routledge is an imprint of the Taylor & Francis Group, an informa business

© 2024 Charles Abraham, Mark Conner, Fiona Jones and Daryl O'Connor

First edition published by Routledge 2008
Second edition published by Routledge 2016

British Library Cataloguing-in-Publication Data
A catalogue record for this book is available from the British Library

Library of Congress Cataloging-in-Publication Data
A catalog record has been requested for this book

ISBN: 978-0-367-77382-3 (hbk)
ISBN: 978-0-367-77381-6 (pbk)
ISBN: 978-1-003-17109-6 (ebk)

DOI: 10.4324/9781003171096

Typeset in Times New Roman
by Apex CoVantage, LLC

CONTENTS

SERIES FOREWORD

Psychology is still one of the most popular subjects for study at undergraduate degree level. As well as providing the student with a range of academic and applied skills that are valued by a broad range of employers, a psychology degree also serves as the basis for subsequent training and a career in professional psychology. A substantial proportion of students entering a degree programme in psychology do so with a subsequent career in applied psychology firmly in mind, and as a result, the number of applied psychology courses available at the undergraduate level has significantly increased over the years. In some cases, these courses supplement core academic areas, and in others, they provide the student with a flavour of what they might experience as a professional psychologist.

The *Topics in Applied Psychology* series consists of eight textbooks designed to provide a comprehensive academic and professional insight into specific areas of professional psychology. These texts cover the areas of clinical psychology, criminal psychology, educational psychology, health psychology, sports and exercise psychology, work and organisational psychology, forensic psychology and counselling psychology, and each text is written and edited by the foremost professional and academic figures in each of these areas.

It's my pleasure to introduce the third edition of the book covering Health Psychology by Charles Abraham, Mark Conner, Fiona Jones and Daryl O'Connor. This new edition has a UK and European perspective but is also relevant to any healthcare system and discusses issues covering both research and practice. It has a substantially revised and updated text throughout, including a comprehensive update on recent research in Health Psychology.

Through successive editions, each textbook is based on a similar academic formula that combines a comprehensive review of cutting-edge research and professional knowledge with accessible teaching and learning features. The books are also structured so they can be used as an integrated teaching support for a one-term or one-semester course in each of their relevant areas of applied psychology. Given the increasing importance of applying psychological knowledge across a growing range of areas of practice, we feel this series is timely and comprehensive. We hope you find each book in the series readable, enlightening, accessible and instructive.

Graham Davey
University of Sussex, Brighton, UK

PREFACE TO THE THIRD EDITION

Health psychology is an area of applied psychological research. It is also a profession in which registered health psychologists offer professional guidance based on health psychology research.

Our beliefs and our interpretations of everyday experiences have direct effects on how our bodies work. For example, stress and worry affects many biological processes including operation of the cardiovascular and immune systems. How we act has major effects on our health. For example, what we eat, how physically active we are and how we sleep have strong effects on health. Psychological research has established *how* cognitions and behaviour patterns affect physiological processes including the cardiovascular, endocrine and immune systems. These physiological processes, in turn, determine symptomatology, morbidity and mortality.

The way we experience everyday life shapes what we do. Perceptions, cognitions and behaviour patterns are strongly influenced by our social interactions. So, health psychology research is inherently biopsychosocial because it concerns psychological, social and biological processes and their interactions.

Health psychology research examines the determinants of *physical* health and illness, as opposed to mental health and illness. Such research is increasingly important. It is clear that health behaviour patterns are critical to health and prevention of illness. It is also clear that, in the absence of effective health promotion, it will become impossible to fund the treatment of those who are ill, including those with long-term illnesses and the elderly. If we cannot encourage populations to look after their health on a daily basis, then comprehensive, and widely accessible health services will become unaffordable.

Health psychology research provides the foundations for future development of health services based on insights into behaviour change and policies that can prompt population-level change. Health services, globally, need to be focused on primary prevention (choosing to act in a way that does not damage health and so avoids illness), secondary prevention (acting to minimise the effects of a health problem, e.g., seeking early diagnosis and adhering to health professionals' advice) and tertiary prevention (when a health problem cannot be cured, acting in a way to minimise increasing physical damage and optimising quality of life).

Health psychology has also developed useful methodological tools to enhance the evidence we can collect from trials of behaviour change and medical treatments. For example, examination of how such interventions work and especially the implications for healthcare professionals' practice. Consequently, there is an increasing need to provide health care professionals with health-psychology-based skills (e.g., knowing how to help people change their behaviour patterns) and to employ health psychologists in healthcare services.

Health psychology is making an important contribution to undergraduate degree programmes (at all levels) and a substantial proportion of undergraduate students (in psychology and applied health) study health psychology.

The purpose of this book is to introduce undergraduate students to health psychology research and to illustrate the links between research and health psychology practice (e.g., in relation to health behaviour change). The book will prepare students for final examinations in health psychology at undergraduate level and provide a solid foundation for students wishing to pursue graduate studies in health psychology. The book has a UK and European perspective but is relevant to any healthcare system. It is divided into five sections: (1) the biological basis of health and illness; (2) stress and health; (3) coping resources: social support and individual differences; (4) motivation and behaviour, focusing on how we can promote motivational and behavioural change and (5) applied health psychology, focusing on professional practice and the delivery of healthcare. Throughout the book, we discuss health-related beliefs and behaviours and explain how psychological processes (e.g., emotional responses) shape health-related behaviour patterns and influence physiological systems such as the immune and cardiovascular systems. These relationships provide the foundation for psychological interventions which can change cognition, motivation, behaviour and physiological functioning.

As with all the books in the *Topics in Applied Psychology* series, this text is written as a support for a one-term or one-semester course. The book contains a range of teaching and learning features such as focus boxes, research methods boxes, activity boxes (supporting students to engage actively with presented material) as well as consideration of issues of contemporary interest (including developments within the UK National Health Service [NHS]). Each chapter also ends with support for further reading, including relevant journal articles and books which will enable the interested student to engage with key topics in more depth.

The aim of this book is to provide the undergraduate, or masters-level, student with a concise, readable, structured introduction to health psychology. We have focused on core topics which define health psychology and linked these so that the text can be read as a continuous course. All of the authors teach health psychology to undergraduates and postgraduates and we hope that, like us, readers will be inspired by the findings of health psychology research and the impact of health psychology practice. The third edition of the book provides an update on this exciting and expanding area of practice and research.

Charles Abraham
Mark Conner
Fiona Jones
Daryl O'Connor
October 2023

1 Introduction

Introduction

This book provides a concise course in health psychology. It is suitable for undergraduate or master's study in psychology or for students of specialist health programmes who want to study evidence-based health psychology and behaviour change.

We discuss the origins and definition of the sub-discipline of health psychology as well as considering evidence identifying processes that affect psychological wellbeing, physiological functioning, health behaviour patterns, behaviour change, health promotion practice, and responses to health services, including adherence to the advice of healthcare professionals. We also envisage new digital health services that may more economically support people to care for their health.

This chapter is divided into five sections.

1. Health Psychology: Brief History and Definition.
2. Research Foundations of Health Psychology: A Biopsychosocial Model of Health.
3. Behavioural Patterns, Lifestyle and Health.
4. Using this Book Effectively.
5. The Structure and Content of this Book.

Learning outcomes

When you have completed this chapter you should be able to:

1. Define and describe the discipline and profession of health psychology.
2. Identify psychological sub-disciplines which contribute to health psychology research and practice.
3. Explain what is meant by the biopsychosocial model of health and illness.
4. Summarise evidence demonstrating the importance of behavioural patterns to individual and public health and explain why this makes the development of effective behaviour-change interventions essential to the maintenance of healthcare systems.
5. Understand how this book is structured and how to study it effectively.

DOI: 10.4324/9781003171096-1

Health psychology: Brief history and definition

Hippocrates is credited with the establishment of the medical professional and the Hippocratic Oath. He was born around 460 BC on the Greek island of Kos and sought to understand the processes that cause a variety of illnesses. While the search for causal processes seems self-evident to us it was a formative step in the development of scientific medicine. Hippocrates also linked behaviour patterns, including diet, to health and emphasised the importance of the relationship between healer (or healthcare professional) and patient. These topics remain active areas of health psychology research today.

More than half a millennium later, in the 2nd century AD, the Greek leader Diogenes commissioned a low wall in the city of Oenoanda in Lycia which was etched with core messages taken from the teachings of the philosopher Epicurus (https://en.wikipedia.org/wiki/Diogenes_of_Oenoanda). The wall included 25,000 words written over 260 square meters and emphasised the importance of quality of life, self-reflection and self-management (see Chapter 11). This wall was a very early public health campaign designed to enhance the quality of life of the general population. Nearly 2,000 years later, we are still designing and evaluating such interventions (see Chapters 8 and 9 on promoting health motivation and behaviour). Of course, today, we have more accessible and interactive media including websites, podcasts and smartphones (see Chapter 11 on digital healthcare services).

William James (1842–1910), was an eminent philosopher who is often credited with the establishment of psychology. He trained as a medical practitioner and taught anatomy at Harvard University. Wilhelm Wundt (1832–1920) was also one of the founders of scientific psychology. He established the first experimental psychological laboratory at the University of Leipzig in 1879. Wundt was trained as a medical practitioner at Heidelberg University. The challenges and concerns which define health psychology are millennia old and are intricately interwoven into the development of medicine and public health.

In the late 20th century, a range of public health studies, undertaken mostly in the USA, began to emphasise the link between behaviour patterns, or lifestyle (e.g., Becker, Drachman & Kirscht, 1974) and the importance of interpersonal relationships to well-being (Horne & Rosenthal, 1997).

Accumulation of such research and a growing interest in applying insights into how psychological processes and behaviour patterns shape health led to the establishment of Division 38 (Health Psychology) of the American Psychological Association (APA), in the USA. Professor Joe Matarazzo was the first president of Division 38. Later, in the UK, following the creation of a Special Group in Health Psychology, a Division of Health Psychology was established within the British Psychological Society (BPS) in 1997, with Professor Charles Abraham as the first chairperson (Quinn, Chater & Morrison, 2020). The European Health Psychology Society (EHPS) was established in 1986 in Tilberg. Many other nations have established professional health psychology organisations and, in some cases, these have led to accredited training courses for practising health psychologists. Today, Health Psychology is both a research sub-discipline of psychology and a distinct practitioner training route, internationally.

The establishment of Health Psychology organisations facilitated high-quality peer-reviewed research and research-based courses to train professional health psychologists worldwide (see Chapter 10 on training in the UK and Europe). These organisations also provide a focus for research and research collaboration by arranging conferences and sponsoring academic journals.

For example, the journal *Health Psychology* is published by the APA, *Psychology and Health*, and *Health Psychology Review*, are published by the EHPS and the *British Journal of Health Psychology* is published by the BPS. Other journals publishing health psychology research include: the *Journal of Behavioral Medicine, Preventive Medicine, Social Science and Medicine, Journal of Health Psychology, Health Education Research, Patient Education and Counselling, Annals of Behavioral Medicine*, and *Psychology, Health and Medicine*.

As president of Division 38, Professor Matarazzo (1982) offered a helpful definition of health psychology which has been used internationally:

> *Health psychology is an aggregate of the educational, scientific and professional contributions of the discipline of psychology to the promotion and maintenance of health, the prevention and treatment of illness, the identification of etiologic and diagnostic correlates of health, illness and related dysfunction and the improvement of the health care system and health policy formation.*

This much-cited definition highlights: (1) the overarching aims of the sub-discipline, namely, promoting health and preventing illness; (2) the scientific focus of research in health psychology, that is, understanding the causes of illness and categorisation of illnesses in terms of underlying psychological, behavioural and biological processes; and (3) the key priorities of professional practice in health psychology, that is, improving healthcare by studying healthcare delivery systems, practising within such services and contributing to health-related policy development.

Health been defined by the World Health Organization as:

> *a state of complete physical, mental and social well-being and not merely the absence of disease or infirmity.*

> (WHO, 1948)

This definition, which has not been amended since 1948, challenges psychologists to define and assess the determinants of "physical, mental and social wellbeing". So, when we discuss "health" in health psychology we rarely focus on physical health alone.

Health psychologists seek to understand the processes which link individual beliefs and behaviours to biological processes which, in turn, result in health and illness. These causal mappings sometimes point to novel ways in which illness can be ameliorated or cured. For example, how a person perceives work demands and copes with them will determine his/her stress levels (see Chapter 3) which, in turn, may affect the functioning of the cardiovascular and immune systems (see Chapter 2). Health psychologists also study social processes including the effect of wider social structure (such as socioeconomic status) and face-to-face interactions with others (e.g., work colleagues) because these social processes shape perceptions, beliefs and behaviour (see Chapters 4 and 10). In addition, health psychologists explore individual processes that shape health outcomes and health behaviour patterns (see Chapters 6 and 7) as well as social processes which influence the effectiveness of health care delivery (see Chapter 10). For example, the way healthcare professionals communicate with their patients influences patient behaviour, including patients' willingness to take medication and adopt health-enhancing behaviours (see Chapters 8 and 10). Most health and medical interventions depend on the behaviour of healthcare professionals and, importantly, on the behaviour of patients and citizens. Behavioural regulation and behaviour change are, therefore, central to health and, importantly, limit the potential of healthcare delivery. A nurse who prescribes an effective medication to a patient with asthma has taken a first step towards helping that patient manage their long-term illness but if they are not persuaded to take the medication the consultation has no impact on the health of the patient (see Chapter 10). The mission begun by Hippocrates remains critical to applied health psychology today.

Research foundations of health psychology: a biopsychosocial model of health

Research facilitates development of an accurate understanding of causal processes. This establishes an evidence base for the design of interventions capable of changing causal processes, including psychological functioning (see Chapter 8) and behaviour patterns (see Chapter 9). This, in turn, enables us to provide guidance that can enhance the effectiveness and cost effectiveness of health care services. Professional health psychologists use research findings to assess individuals and to design and evaluate interventions which can change perceptions, beliefs, behaviours and social relationships. These effects, in turn, shape health-related behaviour patterns, quality of life and physical health. Interventions operate at different levels ranging from those focusing on the individual to those designed to change society; targeting, on the one hand, individual health and, on the other, public health (see Chapter 11).

Modern medicine is founded on basic research that revealed biological processes which constitute health and illness. Painstaking studies of human physiology over many centuries together with key scientific breakthroughs provide the foundation for understanding how the body's systems work. Breakthroughs included understanding the nature of respiration, clarifying that specific bacteria cause particular illness, discovering compounds that kill bacteria, and revealing how vaccination works. Such research continues but we already have good models of how physiological systems (such as the immune and cardiovascular systems) operate. It is these models that allow effective medical intervention through diagnosis and treatment. A good example, was the rapid development of COVID-19 vaccines during the pandemic. These breakthroughs were built on decades of research into immune functioning and the process of vaccine development. This research, in turn, may facilitate faster future development of vaccines (Ball, 2021).

The science of health psychology has important contributions to make to healthcare and public health because we now know that psychological processes and behaviour patterns affect the operation of bodily systems and are important determinants of population-level health and illness.

Health psychology also has its origins in early cognitive and social psychology as well as behaviourism. In the early part of the 20th century, learning theorists including Pavlov, Watson and Skinner established the behaviourist school of psychology which focused on observable behaviour and on learning (e.g., through classical and operant conditioning; Skinner, 1974). The success of behaviourism in explaining behaviour and providing tools with which to change behaviour was critical to the recognition that professional psychology had an important contribution to make to the management of behaviour relevant to mental and physical health. The role of learning theory in health behaviour change interventions remains an interesting topic (Hegel, Ayllon, Thiel & Oulton, 1992).

Wundt studied internal individual processes including attention and use of imagery. Later work clarified that even when explaining how rats learn to run mazes we require a psychology of internal representation. Tolman (1948) found that rats learned mazes even when their behaviour was not reinforced and concluded that they had developed internal cognitive maps. This was an important development in cognitive psychology which seeks to understand how internal representations of reality are necessary to explain people's behaviour and how we process information (e.g., Neisser, 1967).

A key advance in cognitive psychology was the use of computer analogies to understand thought and behavioural regulation. Freud was acutely aware of the operation of the unconscious in directing thoughts and actions but his reliance on analogies with plumbing and hydraulic systems limited his capacity to explain how the unconscious directs action and the nature of inconsistencies between unconscious and conscious action. Thinking of the brain as a kind of computer running planning algorithms allowed much greater flexibility in explaining how psychological process can regulate action (e.g., Miller, Galanter & Pribram, 1960). This computational analogy underpins many cognitive models used in health psychology to understand motivation and behaviour (see Chapter 7). Developing models of how people understand their reality, and in particular their health and illnesses, is central to health psychology research (see Chapters 7 and 8). Of course, it is important to remember that the brain is nothing like any computer we understand. The brain consists of a quadrillion connections and at each synapse marking these connections several hundred different proteins work to organise the precise transfers that occur when the synapse "fires", which may happen many hundreds of times a second. This includes the construction and movement of neurotransmitters such as serotonin. Nonetheless, the more sophisticated analogy to computer programs that generate decision points, priorities and stored plans was an important theoretical advance.

The sub-discipline of social psychology was established when researchers focused on the effects of others on our behaviour (e.g., Triplett, 1898). Social psychologists applied experimental methods to understanding how we perceive and represent others, how others influence us, and how our position in wider society shapes our beliefs, attitudes and behaviour (Allport, 1924; Sherif, 1936). These processes are important to health psychologists because health-relevant perceptions and behaviours are affected by others. For example, interactions with family or work colleagues may cause stress that affect cardiovascular and immune functioning. Similarly, interactions with healthcare professionals may change beliefs and motivations relevant to taking medication (see Chapters 4 and 10). Health psychology must apply social psychological models of interaction to fully understand "health" (in the World Health Organization sense).

Health psychology draws upon the methods and theories of a range of sub-disciplines within psychology including learning theory, psychobiology, cognitive psychology and social psychology. More recently, collaboration between psychologists and neuroscientists has generated new insights (Inagaki, 2020). For example, researchers have developed a standardised way of assessing the extent to which features in a video (such as an advertisement) arouse and engage attention referred to as "message sensation value" (Seelig et al., 2014). Health psychology research applies these various theories and methods in order to better understand how our perceptions, beliefs and behaviour can maintain health or cause illness. The recognition that health (or illness) results from the interaction of biological characteristics and processes (including genetic predispositions and physiological mechanisms), psychological processes (including perceptions, beliefs and behaviours) and social processes and contexts (including social structure, cultural influences and interpersonal relationships) is what is meant by adopting a *biopsychosocial model* (Schwartz, 1982) of health and illness. This biopsychosocial perspective is central to current health psychology research and practice.

Behavioural patterns, lifestyle and health

The Alameda County study followed nearly 7,000 people over 10 years. Results showed that sleep, exercise, drinking alcohol and eating habits predict mortality (Belloc & Breslow, 1972). Similarly, the leading causes of death in the US in 2000 were tobacco use (18.1%), poor diet and physical inactivity (16.6%), and alcohol consumption (3.5%) accounting collectively for almost 40% of all deaths (Mokdad, Marks, Stroup & Gerberding, 2004). Of course, these patterns can change over time, especially as populations age. For example, in the UK in 2001, heart disease was the leading medical cause of death among men and women but, by 2018, this was replaced by dementia (as people lived longer). Cardiovascular disease, dementia and other leading medical causes of deaths are predicted by differences in individual lifestyles.

In the UK, Khaw *et al.* (2008) measured four key health behaviour patterns amongst people with no known cardiovascular disease or cancer. These behaviours were: (1) not smoking; (2) being physically active; (3) only drinking alcohol moderately; and (4) plasma vitamins indicating consumption of five portions of fruit and vegetables a day. Eleven years later more than 20,000 people were followed up. Results showed that, controlling for age, gender, body mass index and socioeconomic status, those engaging in none of the four behaviours were over four times more likely to have died than those engaging in all four. The researchers note that this effect is equivalent to those who engaged in four behaviours having the health of someone 14 years younger than those who engaged in none! Similar findings were reported in Norway using a cohort sample of 37,000 people followed up for 14 years (Krokstad, Ding, Grunseit et al., 2017). Seven behaviour patterns were considered: smoking, excessive alcohol consumption, poor diet, physical inactivity, excessive sitting, too much or too little sleep, and poor social participation. All these behaviour patterns were associated with increased risk of death during follow up, except poor diet. The risk of death during the follow-up study increased from a ratio of 1.37, that is, just over one third above average (1.0) when just one risky behaviour pattern was considered to 6.15 when six risky behaviour patterns were considered. So, a person who reported six of these behaviour patterns was more than six times more likely to die over the 14 years of the study! The most risky behaviours in this cohort were smoking and lack of social participation, that is social isolation. It was also noteworthy that excessive sitting, quite apart from physical activity, and quality of sleep resulted in significant increases in mortality risk. It is important to acknowledge how health risk accumulates as additional health-damaging behaviour patterns are added. What we do day-to-day really matters to our health and to how long we live. For example, we now know that sleeping 7–8 hours a night protects us from cancer and dementia, lowers our risk of heart attacks, stroke and diabetes, makes it less likely that we will get infections and enhances our recovering from infections, reduces food cravings and especially cravings for high-calorie food, and so makes obesity less likely. In addition, 7–8 hours of quality sleep a night enhances memory and is associated with greater creativity, happiness and reduced anxiety and depression (Walker, 2017). So just this one behavioural pattern has diverse effects on psychological functioning and physical health. Improving health is about changing and regulating behaviour patterns.

Health behaviour patterns are not just relevant to our early and middle years but to older people as well. Yates, Djoussé, Kurth, Buring and Gaziano (2008) studied a sample of 2,357 healthy men aged 70 and examined the predictors of mortality over the next 20 years. A healthy 70-year-old had a 54% chance of living to be 90 but this reduced to 44% if he had a sedentary lifestyle, 36% if he had hypertension, 26% if he was obese, and only 22% if he smoked. The percentage living to be 90 dropped to only 14% if three of these factors were present. So, promoting health-enhancing lifestyles amongst 70-year-olds is important because of the years of life that can be gained.

It is not surprising, therefore, that a comprehensive review of the UK National Health Service concluded that its long-term effectiveness and economic viability depended on more successful disease prevention strategies and high levels of public engagement in health care and maintenance. More than 20 years ago Sir Derek Wanless advised the UK government that increasing healthcare demand meant that comprehensive healthcare could not be afforded unless the population became "fully engaged", such that individuals would take responsibility for prevention of health problems (Wanless, 2002). Unfortunately, this "fully engaged" scenario has *not* been established in the UK or elsewhere. For example, the NHS (2023) Health Survey for England recorded increasing rates of obesity with 68% of men and 60% of women being overweight or obese. Obesity is not a disease but exacerbates health problems including the prevalence of diabetes, cardiovascular disease, kidney disease and osteoarthritis, so creating healthcare demand. Perhaps unsurprisingly, countries with higher levels of obesity also recorded higher COVID-19 caseloads and higher COVID-19 mortality rates (Chaudhry et al., 2020).

The economic implications of promoting preventive health behaviours, minimising demands on health services and supporting people coping with chronic illness are substantial. For example, in the UK, in 2021, there were 149 million working days lost due to sickness (https://www.ons.gov.uk/census). The UK spends about 12% of its total economic output on health services but less than 7% of this is spent on preventive behaviour change services. This means that healthcare professionals, including some very highly paid professionals, are sitting in offices waiting for people to arrive with serious health concerns rather than working to prevent these conditions occurring. This is, unfortunately, an illness service not a health service! The prevalence of long-term illnesses and their cost to the national economy necessitate a health service that actively helps people avoid illness and live a healthy life longer into old age. The economic argument has been clear for decades. Research-based interventions have the potential to make a substantial difference to public health, the efficiency of health services and the national economy (Friedman, Sobel, Myers, Caudill & Benson, 1995; Wang & Wang, 2021). Investing appropriately in effective preventive health services is critical to population health, affordable health services and national economic success. Health psychology provides the research background to make these changes. We advocate change by service managers and politicians to implement policies that will facilitate these changes.

Preventive services should focus on changing health-related behaviour patterns that really matter to health including, smoking, alcohol consumption, physical activity, sedentary behaviour, sleep, diet, weight management, stress reduction and social connectedness. Such interventions are the core projects for health psychologists who want to contribute to population health (see Chapters 9 and 11).

Psychological processes can have direct and indirect effects on health and illness. The indirect effects are frequently referred to as behavioural pathways because they provide an explanation as to how psychological factors such as stress influence health through changes in health behaviour patterns (e.g., exercise, diet, smoking). Direct effects are often referred to as psychophysiological pathways because they help us understand how psychological factors can directly impact on the body's physical systems such as the immune or cardiovascular systems (O'Connor, Thayer & Vedhara, 2021; see Chapter 2). Feeling anxious or stressed changes physiological processes and cumulatively these effects can damage physical systems and so compromise health. A number of studies have found that people who frequently exhibit large physiological responses to stress are more likely to develop serious illnesses in the future. For example, the Kuopio Heart Study which followed over 2,500 men for 25 years in Finland, found that men who had large increases in blood pressure or heart rate when they felt stressed at the beginning of the study were more likely to have had a stroke or to have developed hypertension many years later (Everson, Kaplan, Goldberg & Salonen, 1996; Everson et al., 2001). These researchers suggested that the experience of frequent daily stressors over time lead to excessive wear and tear on the cardiovascular system and ultimately to poorer health and earlier death. Psychological processes can also initiate healing processes. These help explain what are referred to as placebo effects and a better understanding of these processes could enable healthcare professionals to harness a patients' own, internal healing processes (see Chapter 11).

The importance of behavioural regulation to well-being and longevity is emphasised by the Lifestyle Medicine movement. Lifestyle Medicine involves a range of healthcare professionals and a wide range of health-related research including health psychology research. For example, the British Society of Lifestyle Medicine (https://bslm.org.uk/ 2023) highlights three principles of care: (1) acknowledgement of the need for action on socioeconomic determinants of health (and thereby reductions in health inequalities), (2) development and application of skills and proven techniques to support people make lifestyle change and (3) knowledge of the six Pillars of Lifestyle Medicine. These six pillars are: (i) healthy eating, (ii) regular physical activity, (iii) good sleep management, (iv) minimising harmful substances, (v) building social supports and (vi) managing mental wellbeing. These behavioural goals echo centuries-old teachings, such as those of Hippocrates and Epicurus and correspond directly to the findings of modern cohort studies. It also offers a way forward for health psychologists to guide their clients to a relatively simple (six pillars) understanding of how feelings and behaviour patterns interact to produce good health or illness.

Research indicates that health-related behaviour change corresponding to the pillars of Lifestyle Medicine can alter common biological pathways for many long-term illnesses that necessitate large-scale, health service, expenditure, including cardiovascular disease, diabetes and auto-immune diseases including arthritis, asthma and hormonal dysregulation. These pathways include inflammation, microbiome depletion, cellular stress and activation of undesirable genetic influence through epigenetic processes. The explanation is that, in all these cases, the route to healing is through lifestyle change that drives biological changes. This, in turn, leads to primary prevention (avoiding illness) and secondary prevention (minimising the consequences of illness). The hope is that even when such illnesses are present their reversal and cure can be effected through lifestyle change that will reduce healthcare and medication usage. A consensus statement reviewing this research has called for targeted research and radical changes to clinical practice to implement this Lifestyle Medicine agenda (Vodovotz et al., 2020). A Lifestyle Medicine approach to healthcare services could result in less expensive, health-promoting services.

From a health promotion perspective, the Lifestyle Medicine approach has the benefit of highlighting six core patterns of behaviour that are readily understood by the lay population. This provides an answer to the often-asked question, "*Where should I begin*"? The answer is provided by assessing *which of these six patterns of behaviour would you most like to improve over the next six months and are most likely to be able to improve*? This provides a foundation for targeted behaviour change interventions (see Chapter 9). Of course, when one has a particular illness, it is critically important to understand the details of effective self-management including adherence to evidence-based medical advice. Many patients with long-term illnesses become expert patients (see

Chapters 8 and 11) because, of course, such self-management is their overriding priority. So, for some people, the six behaviour patterns identified by Lifestyle Medicine may need to be supplemented, for example, with improved diabetes or asthma management. Nonetheless, Lifestyle Medicine provides a simple biologically-based gateway to promoting health, and public health, through behaviour change.

Using this book effectively

In each chapter of this book we have included a brief chapter plan, learning outcomes, lists of terms introduced, individual and/or group exercises and short lists of recommended additional readings. These are designed to help you actively learn as you proceed through the course. In Chapter 8, we note that lasting cognitive change depends on systematic processing of incoming messages involving active engagement with the content. This includes linking content to prior knowledge and, critically, evaluating it in terms of pre-existing standards and principles. In addition, getting a good night's sleep after learning new material makes it easier to recall it better the next day (Walker, 2017). So, in building your expertise in health psychology you are managing your own cognitive development. So how can you facilitate systematic processing of the material in this book?

It is important to read the chapter plans and learning outcomes before reading the chapters to develop an overview of the material. Then at the end of each chapter check that you understand the terms introduced and that you can now do what is specified in the learning objectives. Testing yourself by checking through previous learning objectives and planning essays is also important. Research has found that testing improves retention compared to just studying and that this is true even if the test is never scored (Roediger & Karpicke, 2006). Testing is critical to learning. It is not just an assessment tool. Testing can also work well when students work together in study groups.

You should read papers from our additional reading lists. You should make your own notes on these papers and the chapters in this book. Research has shown that making notes enhances learning and the transfer of learning from one topic to another (e.g., Wittrock & Alesandrini, 1990). Your notes are not just useful for revision. Making them will enhance your learning even if you do not consult them later.

When reading research papers, it may be helpful to think of them as boxes that contain things you want rather than stories that need to be read from beginning to end. You might try reading the abstract first and then the first couple of paragraphs of the discussion to get a good overview of the paper before you decide what else you need to know about it. When reading a paper reporting an empirical study it is useful to check that you can answer the questions highlighted in Activity Box 1.1.

ACTIVITY BOX 1.1

Reading empirical papers

Try reading an empirical paper and answering the questions below. You could try reading the following paper which is highlighted as an additional reading in Chapter 9.

Luszczynska, A., Sobczyk, A. and Abraham, C. (2007). Planning to lose weight: RCT of an implementation intention prompt to enhance weight reduction among overweight and obese women. *Health Psychology*, *26*, 507–512.

What kind of study is reported? For example, is it an experiment, a correlational study (cross sectional or longitudinal), a qualitative analysis of text or interview data, or a review (narrative, systematic or meta-analysis)?

What are the independent variables and which are the dependent variables (or outcome measures)? Are there any mediating or moderating variables (see Research methods Box 3.1)?

How do the measures used relate to measures of these (or similar) constructs in other studies? Are the measures reliable? Do they have good construct and predictive validity?

Are there any confounding variables? Have these been controlled for?

What population is studied? How does this relate to other populations studied in this area?

What are the key findings?

Is the sample size adequate? Is the sample representative? Can we generalise from these findings? If so, what are the limits to this generalisation?

Does the study suggest any new theoretical development/s? What further research should be undertaken to explore questions arising from the results or problems with the study's methodology?

Does the study have practice and/or policy implications?

Does the study need to be replicated?

Planning and writing essays are also effective ways to test and develop your understanding of a topic. You may have a well-developed approach to writing essays but it may be useful to revise the points in Focus Box 1.1 when thinking about your next health psychology essay.

FOCUS BOX 1.1

Essay writing

First make sure you understand the question. The question will direct you towards particular readings and research and perhaps ask you to treat these in a particular way – e.g., "discuss" – "contrast" etc. Make sure you have a good plan which sets out a clear structure for your essay that corresponds to what the question asks. Also try to ensure that you know how your arguments link together (e.g., using a diagram).

In the opening sections ensure your title makes sense to the reader by providing any necessary definitions and explanations. Also outline and explain your objectives in writing the essay – what do you intend to argue and achieve in the essay – how is this linked to previous research? Use appropriate references to anchor your essay to previous research findings.

The main body of your essay will convey your core arguments, which have been outlined in the introduction. Think about the following points.

You should be able to summarise your essay as a series of core arguments or points. It is often helpful to state these explicitly early on in the relevant paragraph. For example, "I will highlight one strength and two weaknesses in this theory . . ." Then for each of these (three) arguments, consider what evidence and illustrations you need.

Be precise about theoretical distinctions and definitions and avoid lapsing into lay psychology.

Know the data you are discussing. Be specific about measures and methods used and illustrate measures where this clarifies a construct or a methodological critique. Support your arguments with data (e.g., means, correlations or effect sizes). This can emphasise the strength or weakness of an association or the effect of an intervention and, thereby, strengthen an argument or critique. However, it is uninformative to provide "p" values alone without references to statistics that convey size of associations, differences or effects.

Note too, that, sometimes, an anecdote or case study can illustrate a point in a concrete way.

Reference claims you make about previous findings using author names and dates. Your essay is about research findings so avoid unsupported claims. Use American Psychological Association (APA) referencing rules, unless told otherwise by your tutor.

Link your arguments. Each paragraph should lead onto the next and the introduction should link clearly to the conclusion. You may want to make this explicit, e.g., "The study by Brown (2003) outlined above also emphasises . . ."

Make links across the reading you have completed for the course.

Provide a short conclusion at the end of the essay. This should summarise your main points and highlight connections between them. In many essays this will also be the opportunity to succinctly state what you think needs to be done next, in terms of further research, intervention, adoption or policy changes (including implications for health care practice and social policy).

You may have been told correctly that your psychology essays are not about your opinion but about research findings. However, a good essay will involve a personal synthesis of research, including your evaluations of findings and your evidence-based conclusions (e.g., the weight of the evidence suggests . . .). Do not be afraid to draw your conclusions – it's your essay.

Finally, make sure you provide a complete set of references (i.e. all papers, books etc. that you have referred to in your text in APA format).

The structure and content of this book

The book is divided into five sections: (1) biological bases of health and illness; (2) stress and health; (3) coping resources: social support and individual differences; (4) motivation and behaviour; and, finally, (5) applied health psychology.

This chapter (led by Charles Abraham) introduces the study of Health Psychology.

Chapter 2 (led by Daryl O'Connor and Fiona Jones) focuses on physiological systems such as the central nervous system, the cardiovascular systema and the immune system. This chapter also considers how these basic biological processes may be influenced by psychological factors such as stress. There is also a brief overview of the role of psychological processes in the experience of pain. The book returns to this topic in relation to behaviour change interventions to reduce opioid use, in Chapter 9.

Chapters 3, 4 and 5 (led by Daryl O'Connor and Fiona Jones) critically appraise research into the nature of stress. These chapters introduce key theories and methodologies used in researching stress and examine the impact of stress on health. Chapter 3 introduces theories which view stress as a physiological phenomenon, before moving to more contemporary approaches examining the impact of major life events and day-to-day hassles on health. Chapter 4 focuses on environmental and contextual factors which have been prominent in stress research and have been shown to affect health, in particular, social inequality and employment factors. Models of work stress are discussed and evidence relating work stress to disease is considered. Chapter 5 focuses on individual differences in coping with stress. Different types of coping strategies are considered and assessed in terms of whether these are consistent across situations (i.e., whether people have their own coping style). The impact of coping styles on health as well as the important impact of social support are examined.

Chapter 6 (led by Mark Conner) focuses on differences between people that affect the way in which environmental factors (such as stress or social inequality) impact health. These factors, particular differences in personality can be said to "moderate" the relationships between the environment and an outcome such as stress. This chapter highlights key models of personality and their relevance for health behaviour patterns and health. Much of the research discussed focuses on the "big five" dimensions of personality: openness, conscientiousness, extraversion, agreeableness and neuroticism. Several of these personality dimensions have important consequences for health including how long we can expect to live. A key issue addressed in this chapter is the way in which personality factors influence health outcomes. So, for example, the personality trait of conscientiousness appears to affect health by promoting engagement with preventive health actions.

Chapter 7 (led by Mark Conner) examines models which identify beliefs, attitudes and intentions (that is, *cognitions*) which predict individual behaviour. Critical appraisal of research highlights the success of these models in predicting behaviour using prospective surveys and objective measures. These models identify potentially modifiable determinants of behaviour patterns. For example, if we change attitudes and motivation can we promote healthy behaviour patterns?

Chapter 8 (led by Charles Abraham) examines methods used to change cognitions including use of information provision, persuasive communication, fear appeals and social influence. The chapter identifies some of the pitfalls that health educators should avoid in using these methods and offers best practice recommendations. The chapter illustrates how to best change attitudes and motivation using persuasive methods and also discusses how self-efficacy can be enhanced. Self-efficacy (believing that you can succeed) is an important antecedent of motivation and action.

Chapter 9 (led by Charles Abraham) explains what is involved in evidence-based health promotion. In particular, how tailoring messages to particular target audiences is critical to persuasion. The chapter also considers the usefulness and hazards of using fear to motivate behaviour change. In addition, this chapter considers how we design and evaluate behaviour-change interventions. Finally, the chapter considers how we need to look beyond individual-level intervention to promote population health.

Chapter 10 (led by Charles Abraham) focuses on practice in healthcare services. How can we encourage people to consult services when they have a health problem? How can healthcare professionals (whether health psychologists, nurses or medical practitioners) communicate with patients so as to optimise the impact of consultations? What do health psychologists contribute to healthcare services in practice? These questions are answered drawing on relevant research.

Chapter 11 (led by Charles Abraham) focuses on how health psychology research can be applied in practice. We consider the special needs of people with long-term illnesses. We explore how the group consultations and self-help groups could contribute to future health services. We also explore the role of complementary therapies and how placebo effects shape the effectiveness of all consultations between healthcare professionals and their clients. Finally, we consider how healthcare services may evolve as digital services become commonplace.

Key terms introduced in Chapter 1 (in order of appearance)

- Public health campaigns
- World Health Organization
- American Psychological Association
- European Health Psychology Society
- British Psychology Society
- Promoting health and preventing illness
- Professional practice
- Health behaviour patterns
- Classical and operant conditioning
- Cognitive maps
- Social influence
- Biopsychosocial model
- Direct and indirect effects on health
- Behaviour change
- Lifestyle Medicine
- Testing
- Making notes
- Essay writing

Summary of main points addressed in Chapter 1

Health psychology aims to promote health and prevent illness through scientific research that elucidates psychological processes linked to health. Evidence-based causal models provide the basis for effective interventions that may enhance health by changing psychological processes. Interventions designed to change demand for health services can have substantial effects on the cost effectiveness of services. Emotional responses and health behaviours have been shown to have important measurable effects on morbidity and mortality. Behavioural effects are referred to as indirect effects whereas psychological processes which affect health through psychophysiological pathways are referred to as direct effects.

The origins of health psychology research can be seen in the teaching of ancient Greek philosophers and more recently in the application of learning theory, cognitive theories and social

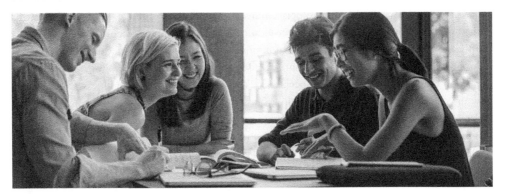

Figure 1.1 Structured learning makes studying easier.
Source: Copyright jacob lund/shutterstock.com.

psychological theories of health and health behaviour. The biopsychosocial model incorporates biological, psychological and social processes.

You will learn more effectively if you: (1) read chapter plans and learning outcomes before reading chapters; and (2) check that you understand terms introduced and check that you can do what is specified in the learning objectives. Taking notes, reading recommended additional readings and writing essays will also consolidate your learning.

Illustrative essay titles

Discuss the main theoretical concepts that underpin research and practice in health psychology today.

Explain how health psychology is distinct form psychology more generally and discuss how health psychology is relevant to modern health services.

Recommendations for further reading

Journal articles

Adler, N. & Matthews, K. (1994). Health psychology: Why do some people get sick and some stay well? *Annual Review of Psychology*, *45*, 229–259. https://doi.org/10.1146/annurev.ps.45.020194.001305

Schwartz, G. E. (1982). Testing the biopsychosocial model: The ultimate challenge facing behavioral medicine? *Journal of Consulting and Clinical Psychology*, *50*(6), 1040–1053. https://doi.org/10.1037/0022-006X.50.6.1040

Website

Ulster University Blog (2022). *What is Health Psychology? 2022 Guide*. https://online.ulster.ac.uk/blog/what-is-health-psychology/

PART 1

Biological bases of health and illness

2 Biopsychosocial pathways to health and illness

Biopsychosocial pathways to health and illness

In Chapter 1, we introduced health psychology as a discipline, the biopsychosocial model of health and illness, the context in which health psychology research takes place and areas studied. In this chapter we consider the main psychophysiological pathways through which psychological factors impact on physical health and illness.

We discuss the body's physical systems including the central nervous system, the endocrine system, the cardiovascular system and the immune system. We then consider how these basic biological processes may be influenced by psychological factors such as stress. In particular, we will describe how activation of the hypothalamic–pituitary–adrenal (HPA) axis and the sympathetic adrenal medullary (SAM) system are linked to increased cardiovascular disease. Next, we present a brief overview of the role of psychological factors in the experience of pain and gate-control theory. Finally, we introduce important developments in the area of psychoneuroimmunology and discuss how psychological factors can affect the immune system within the context of susceptibility to upper respiratory illness and the speed of wound healing.

The chapter is composed of five sections:

1. Basic Features of the Nervous System.
2. The Stress Response.
3. Biopsychosocial Aspects of Pain.
4. Psychoneuroimmunology.
5. Stress and the Immune System.

> ### Learning outcomes
>
> When you have completed this chapter, you should be able to:
>
> 1 Describe the basic features of the central nervous system.
> 2 Explain how activation of the hypothalamic–pituitary–adrenal (HPA) axis and the sympathetic adrenal medullary (SAM) system links to stress and health.
> 3 Understand the role of psychological factors in the experience of pain.
> 4 Discuss how psychoneuroimmunology (PNI) plays a role in illness processes.
> 5 Design an experiment to examine the effects of psychological stress on health outcomes within a laboratory setting.

DOI: 10.4324/9781003171096-3

What is the biopsychosocial perspective on health and illness?

As outlined in Chapter 1, the biopsychosocial model postulates that health and illness are influenced by psychological factors (e.g. cognition, emotion, personality), social factors (e.g. people in your social world, social class, ethnicity) and biological factors (e.g. viruses, lesions, bacteria). Within this context, there is increasing evidence that psychological factors such as stress affect health directly, through autonomic and neuroendocrine responses (e.g. blood pressure and hormonal changes), but also indirectly, through changes to health behaviours (e.g. exercise, diet, smoking). The direct effects of stress on health are often referred to as psychophysiological pathways because they help us understand how psychological factors can directly impact on physiological disease-related processes. The indirect effects are frequently referred to as behavioural pathways as they provide an explanation as to how psychological factors can indirectly influence disease-related processes by producing negative changes in health behaviours. This chapter describes the main psychophysiological pathways that may influence health and illness, while the key behavioural pathways are considered in Chapter 3. Before the direct effects are considered in more detail, we introduce you to the basic features of the nervous system. It is paramount that you understand some of the basic biological processes constituting the human body in order to gain a good understanding of the psychophysiology of health and illness. Throughout this book we use activity boxes to consolidate your learning, and there is one just beyond the next section so read carefully!

Basic features of the nervous system

The role of the nervous system is to allow us to adapt to changes within our body and environment by using our five senses (touch, sight, smell, taste, sound) to understand, interpret and respond to internal and external changes quickly and appropriately. The nervous system consists of the brain, the spinal cord and the nerves (bundles of fibres that transmit information in and out of the nervous system). The brain is the central part of the nervous system and it helps control our behaviour. It receives and sends messages for the rest of the body through the spinal cord. The brain has three major anatomic components: the forebrain, the midbrain and the hindbrain.

The anatomy of the brain

The forebrain consists of dense, elaborate masses of tissue and has two main subdivisions:

1.   The telencephalon, which is composed of the cerebrum and limbic system.
2.   The diencephalon, which comprises the thalamus and hypothalamus.

The cerebrum is the largest part of the human brain and is divided into the two halves – the left and right cerebral hemispheres – that are connected in the middle by a bundle of nerve fibres called the corpus callosum. The upper part of the cerebrum is the cerebral cortex (its outermost area). This is subdivided into the frontal, parietal, occipital and temporal lobes and controls higher processes such as speaking, reasoning, memory, etc. (see Figure 2.1). More specifically, the frontal lobe (located towards the front of the cerebrum) is involved in speech, thought and emotion. Behind this is the parietal lobe which perceives and interprets sensations like touch, temperature and pain. The occipital lobe is at the centre back of the cerebrum and detects and interprets visual

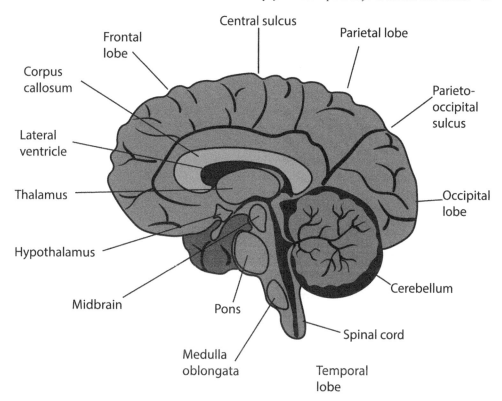

Figure 2.1 Anatomical Structure of The Brain
Copyright of Sofia Bessarab/Shutterstock

images. Finally, the temporal lobes located on either side are involved in hearing and aspects of memory storage. The limbic system is evolutionarily older than other parts of the brain and consists of the amygdala and hippocampus among other structures (not described above). This system interacts with the endocrine system (a network of glands that secrete hormones throughout the body described later) and the autonomic nervous system (ANS) and plays an important role in motivational and emotional aspects of behaviours such as sex, eating, drinking and aggression. It is also involved in aspects of memory processes.

The second major division of the forebrain is the diencephalon. Its two most important structures are the thalamus and the hypothalamus (see Figure 2.1). The thalamus is thought to have multiple functions and plays an important role in regulating states of sleep, arousal and consciousness. The hypothalamus is located below the thalamus and although it is a relatively small structure it is very important as it regulates the ANS and the endocrine system and, as we will see later in this chapter, it controls how individuals respond to stressful encounters. In short, it oversees the basic behaviours associated with the survival of the species: fighting, feeding, fleeing and mating, often referred to as the four Fs!

The midbrain consists of two major parts: the tectum and the tegmentum.

Broadly speaking, the midbrain, including the brain stem, regulates critical bodily functions such as breathing, swallowing, posture, movement and the rate at which the body metabolizes foods.

The hindbrain has two major divisions: the metencephalon and the myelencephalon. The former comprises the cerebellum and the pons and the latter contains one major structure, the medulla oblongata (usually referred to simply as the medulla). The cerebellum is involved in coordinating the body's movements and the pons has been implicated in sleep and arousal. The medulla controls vital functions linked to the regulation of the cardiovascular system and respiration.

ACTIVITY BOX 2.1

You have just read that the brain has three major anatomical components and each has a number of subdivisions. Can you list them? If not, it might be useful as a revision aid to draw a diagram of each component and its subdivisions.

The spinal cord and nerve cells

The spinal cord is a long, delicate structure that begins at the end of the brain stem and continues down to the bottom of the spine. It carries incoming and outgoing messages between the brain and the rest of the body. The brain communicates with much of the body through nerves that run up and down the spinal cord. As you will see later, the spinal cord plays an important role in responding to pain stimuli. The nervous system contains 100 billion or more nerve cells that run throughout the body. A nerve cell, called a neuron, is made up of a large cell body and a single, elongated extension (axon) for sending messages. Neurons usually have many branches (dendrites) for receiving messages. Nerves transmit messages electrically from the axon of one neuron to the dendrite of another (at the synapse) by secreting tiny amounts of chemicals called neurotransmitters. These substances trigger the receptors on the next neuron's dendrite to start up a new electrical impulse.

Central nervous system and peripheral nervous system

The nervous system is classified into various different subsystems and subdivisions but these different components are all part of an integrated system and do not operate independently.

The nervous system has two distinct parts:

1.   The central nervous system.
2.   The peripheral nervous system.

The central nervous system (CNS) comprises the brain and spinal cord and is protected by bone. The brain is encased in the cranial subcavity within the skull and the spinal cord is enclosed in the spinal cavity and protected by the vertebrae. Both the brain and the spinal cord do not come into direct contact with the skull or the vertebrae as they are further enclosed by a three-layered set of membranes called the meninges. Instead, they float in a clear liquid called cerebrospinal fluid.

The peripheral nervous system (PNS) is a network of nerves that connects the brain and spinal cord to the rest of the body. The PNS is further subdivided, according to its function, into the:

1.   Somatic nervous system (SNS).
2.   Autonomic nervous system (ANS).

The SNS is concerned with coordinating the 'voluntary' body movements controlled by the skeletal muscles. The ANS regulates internal body processes that require no conscious awareness, for

PARASYMPATHETIC AND SYMPATHETIC NERVOUS SYSTEMS

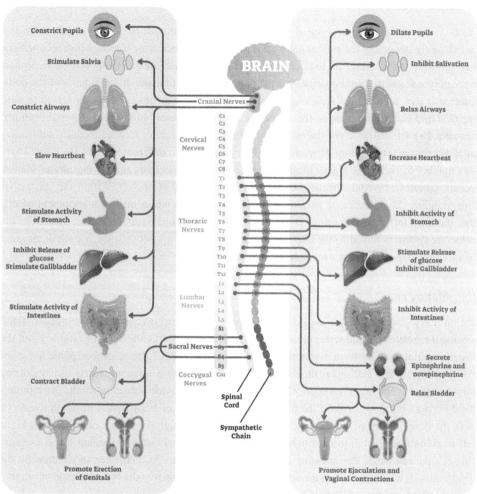

Figure 2.2 The sympathetic nervous system (solid lines) and the parasympathetic nervous system (broken lines).
Copyright of VectorMine/Shutterstock.

example, the rate of heart contractions and breathing, and the speed at which food passes through the digestive tract.

The ANS is subdivided into the:

1. Sympathetic division.
2. Parasympathetic division.

As shown in Figure 2.2, the sympathetic division mobilizes the body by increasing heart rate and blood pressure among other physiological changes, whereas the parasympathetic division generally restores the body's energy by reducing heart rate and respiration while increasing the rate of digestion. The changes in each of the divisions occur when the ANS triggers the endocrine system to react in the face of stress.

Endocrine system

The endocrine system is an integrated system of small glands that work closely with the ANS and are extremely important for everything we do! In particular, endocrine glands, which secrete their chemicals into the bloodstream to be carried to their point of use, are most important here. Similar to the nervous system, the endocrine system communicates with many different parts of the body, however, it uses a different 'signalling system'. Whereas the nervous system uses nerves to send electrical and chemical messages, the endocrine system only uses blood vessels to send chemical messages. In particular, each of the endocrine glands, once activated, secretes chemical substances called hormones into the bloodstream which carry messages to different parts of the body. There are a number of endocrine glands located throughout the human body such as the adrenal glands, gonads, pancreas, thyroid, thymus and pituitary gland (see Figure 2.2). Within the context of understanding the influence of psychological factors, such as stress, on the development of disease, the most important glands to consider are the adrenal and pituitary glands. Moreover, the endocrine system is linked to the nervous system by connections between the hypothalamus and the pituitary gland, the latter of which is discussed next.

The pituitary gland

The pituitary gland is located just below the hypothalamus and is considered the 'master' gland because it regulates the endocrine gland secretions. It has two parts: the anterior pituitary and the posterior pituitary. The former secretes growth hormone (GH), adrenocorticotrophic hormone (ACTH), thyroid stimulating hormone (TSH), follicle stimulating hormone (FSH) and luteinizing hormone (LH). The latter component releases oxytocin and vasopressin. Overall, the pituitary gland plays an important role in the regulation of the growth of body tissues (through release of GH), the development of the gonads, ovum and sperm (through the release of FSH and LH) as well as stimulating lactation (through the release of oxytocin) and maintaining blood pressure (through the release of vasopressin). However, it also releases ACTH (after stimulation by the hypothalamus) which stimulates the adrenal cortex – this is known as the hypothalamic–pituitary–adrenal (HPA) axis response. This is a most important response system which we will consider in some detail shortly.

The adrenal glands

There are two adrenal glands located on the top of each kidney. The adrenal glands are best considered as being two glands within one. Each has a central core, called the adrenal medulla, which secretes the hormones adrenaline and noradrenaline (also known as epinephrine and norepinephrine), which act on the visceral organs in the same way as neurons in the nervous system. In other words, they increase heart rate and mobilize glucose into the blood among other things. Collectively, adrenaline and noradrenaline (and dopamine) are known as catecholamines. The outer portion of the adrenal gland, called the adrenal cortex, produces mineralocorticoids and glucocorticoids. The former hormones act on the kidneys to conserve salt and water by returning them to the blood during urine formation. The latter are secreted when we encounter stressors in order to help the body respond appropriately. One of the most important glucocorticoids is cortisol (corticosterone in rodents) and as such it is frequently referred to as the 'stress hormone' and measured in studies of psychological stress.

Cardiovascular system

The central function of the cardiovascular system is to ensure that oxygen (with other nutrients) is transported to all the organs of the body and that carbon dioxide (as well as other waste products) is removed from each of the body's cells. The blood is the vehicle that transports the oxygen with the heart and blood vessels allowing the blood to be carried around the body. The heart, the centre of the cardiovascular system, is made of muscle and 'beats' or 'pumps' approximately 100,000 times per day. The main muscular outer part of the heart, which contains the cardiac veins and arteries, is called the myocardium. The heart has four chambers: the two upper chambers are known as atriums and the two lower ones are called ventricles. In the cardiovascular system, veins carry blood to the heart and myocardium and the arteries carry blood away from the heart and myocardium.

We can follow the journey of blood flow by considering where it enters the heart. Blood enters the right atrium deficient of oxygen and full of waste products (carbon dioxide) and is bluish in colour. Once the atrium is full, the blood is pushed into the right ventricle, which then contracts, thus pumping the blood from the heart towards the lungs, where it becomes oxygenated (and red in colour). Once oxygenated, the blood travels to the left atrium in the heart and is passed into the left ventricle before it is pumped into the general circulation via the aorta (a large artery). Before returning to the heart, some of the blood is cleansed of waste products by passing through the kidneys (where the waste products are filtered out and excreted in urine) and the liver (where nutrients, e.g. simple sugars, are stored and harmful bacteria are removed).

The cardiovascular system is a closed system and therefore it always contains some pressure. Blood pressure is the force exerted by the blood on the artery walls and has two components:

1.   Diastolic blood pressure is the resting level in the arteries in between contractions.
2.   Systolic blood pressure is the maximum pressure in the arteries when the heart pumps.

An individual's blood pressure is described using two numbers representing both the systolic and diastolic components and is expressed in units known as millimetres of mercury (mmHg; e.g. 126 over 70 or 126/70 mmHg). A number of factors increase blood pressure including temperature, weight, posture and food intake. Psychological factors, such as chronic stress, have also been found to be associated with the development of high blood pressure (or hypertension), which is known to damage the heart and the arteries. We will consider the links between stress, blood pressure and cardiovascular disease in more detail later.

The stress response

What happens when you experience stress? Two systems are activated. The first and easiest to activate is the sympathetic adrenal medullary (SAM) system; the second is the hypothalamic–pituitary–adrenal (HPA) axis. To borrow an analogy from Clow (2001: 53) activating the SAM system

> can be likened to lighting a match whereas activating the HPA axis is like lighting a fire. Lighting a match is easy, has an instant effect and the effect does not last long, whereas lighting a fire takes a lot more effort and its effects last much longer. The HPA axis is only activated in extreme circumstances.

Each of these systems is considered in more detail in the following sections. In addition, later we consider how researchers induce the stress response in the laboratory using the Trier Social Stress Test (see Research methods box 2.1).

The sympathetic adrenal medullary (SAM) response system

When an individual is suddenly under threat or frightened, their brain instantly sends a message to the adrenal glands which quickly release noradrenaline that in turn activates the internal organs. This is the basic ANS sympathetic division response to threat. However, at the same time, the adrenal medulla releases adrenaline which is rapidly transported through the bloodstream in order to further prepare the body for its response. This system is known as the sympathetic adrenal medullary (SAM) system (see Figure 2.3). Within moments adrenaline and noradrenaline have the entire body on alert, a response sometimes called the fight or flight response. As outlined earlier, as a result breathing quickens, the heart beats more rapidly and powerfully, the eyes dilate to allow more light in, and the activity of the digestive system decreases to permit more blood to go to the muscles. This effect is both rapid and intense.

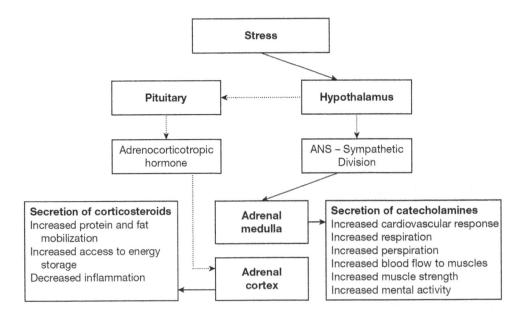

Figure 2.3 Stress response. Hypothalamic-pituitary-adrenal (HPA) axis response system (dashed line) and the sympathetic adrenal medullary system (SAM) response system (solid line).

The hypothalamic–pituitary–adrenal (HPA) axis response system

In addition to the SAM response, when an individual experiences an unpleasant event in their environment that they perceive as stressful, the hypothalamus (the H in HPA) releases a chemical messenger called corticotrophin releasing factor (CRF). Once released, CRF is transported in the blood supply to the pituitary gland (the P) where it stimulates the release of adrenocorticotrophic hormone (ACTH). Subsequently, the latter hormone travels through the circulatory system to the adrenal (the A) cortex where it stimulates production of the glucocorticoid, cortisol – known as the 'stress hormone' (see Figure 2.3).

Why is cortisol released in response to stress? One of the central functions of cortisol is to increase access to energy stores, increase protein and fat mobilization, and decrease inflammation. Therefore, when an individual experiences stress, the release of cortisol triggers excess energy stored in the muscle and liver as glycogen to be liberated and broken down into glucose ready for utilization by the muscles and brain.

The stress response and cardiovascular disease

In evolutionary terms, these stress response processes are adaptive and help ensure survival. Nevertheless, they are only adaptive in so much as they are short lived and the body's systems swiftly return to normal. Our ancestors may well have encountered acute stressors in the form of wild animals while hunting which made such 'flight or fight' responses adaptive. The SAM and HPA response systems would prepare the body appropriately. However, the stress of modern-day life rarely affords such infrequent, acute, life-threatening stressful encounters. Instead, we are exposed to frequent daily hassles as well as long-lasting, chronic stressors. As a result, the stress response system is repeatedly activated and the cardiovascular system is potentially exposed to excessive wear and tear. Over time, such repetitive activation may contribute to future ill health by increasing cardiovascular disease risk (see Steptoe & Kivimaki, 2013; O'Connor, Thayer & Vedhara, 2021).

This may result in the development of atherosclerosis, that is, the build-up of fatty plaques in the inner lining of the blood vessels which leads to the occlusion (narrowing) of the arteries. The increase in blood pressure as a result of the repeated activation of the SAM system may cause damage to the lining of the blood vessels, thus allowing access to fatty acids and glucose. At the same time, activation of the HPA axis leads to the release of cortisol which increases the liberation of glucose from glycogen stores. These processes taken together increase the likelihood that chronic stress may lead to a build-up of plaque. The development of plaque can have serious health consequences. The first symptom of a narrowing artery may be pain or cramps at times when the blood flow cannot keep up with the body's demands for oxygen. During exercise, an individual may feel chest pain (angina) because of the lack of oxygen reaching the heart. In addition, this person may experience leg cramps because of lack of oxygen to the legs. However, more seriously, if the coronary arteries supplying the heart become 'blocked', which may happen if increased blood pressure in a narrowed artery sheers off a section of plaque, this can lead to a myocardial infarction (or heart attack) where part of the heart muscle (deprived of oxygen) dies. If blood flow to the brain is obstructed, this can result in a stroke where part of the brain dies.

We will consider evidence linking stress with cardiovascular disease in more detail in Chapter 3. Research has found that acute (i.e. short-lived) and chronic (long-lasting) stress are both associated with the development of cardiovascular disease. For example, Wang et al. (2021) investigated the effects of psychosocial stressors including job strain, stressful life events and social strain on the incidence of coronary heart disease (CHD) in women in a large scale 14.7-year follow-up study. The authors found that women who had high stressful life events scores and high social strain were at greater risk of having developed CHD at follow-up. These findings are consistent with a recent review of studies that explored the association between work stressors and CHD mortality (Spittal, LaMontagne & Milner, 2020). Across 45 studies, the review found that workers in jobs with low job control (a key component of job strain) were at increased risk of CHD mortality compared to workers with high job control. In terms of more acute, short-lived stressors an earlier, but notable study investigating the impact of an acute stressor found that admissions to hospitals in England increased on the day following England losing to Argentina in a penalty shoot-out in the 1998 Football World Cup (Carroll et al., 2002). The authors argue that their results suggest myocardial infarction can be triggered by emotional upset, such as watching your football team lose an important match. It is very possible that there were similar consequences following England's defeat against Italy in another penalty shoot-out in the Euro 2020 football final! Correspondingly, a meta-analysis of five studies showed that the risk of having a cardiac event was increased 2.5 times if preceded by a period of emotional stress (Steptoe & Kivimaki, 2013). Another study by Mostofsky and colleagues (2012) reported that the risk of having an acute myocardial infarction increased 21-fold following the death of a significant person in one's life (see also Cohen, Murphy & Prather, 2019).

RESEARCH METHODS BOX 2.1

How to induce stress in the laboratory: The Trier Social Stress Test (TSST)

The Trier Social Stress Test (TSST) was developed in 1993 by Kirschbaum, Pirke and Helhammer at the University of Trier. The aim was to develop a stress paradigm which would reliably stimulate the HPA axis. Previous techniques had yielded inconsistent results, therefore a standardized protocol was deemed necessary.

After arriving in the laboratory (room A), participants rest for between 10 and 30 minutes depending on whether hormones are being measured in saliva (using salivettes) or in blood (using an intravenous catheter). Participants are then taken to a different room (room B) where they are introduced to three individuals sitting in a panel and asked to stand by a microphone. Next the investigator explains that the participant is to take the role of a job applicant who will be interviewed by the panel. As part of the interview process, the participants are given ten minutes to prepare a five-minute free speech in which they must convince the interview panel that they are the perfect applicant for the vacant position. The participant is informed that the presentation will be video-taped and evaluated for non-verbal behaviour and voice frequency and that a video analysis of the participant's performance will also be conducted. The anticipation of giving such a presentation is the stressor that stimulates the HPA axis. Following receipt of the instructions, participants return to room A to prepare a speech with the aid of paper and a pen. After ten minutes, the participant returns to room B to deliver the speech in front of the panel. If the speech falls short of five minutes, the participant is told 'You still have some time left. Please continue!'. After 15 minutes, the panel asks the participant to start to serially subtract the number 13 from 1022 as quickly and accurately as possible. If an error is made, one of the panel requests that the participant start again at 1022. After 20 minutes, the task is ended and the participant returns to room A to rest and be debriefed about the nature of the experiment and be informed that no voice and video analysis of their performance will be conducted. The rest period may last between 30 and 70 minutes depending on which hormones are being monitored.

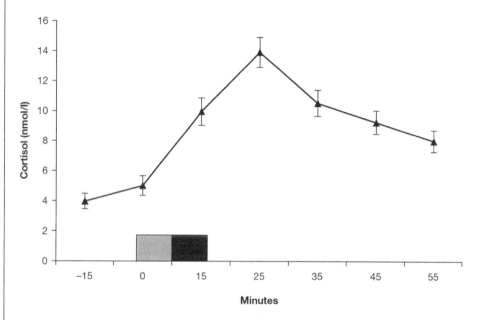

Figure 2.4 Typical cortisol profile following the TSST.

The TSST has been widely used by health psychologists because it is simple to administer and researchers can easily monitor changes in a wide range of cardiovascular (e.g. heart rate, blood pressure) and neuroendocrine (e.g. cortisol, ACTH) parameters during the paradigm. Changes in salivary and serum (in the blood) cortisol levels have probably received the most attention in the literature. A typical cortisol profile (using salivettes) in response to the TSST is shown in Figure 2.4. Two characteristics of the profile are worth noting: the extent to which cortisol increases in response to the stressor (i.e. stress reactivity) and the length of time it takes for cortisol levels to return to baseline (stress recovery). Stress reactivity and stress recovery are discussed further in Chapter 3.

Biopsychosocial aspects of pain

Psychological factors have been found to affect many different biological processes too numerous to describe here. However, one area in which psychology has made a substantial impact is in understanding the experience of pain and the management of pain.

Early theories of pain did not incorporate a role for psychological factors in explaining how we experience pain. This is surprising given that we can all think of episodes when someone's perception of pain has been influenced by cognitive, emotional or social factors. For example, we are less likely to experience pain when we are distracted by the demands of taking part in a competitive sporting event.

The role of meaning in pain

The meaning an individual attributes to pain has been found to affect their experience of it. Beecher (1956) provided striking evidence of the important role of the meaning of pain during the Second World War. As a physician he treated many soldiers who had been badly wounded and found that 49% reported being in 'moderate' or 'severe' pain with only 32% requesting medication when it was offered. However, several years later when he was treating civilians with similar if not less severe wounds after having undergone surgery, he found that 75% of the civilians reported being in 'moderate' or 'severe' pain with 83% requesting medication. Beecher accounted for these stark differences in terms of the meaning the injuries had for the soldiers compared to the civilian surgical patients. For the soldiers their injuries represented the end of their war and they could look forward to resuming their lives away from the dangerous battleground. In contrast, for the civilians, the surgery represented the beginning of a long and challenging disruption to their lives.

Two of the early dominant theories of pain perception are specificity theory and pattern theory. The former theory takes a very mechanistic view and assumes that we have a separate sensory

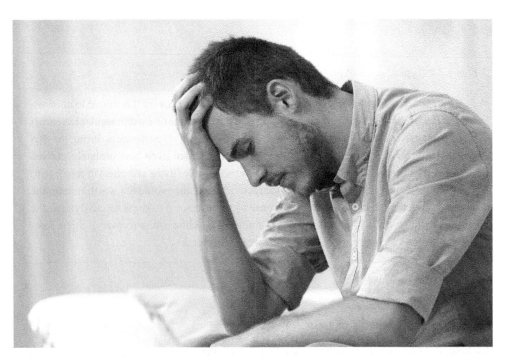

Figure 2.5 Anxiety and worry can open the gate leading to the experience of greater pain.
Copyright Antonio Guillem/Shutterstock.

system for perceiving pain similar to hearing and vision. Moreover, specificity theory posits that the 'pain system' has its own set of special pain receptors for detecting pain stimuli and its own peripheral nerves which communicates via a separate pathway to a designated area in the brain for the processing of pain signals.

Pattern theory offers a competing view. It suggests that a separate sensory system does not exist but instead receptors for pain are shared with the other senses. Central to this view is the notion that an individual will only experience pain when a certain pattern of neural activity reaches a critical level in the brain. Moreover, given that mild and strong pain stimulation uses the same sense modality, this theory suggests that only intense stimulation will produce a pattern of neural activity that will result in pain.

Nevertheless, as outlined above, none of these early theories can explain the role of psychological factors in pain perception. For example, they cannot account for how cognitive, emotional and social factors such as the meaning of pain can influence the experience of pain.

Gate-control theory of pain

In 1965, Melzack and Wall introduced the gate-control theory of pain perception. This theory was innovative as it incorporated important aspects of earlier theories but at the same time provided a detailed description of the physiological mechanisms through which psychological factors could influence an individual's experience of pain. In a nutshell, gate-control theory proposes that a neural gate in the spinal cord can modulate incoming pain signals and that a number of factors influence the opening and closing of the gate. Broadly speaking, these are:

1. The amount of activity in pain fibres.
2. The amount of activity in other peripheral fibres.
3. Messages that descend from the brain (or central nervous system).

When the neural gate receives information from each of these sources it decides whether to open or close the gate. When the gate is open, pain is experienced.

The theory postulates that the gating mechanism is located in the substantia gelatinosa (i.e. the grey matter that extends along the length of the spinal cord) of the dorsal horns in the spinal cord. When we are exposed to a painful stimulus the gating mechanism receives signals from pain fibres (A-delta and C fibres) located at the site of the injury, other peripheral fibres (A-beta fibres) which transmit information about harmless stimuli, and the brain (or central nervous system) to open the gate. The pain fibres then release a neurotransmitter called substance P that passes through the gating mechanism (substantia gelatinosa) and stimulates transmission cells that in turn transmit impulses to specific locations in the brain (e.g. thalamus, limbic system, hypothalamus). When the activity of the transmission cells reaches a critical threshold level we experience pain with greater pain intensity associated with greater activity. Once the pain centres in the brain have been activated, we are able to respond quickly to remove ourselves from danger. It is worth noting that the brain produces its own pain-relieving chemicals in the form of endorphins (i.e. a chemical similar to opiates) that inhibits the pain fibres from releasing substance P which subsequently reduces the experience of pain. This is why endorphins are often described as being associated with a 'jogger's high'.

Moreover, pain sensations from the injury site are transmitted to the gating mechanism by pain fibres (or nerves) known as nociceptors. This is known as an afferent pathway because it indicates information is travelling towards the CNS. As outlined above, in addition to A-beta fibres two other key fibre types have been identified:

- A-delta fibres (types I and II).
  Transmit information about sharp, brief pain.
  Wrapped in layers of 'fatty' cell membranes (i.e. myelinated) which increases the speed of action.
- C-fibres.
  Transmit information about dull, throbbing pain.
  - Not wrapped in 'fatty' cell membranes, therefore they have a slower speed of action.

Each of the three types of nociceptors is important as stated by Melzack and Wall (1965: 975) 'The degree to which the gate increases or decreases sensory transmission is determined by the relative activity in large diameter (A-beta) and small diameter (A-delta and C) fibres and by descending influences from the brain'. The other group of nerves that transmit information to the gating mechanism are the other peripheral fibres. In particular, A-beta fibres carry information about harmless stimulation or mild irritation, such as gentle touch or stroking or lightly scratching the skin, to the spinal cord. When A-beta fibres are stimulated the gate is likely to close and pain perception is inhibited, explaining why people experience a reduction in pain during a gentle massage or when heat is applied to aching limbs.

The final factor that influences the opening and closing of the gate is the impact of messages descending from the brain. Neurons in different parts of the brain send impulses, via what are known as efferent pathways (i.e. indicating they lead away from the CNS or are descending from the brain), to the spinal cord. Various brain processes such as anxiety, distraction, hypnosis and excitement have the capacity to influence this neural activity by releasing chemicals such as endorphins and therefore the opening and closing of the gate. From a biopsychosocial point of view, this is the most important component of gate-control theory as it provides a clear route through which cognitive, emotional and social factors can influence pain perception. Focus box 2.1 provides an overview of various conditions that individuals may experience that may open and close the gate. Since the introduction of this theory, researchers have been inspired to investigate the efficacy of psychological and behavioural approaches to pain management. We will consider these approaches in Chapter 10.

FOCUS BOX 2.1

Conditions that can open and close the pain gate

Conditions that open the gate:

Physical conditions

- – Extent of the injury
- – Inappropriate activity level

Emotional conditions

- – Anxiety or worry
- – Tension
- – Depression

Mental conditions

- – Focusing on the pain
- – Boredom; little involvement in life activities

Conditions that close the gate:

Physical conditions

- – Medication
- – Counterstimulation (e.g. heat or massage)

Emotional conditions

- – Positive emotions (e.g. happiness or optimism)
- – Relaxation
- – Rest

Mental conditions

- – Intense concentration or distraction
- – Involvement and interest in life activities

Source: Adapted from Sarafino (2008)

Neuromatrix theory of pain

Melzack (1999) extended his gate-control theory of pain during the 1980s and 1990s. The primary reason for this was the original theory's inability to explain the phenomenon known as phantom limb pain (i.e. experiencing pain in a limb that no longer exists). This new model has suggested a stronger and more dominant role for the brain. The central tenets of the theory are:

1. The areas of the brain linked to particular parts of the body continue to be active and receive inputs even if a body part no longer exists.
2. We can still experience the qualities of the human condition, including pain, without receiving input from the body, indicating that the origins of the patterns of activation that bring about these qualities of experience must be located in neural networks in the brain.
3. Conscious awareness of 'body' and 'self' is generated in the brain via patterns of input that can be modified by different perceptual inputs.
4. A network of neurons, known as the neuromatrix, is distributed throughout the brain to process all incoming sensory information including pain signals (known as the body-self neuromatrix). This neural network consists of cyclical, feedback loops between three of the

brain's main neural circuits: the thalamus, limbic system and the cortex. The neuromatrix can process 'experiences' such as pain without receiving direct input from the body.

5. When the neuromatrix receives sensory inputs, they are processed (synthesized) and become imprinted on the matrix creating what is known as a neurosignature. The neurosignature is projected to areas of the brain – the sentient neural hub – where the flow of nerve impulses is transformed into a constantly changing stream of awareness.

6. An action neuromatrix is then activated to signal appropriate movements when pain is experienced (e.g. remove hand from hot iron).

7. The neuromatrix is genetically determined, however, it is modified through sensory inputs such as pain experiences.

As you will have gathered, this is a complicated theory and further work is required before researchers fully understand issues like phantom limb pain (e.g. Pacheco-Barrios, Meng & Fregni, 2020). For example, recent advances of the theory have suggested that exploration of how the stress response systems interact and provide additional inputs into the neuromatrix is required. Nevertheless, the developments presented by Melzack's neuromatrix theory of pain have provided valuable insights into the mechanisms underlying this phenomenon (Jensen & Turk, 2014).

Psychoneuroimmunology

Have you ever wondered why a relatively large number of students report having the common cold around the time of important examinations? Is this simply bad luck, all in the mind, or is there a biological explanation? A growing body of evidence indicates that there is a link between social and psychological factors and susceptibility to respiratory infectious illness. This is noteworthy given that historically these two realms were considered quite distinct (i.e. the mind versus body debate).

The term psychoneuroimmunology or PNI was coined by Robert Ader and Nicholas Cohen of the University of Rochester in the USA to describe this new area of science that explored the interaction between psychological processes and the nervous and immune systems. Ader and Cohen were at the forefront of this area and demonstrated the link between the brain and the immune system early on (Ader & Cohen, 1975). Using a paradigm called conditioned immuno-suppression, based upon Pavlov's classical conditioning, they discovered that the immune system of rats could be conditioned to respond to external stimuli unrelated to immune function. They found that after an artificially flavoured drink was paired with an immune suppressive drug in rats, the presentation of the drink alone was sufficient to suppress immune functioning. Studies such as this one have provided the starting point for researchers to examine the effects of various psychological factors on human immunity. Over the last 25 years or so, a large amount of research effort has concentrated on exploring the extent to which psychological stress may influence different aspects of the immune system. Two areas that have received particular attention are respiratory infectious illness and wound healing (cf., Cohen, 2005; Kiecolt-Glaser et al., 1998; O'Connor, Thayer & Vedhara, 2021). However, in order to understand the link between stress, the common cold and wound healing, we need to appreciate how the immune system works. Therefore, the next section provides a basic introduction to the immune system.

The immune system

The function of the immune system is to defend the body against invaders. Microbes (germs or microorganisms), cancer cells and transplanted tissues or organs are all interpreted by the immune system as 'non-self' against which the body must be defended. Although the immune system is incredibly complex, its basic strategy is straightforward: to recognize the enemy, mobilize forces and attack. Amazingly, the immune system can distinguish between 'self' and 'non-self' and learns to remember the distinctive cellular features of invaders. Moreover, it is able to form an immunological memory of infectious agents and so mount a more effective response the next time the invader attacks. It is this process that is exploited when a person is vaccinated with a mild dose of an infectious agent – the body becomes primed for a real invasion.

What are the basic features of the immune system? Broadly speaking, the human body has the capacity to mount two types of immune defence:

1. Cell-mediated immunity.
2. Antibody-mediated immunity.

In both cases, the basic immune response is brought about by the actions of two types of white blood cells known as lymphocytes and monocytes. Importantly, there are two types of lymphocytes with different functions: T (for thymus) cells and B (for bone) cells. Both types are formed in the bone marrow, but the T cells migrate to the thymus to mature while the B cells remain in the marrow. B cells produce antibodies (i.e. large proteins that will recognize and bind to invading infectious agents), whereas T cells do not. It is also worth noting that there are a number of different kinds of T cells including T helper cells, natural killer cells, T suppressor cells and cytotoxic killer cells.

T and B cells operate very differently when attacking infectious agents. The former bring about cell-mediated immunity while the latter bring about antibody-mediated immunity (see Table 2.1 for an overview of the roles of T and B cells). In the former case, when an infectious agent enters the body, it is recognized by a type of monocyte called a macrophage, which presents the infectious agent to a T helper cell and releases interleukin-1 (IL-1; a type of cytokine released from cells to influence the activity of other cells), this in turn stimulates T-helper cell activity. As a result, the T helper cells then release interleukin-2 (another cytokine) which triggers the proliferation of T cells and eventually the release of cytotoxic killer cells which attack and destroy the infectious agent.

Table 2.1   Comparison of the roles of T and B cells

Cell-mediated immunity: T cells	Antibody-mediated immunity: B cells
Work directly at cell level	Work via the bloodstream
A type of lymphocyte (white blood cell)	A type of lymphocyte (white blood cell)
Formed in the bone marrow, but matured in thymus (T)	Formed and matured in the bone (B) marrow
Attack and destroy infectious agents by triggering release of cytotoxic killer cells	Attack and destroy infectious agents by stimulating the release of antibodies

In antibody-mediated immunity, the initial stages are similar, such that there is collaboration between macrophages and T helper cells. However, in this case, the T helper cells stimulate the proliferation of B cells leading to the secretion of antibodies which identify and bind to specific features of the infectious agent. The antibodies then immobilize and destroy the pathogen.

Stress and the immune system

Can stress alter immune functioning? There is evidence to show that stress can suppress cell-mediated immunity, although the data relating to the antibody response and B cell function in particular are less clear. For example, many studies have shown that increased secretion of stress hormones such as cortisol can alter the production of cytokines. As we already know, cytokines are important in the activation of T cells as well as in mediating the pro-inflammatory response (this process is explained further in a later section). Therefore, stress-induced changes in the production of cytokines may represent an important mechanism through which stress compromises the body's response to infectious illness. An important study by Kunz-Ebrecht and colleagues (2003) showed that cortisol responses to psychological stress were inversely associated with the production of two cytokines (IL-6 and IL-1ra), indicating that psychological factors can influence important components of immune functioning. Moreover, there is robust evidence to suggest that psychological stress, suffered as a result of adverse early experiences, is likely to increase people's vulnerability to immune dysregulation in adulthood (O'Connor, Thayer & Vedhara, 2021; Kraynak et al., 2019). For example, a recent study found that adults in middle age who reported childhood physical abuse had elevated pro-inflammatory responses (i.e. increased IL-6) and decreased functionality connectivity between key parts of the brain compared to those who did not report childhood physical abuse (Kraynak et al., 2019).

Stress and respiratory infectious illness

Over the last 35 years, Sheldon Cohen, a psychologist at Carnegie Mellon University in the USA, has explored the extent to which psychological and social factors influence susceptibility to infectious illnesses such as the common cold (see Cohen, 2005, for a review). As part of this work, Cohen and his colleagues have developed a unique prospective study design in which healthy participants are exposed to a virus that causes the common cold. Participants are then monitored following exposure in order to determine who develops a respiratory illness and reports cold-like symptoms. At baseline, participants also normally complete a range of psychological measures to assess their current level of perceived stress, their mood and any recent stressful life events.

In 1991, Cohen and his colleagues published a seminal paper, in the prestigious journal, the *New England Journal of Medicine*, in which they demonstrated for the first time that increases in psychological stress are associated with increases in risk for developing a cold after exposure to a cold virus. If this is not impressive enough, they also demonstrated that this association was independent of the participants' baseline levels of specific antibody, age, sex, education, allergic status and body mass index, and the season of the year. In addition, they also explored whether the increased susceptibility was related to changes in stress-related health behaviours such as smoking, exercise and diet. None of these variables explained the relationship.

In a subsequent study, Cohen and colleagues (1998) concentrated on identifying the types of stressful life events that were most predictive of increased susceptibility to infectious illness. In order to do this, these researchers conducted detailed interviews with each of the participants who took part in their standard prospective design and found two types of stressful life events were most strongly related to susceptibility. The first type of event was enduring (one month or longer) interpersonal problems with family and friends. The second type were enduring problems associated with work (such as under- or unemployment). They also found that the longer the stressful event had lasted, the greater was the risk of developing an infectious illness.

Similar to their earlier study, the authors again examined which psychological and biological factors may be mediating the effects of psychological stress on increased susceptibility (see Research methods box 5.2). Interestingly, they found that regular exercise, non-smoking and greater sleep efficacy (percent of time in bed sleeping) were associated with lower susceptibility to developing a common cold. In addition, they also found that higher levels of adrenaline and noradrenaline (in the urine in the past 24 hours) were related to greater susceptibility. However, surprisingly, the effects of these factors were independent of the relationship between psychological stress and risk of developing a cold.

In the last 20 years, research has turned its attention to exploring the role of pro-inflammatory cytokine regulation in explaining the mediating pathways between psychological stress and the common cold. You will recall from earlier that cytokines are produced in response to infection. They are also believed to trigger symptoms associated with upper respiratory infections such as the common cold and the influenza virus (Cohen, 2005; 2021). Therefore, using a more complex study design, Cohen, Doyle and Skoner (1999) investigated whether psychological stress influenced cytokine production in participants after receiving an influenza virus. Specifically, they tested whether stress had the capacity to interfere with the body's ability to regulate cytokine production. Normally, when a virus is detected, the body produces enough cytokines to remove the virus. However, Cohen et al. found that stress short-circuited the body's ability to switch off the cytokine response. Individuals who had previously experienced high stress prior to receiving the virus were found to have higher IL-6 (cytokine) levels and greater symptom scores in response to the viral challenge. In a subsequent study, these researchers replicated their findings and demonstrated that prolonged stress influences susceptibility to infectious illness by decreasing cortisol's effectiveness in regulating the pro-inflammatory cytokine response, leading to increased production of IL-6 and greater illness expression (Miller, Cohen & Ritchey, 2002). Taken together, these findings bring us to a surprising conclusion: psychological stress does not influence upper respiratory illness by suppressing the immune system. On the contrary, stress experienced over an extended period of time results in the immune system over-responding, which in turn activates and extends the symptoms of upper respiratory infections.

There have been a number of exciting developments in the area of stress and the common cold. Of particular note is the investigation of the relationship between telomeres and the development of upper respiratory infections (Cohen et al., 2013a;b). Telomeres are 'caps' at the end of chromosomes which get shorter as we get older and it has been suggested that these are biomarkers (or indicators) of good or bad aging. For example, shorter telomeres have been linked with the development of diseases such as cardiovascular disease, cancer and can confer risk of degenerative diseases (Lin & Epel, 2022). Moreover, a study has shown that people with shorter telomeres were at greater risk of developing an upper respiratory infection after receiving the common cold virus in the laboratory (Cohen et al., 2013a). In addition, in a related investigation, these authors also found that participants from lower socioeconomic backgrounds were also more likely to be infected by the cold virus and that this was explained, in part, by having shorter telomeres (Cohen et al., 2013b).

Recently, Cohen (2021) has turned his attention to consider the implications of his body of work on stress and respiratory illnesses for understanding susceptibility to the Coronavirus Disease 2019 (COVID-19). He has theorized that greater risk of respiratory illnesses after exposure to a virus will be associated with smoking, lower levels of vitamin C intake and of course higher levels of chronic psychological stress. Furthermore, he has suggested, based on their previous research that physical activity, better social support and integration, adequate and efficient sleep and moderate alcohol intake will be associated with decreased risk of susceptibility. Interestingly, a new study has begun to confirm these predictions. This prospective cohort investigation found that individuals who experienced elevated levels of psychological distress earlier in the COVID-19 pandemic were more likely to report COVID-19 infection and more severe symptoms eight months later (Ayling et al., 2022).

Stress and wound healing

In 1995, Janice Kiecolt-Glaser and colleagues from Ohio State University published a seminal study that provided evidence, for the first time, that psychological stress slowed wound healing. Similar to Cohen and his co-investigators, Kiecolt-Glaser and her colleagues developed an unusual research design to investigate the links between stress and immune functioning. Using a punch biopsy, a 3.5 mm full thickness wound was created on the non-dominant forearm, approximately 4 cm below the elbow, in each of the study participants. Levels of perceived stress were then measured using questionnaires and the wound was photographed every day until it completely healed. A wound was considered fully healed when it no longer foamed after hydrogen peroxide was applied! In this study the researchers were interested in the effects of chronic stress on immune function and wound healing. Therefore, participants who were caring for a relative with Alzheimer's disease (high stress group) were compared to control participants (low stress group) matched for age and family income. The results of the study showed that complete wound healing took an average of nine days or 24% longer in the caregiver group compared to the controls. They also found differences between the groups in the production of an important cytokine (interleukin-1ß) suggesting this as one of the immunological mechanisms underlying the observed effects.

Next, this research group investigated whether a relatively minor, commonplace stressful event such as an examination had the potential to similarly influence wound healing. In this study, Marucha et al. (1998) placed a 3.5 mm punch biopsy wound in the mouths (i.e. on the hard palate) of a sample of dental students, once during the summer vacation and again three days before a major examination. This repeated measures design allowed the participants to act as their own controls. Again, two independent methods assessed wound healing (daily photographs and a foaming response to hydrogen peroxide). Surprisingly, all students took longer to heal in the examination condition compared to control conditions with complete healing taking an average of three days (or 40%) longer in the examination condition. These data suggest that even short-lived, predictable and relatively benign stressors can have significant consequences for wound healing. More importantly, these findings have important implications for understanding recovery from surgery. Evidence suggests that a more negative psychological response to surgery is associated with a slower and more complicated post-operative recovery, greater pain, longer hospital stay and worse treatment adherence (for more detailed discussion see Kiecolt-Glaser et al., 1998). Moreover, these results indicate that if patients are psychologically better prepared for surgery they are likely to experience significant health benefits. This is consistent with an investigation of recovery from total knee replacement surgery that showed that higher levels of anxiety and depression pre-operatively were associated with poorer recovery one year later (Hanusch, O'Connor, Ions, Scott & Gregg, 2014). A recent review found that psychological interventions aimed at reducing stress and anxiety before abdominal surgery were successful in reducing the pain and anxiety experienced, and the authors speculated that these improvements may positively influence neuroendocrine and inflammatory response to surgical stress outcomes (Villa et al., 2020).

Psychological influences on recovery from surgery

Using this work as a starting point, Kiecolt-Glaser and colleagues (1998: 1209) have developed a model of psychological influences on surgical recovery. They suggest that psychological factors can impact wound healing, a key variable in short-term post-surgical recovery, via three key pathways:

1. Emotions have direct effects on 'stress' hormones, and they can modulate immune function.
2. The patient's emotional response to surgery can influence the type and amount of anaesthetic, and anaesthetics vary in their effects on the immune and endocrine system.
3. Individuals who are more anxious are also more likely to experience greater post-surgical pain, and pain can suppress immune functioning.

Summary

In this chapter we have considered several of the key psychophysiological pathways through which psychological factors (and particularly stress) may influence health and illness processes. Chapter 3 describes the key theoretical approaches to stress and evaluates the research evidence concerning the links between stressors and illness and between stressors and health behaviour. Psychological factors such as stress can affect health directly, through autonomic and neuroendocrine changes but also indirectly, through changes in health behaviours. The direct effects of stress on health outcomes are known as psychophysiological pathways, while the indirect effects are known as behavioural pathways.

The role of the nervous system is to allow us to adapt to changes both within our body and our environment. It consists of the brain, the spinal cord and billions of nerves. The brain is the central part of the nervous system and consists of three major components: the forebrain, the midbrain and the hindbrain. The forebrain is divided into two main subdivisions: 1) the telencephalon which comprises the cerebrum and the limbic system; and 2) the diencephalon which is composed of the thalamus and hypothalamus. The midbrain consists of two major parts: the tectum and the tegmentum. Similarly, the hindbrain has two major divisions: the metencephalon and the myelencephalon.

The nervous system is divided into the central nervous system (CNS) and the peripheral nervous system (PNS). The CNS comprises the brain and spinal cord whereas the PNS is a network of nerves that connects the brain and spinal cord to the rest of the body. An important part of the

PNS is the autonomic nervous system (ANS) that has a sympathetic division and a parasympathetic division. The former mobilizes bodily processes (e.g. increases heart rate), whereas the latter restores the body's energy resources.

Two response systems are activated when we experience stress. The first and easiest to activate is the sympathetic adrenal medullary (SAM) system; the second is the hypothalamic–pituitary–adrenal (HPA) axis response system. The SAM system leads to the release of the adrenaline and noradrenaline that put the body on alert; the HPA axis response system leads to the release of the stress hormone, cortisol. The stress response has been found to impact negatively on a number of health outcomes such as cardiovascular disease. Excessive wear and tear of the cardiovascular system through repeated activation of the stress response may increase the development of atherosclerosis and increase the likelihood of myocardial infarction and stroke.

Psychological factors can play a role in the perception of pain. Early theories of pain were mechanistic and did not account for the influence of cognitive, emotional and social factors. Gate-control theory, introduced by Melzack and Wall (1965), proposes that a neural gate in the spinal cord receives signals from pain fibres at the site of injury, other peripheral fibres and messages descending from the brain. The degree to which the gate opens (leading to experience of pain) is determined by the combined effects of these three factors. Gate-control theory was extended by Melzack and is known as the neuromatrix theory of pain. This theory contends that the pain experience is governed by the body-self neuromatrix.

The human body has the capacity to mount two types of defence known as cell-mediated immunity and antibody-mediated immunity. Psychological factors such as stress have been found to influence these immune functions. A number of researchers have shown stress to be associated with increased susceptibility to infectious illnesses and the slowing down of wound healing.

Key concepts and terms

- Antibody-mediated immunity
- Autonomic nervous system
- Cardiovascular system
- Cell-mediated immunity
- Central nervous system
- Endocrine system
- Gate-control theory
- Hypothalamic–pituitary–adrenal (HPA) axis response system
- Limbic system
- Neuromatrix theory of pain
- Parasympathetic nervous system
- Peripheral nervous system
- Psychoneuroimmunology
- Psychophysiological pathways
- Somatic nervous system
- Sympathetic adrenal medullary (SAM) response system
- Sympathetic nervous system
- Trier Social Stress Test

Sample essay titles

- To what extent can psychological factors influence health and illness processes?
- Cognitive, emotional and social factors affect pain. Discuss this statement with reference to recent psychological theory.
- Social and psychological factors are linked to susceptibility and respiratory infectious illness. Discuss.
- What are the pathways through which stress can alter immune functioning?

Further reading

Books

Darnall, B.D. (2019). Psychological treatment for patients with chronic pain. American Psychological Association.

Kalat, J.W. (2018). *Biological psychology*. New York: Thomson Wadsworth.

Lovallo, W.R. (2015). *Stress and health: Biological and psychological interactions*. Los Angeles: Sage.

Yan, Q. (2018). *Psychoneuroimmunology: Methods and protocols*. New York, NY: Humana Press.

Journal articles

Burgin, D., O'Donovan, A., d'Huart, D., di Gallo, A., Eckert, A., Fegert, J., Schmeck, K., Schmid, M. & Boonmann, C. (2019). Adverse childhood experiences and telomere length a look into the heterogeneity of findings—A narrative review. *Frontiers in Neuroscience, 13*. https://doi.org/10.3389/fnins.2019.00490

Cohen, S. (2005). The Pittsburgh common cold studies: Psychosocial predictors of susceptibility to respiratory infectious illness. *International Journal of Behavioral Medicine, 12*, 123–131. https://doi.org/10.1207/s15327558ijbm1203_1

Cohen, S., Murphy, M.L.M. & Prather, A.A. (2019). Ten surprising fact about stressful life events and disease risk. *Annual Review of Psychology, 70*, 577–597. https://doi.org/10.1146/annurev-psych-010418-102857

Jensen, M.P. & Turk, D.C. (2014). Contributions of psychology to the understanding and treatment of people with chronic pain: Why it matters to ALL psychologists. *American Psychologist, 69*, 105–118. https://doi.org/10.1037/a0035641

O'Connor, D.B., Thayer, J.T. & Vedhara, K. (2021). Stress and health: A review of psychobiological processes. *Annual Review of Psychology, 72*, 663–688. https://doi.org/10.1146/annurev-psych-062520-122331

PART 2

Stress and health

3   Stress theory and research

Stress theory and research

Stress is widespread and media coverage suggests that it causes illness. In this chapter we will examine how stress is studied and how it is linked to disease. Evolutionary perspectives on stress in preparing humans for fight or flight will be considered as well as more contemporary views. Building on Chapter 2, we discuss a model of physiological responses to stress leading to the long-term health impact of stress, known as allostatic load. We then explore different measures of stress including life events such as marriage, divorce or bereavement and daily hassles such as losing one's keys. We discuss these in terms of Lazarus' Transactional Theory of Stress (1966, 1999; Lazarus & Folkman, 1984). Finally, we discuss Conservation of Resources theory (Hobfoll, 1989, 2001).

This chapter will highlight the pathways by which stress impacts on health. Stress affects health through biological processes (e.g. blood pressure, release of stress hormones, immune functioning) and (indirectly) through health behaviours (e.g. exercise, diet, smoking). We consider evidence for both pathways when discussing the impact of life events and daily stressors on health outcomes. In the final section of this chapter, we consider why some people become ill in response to stressful situations and others do not.

The chapter has five sections:

1. What is stress?
2. Early approaches to stress.
3. Contemporary approaches to stress – allostatic load and health.
4. Contemporary psychological approaches.
5. Why do some people get ill in response to stressors and others do not?

Learning outcomes

When you have completed this chapter you should be able to:

1   Describe what is meant by stress. Discuss whether stress is a growing problem.
2   Describe and evaluate key theoretical approaches to stress.
3   Describe and evaluate key ways in which stress has been measured.

DOI: 10.4324/9781003171096-5

4   Discuss and evaluate research evidence concerning the links between stressors and a) illness, and b) health behaviour.
5   Describe the impact of individual differences in responses to stressors.

What is stress?

The increase in press and television coverage of stress over few decades has corresponded to a growth in research and public awareness. Indeed, stress is now the most common cause of long-term sick leave and is frequently shown to be a very important factor accounting for in excess of 10 million working days lost per annum in the UK (HSE, 2017). In 2021/22, work-related stress, depression and anxiety accounted for 50% of all cases of work-related illnesses in the UK (i.e. 822,000 cases of work-related stress, depression or anxiety). In the United States, the impact of stress is also far reaching, with 76% of Americans reporting that stress has had an impact on their health and 76% reported that the future of their nation was a significant source of stress (American Psychological Association, 2022).

We can all empathize with feeling stressed. However, it is not always clear what we mean by 'stress' (Segerstrom & O'Connor, 2012). Over centuries, 'stress' has come to mean pressure or strain. Scientific interest dates back to the early part of the 20th century. For example, First World War concerns about industrial efficiency led to studies of fatigue in wartime munitions factories and the war focused attention on 'shellshock' which was subsequently acknowledged as a manifestation of post-traumatic stress disorder (Lazarus, 1999).

There have been three different approaches to the study of stress: the stimulus-based or engineering approach; the response-based or medico-physiological approach; and the psychological 'interactional-appraisal' approach. The engineering approach views stress as a demand on an individual from their environment which produces a strain reaction: the greater the strain, the larger the reaction. This approach assumes that undemanding situations are not stressful. However, monotonous undemanding work environments very often are stressful. The engineering analogy is also problematic because it makes the assumption that individual's function both unconsciously and automatically; no consideration is given to the mediating psychological processes (e.g. cognitive appraisal) but such processes are very important. The response-based approach mainly considers stress in terms of the general physiological reaction to noxious events in a person's environment such as changes in blood pressure, heart rate and stress hormones. Again, this approach does not account for individual psychological processes. More recent work has adopted an interactional-appraisal (or transactional) approach in order to explain the stress process. Such theories have contributed to our understanding of the variation in responses to similar noxious (or stressful) stimuli by emphasizing the importance of the intervening psychological processes.

The development of the transactional approach owes much to the work of Richard Lazarus and his colleague Susan Folkman (Lazarus & Folkman, 1984). They define stress as 'a particular relationship between the person and the environment that is appraised by the person as taxing or exceeding his or her resources and endangering his or her well-being' (Lazarus & Folkman, 1984: 19). This means that researchers need to look at the environment, the individual's reaction to the environment and the outcome (which might be in terms of physiological or psychological well-being). Perhaps because of the breadth of issues encompassed within this concept of stress, Lazarus also suggested that the most useful approach would be to regard stress not as a single variable but as a 'rubric consisting of many variables and processes' (Lazarus & Folkman, 1984: 12). Thus, stress may be viewed as an umbrella term covering a general field of study. Within this field there are many diverse areas of research which look at relationships between objective or perceived antecedents (or stressors) and a range of physiological, psychological or behavioural outcomes (often referred to as strains). The latter may include the kind of physiological measures (e.g. cortisol, blood pressure) discussed in Chapter 2, as well as illness outcomes (like the occurrence of cancer or heart disease), measures of work performance or health behaviours or, perhaps most frequently, self-ratings of satisfaction or anxiety.

The usefulness of the concept of stress has been called into question by Jerome Kagan (2016). He argued that the overly permissive use of classifying any event as a stressor just because it leads to biological or behavioural change limits its usefulness. Instead, he argues that the concept of stress should only be applied to events that ultimately pose a serious threat to an organism's well-being. Despite these concerns, leading theorists and stress researchers have challenged this view and it is clear that the cumulative science linking stress to negative health outcomes is robust (see O'Connor, Thayer & Vedhara, 2021). Perhaps because of the vagueness of the concept there is sometimes disagreement about basic issues such as whether a certain amount of stress is good for you. This clearly depends on the definition you use. For example, taking a stimulus-based approach, up to a certain point, stimuli such as work pressures may certainly be motivating and beneficial. However, using Lazarus' popular definition given above, which views stress in terms of a process involving threats to our well-being, it is harder to see how this can be construed as beneficial! A number of different approaches to stress are considered in the following sections.

FOCUS BOX 3.1

Is stress increasing?

There is a widespread view, often reflected in the media, that the amount of stress in society, both within the family and the workplace, has increased greatly in recent decades. This has been attributed to the breakdown of the nuclear family, the loosening of extended family bonds caused by the widespread mobility in the community and rapid changes in the workplace. What do you think? Is life really much more stressful than it was 50 years ago? Discuss this topic in groups, taking into account the increased public awareness of psychological responses to stressors and changes in people's expectations.

Consider also what variables you would need to consider in making an assessment of whether stress had increased. This could include increases in stressors such as wars, poverty, unemployment or work stressors. It could also include increases in outcomes such as psychiatric illness or stress-related disease.

Early approaches to stress

Two theorists who had a great influence in terms of popularizing the concept of stress were both physiologists: Walter Cannon and Hans Selye. Cannon (1932) wrote about the 'fight-or-flight' reaction to describe the human response to threats. Cannon believed that when faced with danger, such as a predator, the human being feels the emotions of fear or anger, the former being linked to an instinct to run away and the latter with the urge to fight. These reactions served to prepare the body for action as outlined in Chapter 2.

Hans Selye built on Cannon's work and described a reaction pattern called the general adaptation syndrome (GAS; Selye, 1956). Selye wrote that 'Adaptability and resistance to stress are fundamental prerequisites for life, and every vital organ participates in them' (Selye, 1950: 1383). He believed that the basic physiological reaction was always the same regardless of the stressor and that an understanding of this phenomenon depended on many branches of physiology, biochemistry and medicine. He even stated that the phenomenon would never be really understood 'since the complete comprehension of life is beyond the limits of the human mind' (Selye, 1950: 1383). It is difficult to do justice to this complex theory in a brief paragraph! However, in essence it comprises three stages:

- Alarm. This is the immediate reaction whereby stress hormones are released to prepare the body for action (fight or flight).
- Resistance. If stress is prolonged, levels of stress hormones remain high. However, during this period the individual seems superficially to adapt to the stressor but will still have heightened susceptibility to disease.
- Exhaustion. If the stress continues long enough the body's defensive resources are used up leading to illness and, ultimately, death.

In summary, according to Selye, prolonged exposure to a strong stressor will increase an individual's risk of developing health problems which he described as diseases of adaptation (e.g. ulcers, high blood pressure). Moreover, he suggested that repeated and long-term exposure to stress will lead to dysfunction of a number of the body's basic systems such as the immune and metabolic systems.

Selye's early approach focused on stress as a physiological reaction and his theory influenced many subsequent researchers. However, Mason (1971) questioned the generality of this approach, arguing that some noxious (stressful) physical conditions do not produce the predicted three-stage alarm, resistance and ultimately exhaustion responses (e.g. exercise, fasting, heat). More recent approaches have tended to emphasize psychological process and impacts and have recognized that individuals may respond differently to the same stressful events.

RESEARCH METHODS BOX 3.1

How is stress measured?

There are three main types of measures used to study stress: (1) generic measures of perceived stress, (2) event measures and (3) cognitive appraisal measures. These are not mutually exclusive. Generic measures of perceived stress aim to capture appraisals of non–event-specific perceptions of stress over the recent past. Event measures examine the experience of major life events, hassles and single acutely stressful events. Cognitive appraisal measures assess primary (the extent to which an event is appraised as threatening, challenging or likely to lead to loss) and secondary appraisals (e.g. the extent to which an event is appraised as controllable).

Generic measures of perceived stress

The most popular global measure of stress is the Perceived Stress Scale (PSS) developed by Cohen, Kamarck and Mermelstein (1983). This measure was designed to evaluate the degree to which situations in general in one's life are appraised as stressful. This scale asks participants to report about their feelings and thoughts during the *last month* in relation to non-specific events. For example, in the last month, 'how often have you been upset because of something that happened unexpectedly', and 'how often have you been able to control irritations in your life?' Other generic measures of stress have been developed such as the Stress Arousal Checklist (SACL; Cox & Mackay, 1985) and more recently the Trier Inventory of Chronic Stress has been introduced (TICS; Schulz, Schlotz & Becker, 2011)

Event measures of stress

These types of measures aim to capture participant's responses to significant life events (e.g. divorce), a single acutely stressful event (e.g. examination) and daily hassles (e.g. being late for a meeting). This may be achieved by the use of a questionnaire or by a structured interview. These may be generic life events as in the original Holmes and Rahe (1967) work (described later) or developed to focus on specific groups such as children. Event measures also include assessments of 'hassles', minor daily stressful events or annoyances as conceptualized by the original Hassles Scale (Kanner et al., 1981).

Cognitive appraisal measures of stress

Appraisal measures of stress are informed by the transactional model of stress (Lazarus & Folkman, 1984). As outlined earlier, cognitive stress appraisals are the interpretations of events in terms of their benefit or harm for the individual and the theory posits two dimensions: primary and secondary appraisals (Lazarus & Folkman, 1984). For example, the Appraisal of Life Events (ALE; Ferguson, Matthews & Cox, 1999) scale consists of three primary appraisal scales: Threat, Challenge and Loss. The 'Threat' scale assesses how threatening and anxiety provoking the situation is; 'Challenge' assesses the potential for growth and learning from the situation, and 'Loss' how sad and depressing the situation is.

Gartland, O'Connor and Lawton (2012) developed a Stressor Appraisal Scale (SAS) that can be used to assess stressor appraisals in relation to the most stressful hassle in the past seven days and it can be used in a daily diary format (see Gartland et al., 2014). This scale comprises ten items tapping primary appraisal and secondary appraisal.

Contemporary physiological approaches to stress – allostatic load and health

Building on the work of Selye is an important contemporary approach to stress, introduced by McEwen and Stellar (1993), that helps us understand how stress can cause illness over a lifetime. This approach attempts to provide a complete physiological account of the various bodily systems which may be affected by stress and how different stressful situations may impact on health. McEwen (1998) proposed that the long-term impact of stress, known as allostatic load affects the body at cardiovascular, metabolic, neural, behavioural and cellular levels. Similar to basic homeostatic systems such as body temperature, the HPA axis, the autonomic nervous system and the cardiovascular, metabolic and immune systems protect the body by adapting to internal and external stress. This is known as allostasis. However, if the activation of these systems is repeated and prolonged, allostatic load will be experienced in the form of increased release of stress hormones, immune cells, brain activity and cardiovascular response. It is suggested that if a person experiences allostatic load for a long time, they are at increased risk of developing disease because the bodily systems will stop working as effectively (for a full account see McEwen, 1998). A recent systematic review and meta-analysis investigated the relationship between allostatic load and mortality (Parker et al., 2022). Across 17 studies, this review found that high allostatic load was associated with an increased mortality risk of 22% for all-cause mortality and 31% for cardiovascular disease mortality. Another recent narrative review found that allostatic load was also associated with a range of psychiatric disorders (Finlay et al., 2022).

In terms of allostasis, when we encounter a psychological or physical stressor (e.g. giving a speech or encountering an infection or a physical threat), our body has a twofold response. First, it initiates an allostatic response that activates the stress response (as described in Chapter 2). Second, when the stressor has passed, the allostatic response is terminated. As you already know, activation of these systems leads to the release of several stress hormones including cortisol and changes in blood pressure and heart rate, which normally return to baseline levels when the stressful encounter has ended. However, if the allostatic response is not shut off but is maintained over time, due to inadequate coping, this will result in allostatic load, thus placing excessive pressure on our bodily systems.

McEwen has suggested that four situations are associated with allostatic load. Each situation differs in terms of how often we encounter stressful situations and whether we can cope with them:

1. Repeated 'hits' from multiple stressors.
2. Lack of adaptation.
3. Prolonged response.
4. Inadequate response.

As shown in Figure 3.1, the first situation is when we experience frequent stressors. If these are sustained over long periods of time they can trigger repeated elevations in blood pressure thereby increasing the risk of having a heart attack or speeding up the early stages of heart disease. The second is where we are unable to cope with or to adapt to the same type of stressor, and as a result our body is exposed to stress hormones for a long period of time. The third condition is when our bodily systems are exposed to the stress response over an extended episode due to a delayed shutdown of the body's response. The fourth is when an inadequate stress response causes the body to release extra, unnecessary hormones and other chemical messengers which may be harmful to health. As you can see, this approach deals primarily with the physiological changes that accompany stress. Contemporary psychological approaches are considered in the next section.

Contemporary psychological approaches to stress

In parallel with the development of physiological explanations of the stress process, psychologists have focused on stress as a predominantly psychological phenomenon and produced definitions and theories which concentrate on the psychological precursors and processes (O'Connor, Thayer & Vedhara, 2021). The three approaches described in this section have all been influential but approach the conceptualization and study of stress in different ways. For each approach the evidence linking them to disease is considered.

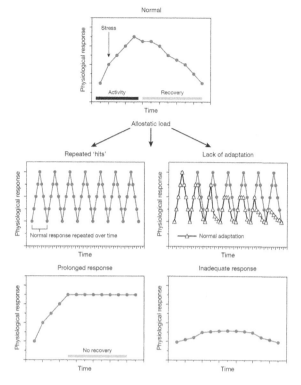

Figure 3.1 Three types of allostatic load. Top, the normal allostatic response in which a response is initiated by a stressor, sustained for an appropriate interval, and then turned off. The other four panels illustrate four conditions that lead to allostatic load: repeated 'hits' from multiple stressors; lack of adaptation; prolonged response due to delayed shut-down; and inadequate response that leads to compensatory hyperactivity of other mediators (e.g. inadequate secretion of glucocorticoids, resulting in increased concentrations of cytokines that are normally counter-regulated by glucocorticoids). Adapted from McEwen, 1998.

Life events

The study of major life events is perhaps the earliest, as well as most enduring, approach to measuring stressors. The idea that emotionally distressing events might be associated with disease and particularly cancer goes back at least as far as the 19th century where many anecdotal reports of links between negative events such as bereavement and cancer can be found in the medical literature. The first statistical study of this association is attributed to Snow (1893) who studied 250 cancer patients in London and found that in over 60% of them there had been some problem before the onset of the disease. Frequently this was the death of a close relative.

More formal measurement approaches to studying life events originated in the 1960s when Holmes and Rahe (1967) published a checklist of life events called the Social Readjustment Rating Scale which is reproduced in Table 3.1. The idea of a change being stressful and requiring adaptation is central to the approach. Thus, life events were changes rather than persistent states. Furthermore, they were objectively verifiable events.

Table 3.1 Social Readjustment Rating Scale (Holmes & Rahe, 1967)

Rank	Life events	LCU* score
1	Death of spouse	100
2	Divorce	173
3	Marital separation	165
4	Jail term	163
5	Death of close family member	163
6	Personal illness or injury	153
7	Marriage	150
8	Fired at work	147
9	Marital reconciliation	145
10	Retirement	145
11	Change in health of a family member	144
12	Pregnancy	140
13	Sex difficulties	139
14	Gain of a new family member	139
15	Business readjustment	139
16	Change in financial state	138
17	Death of a close friend	137
18	Change to a different line of work	136
19	Change in number of arguments with spouse	135
20	Mortgage over $10,000	131
21	Foreclosure of mortgage or loan	130
22	Change in responsibilities at work	129
23	Son or daughter leaving home	129
24	Trouble with in-laws	129
25	Outstanding personal achievement	128
26	Wife begin or stop work	126
27	Begin or end school	126
28	Change in living conditions	125
29	Revision of personal habits	124
30	Trouble with boss	123
31	Change in work hours or conditions	120
32	Change in residence	120
33	Change in schools	120
34	Change in recreation	119
35	Change in church activities	119
36	Change in social activities	118
37	Mortgage or loan less than $10,000	117
38	Change in sleeping habits	116
39	Change in number of family get-togethers	115
40	Change in eating habits	115
41	Vacation	113
42	Christmas	112
43	Minor violations of the law	111

Source: Reprinted from Holmes and Rahe (1967), with permission from Elsevier
Note: * LCU = Life change unit

In the initial research to establish this measure, Holmes and Rahe drew on their clinical experience to list 43 events. A sample of 394 people were asked to rate these for the degree of 'social readjustment' they required. Marriage was given an arbitrary value (50 in the final scale) and they were asked to assign numeric values to all the other events based on how much more (or less) adjustment the event required than marriage. The sum of ratings for events an individual experiences in the last year is known as their life change unit (LCU) score. Holmes and Masuda (1974) described an LCU score of over 150 in one year as a life crisis, (150–199 is a mild crisis, 200–299 a moderate crisis and over 300 a major crisis). They also reported an early study which indicated that life crises were linked to deterioration in health. For example, 37% of those whose scores indicated they had experienced a minor crisis, and 79% of those with a major crisis, reported changes in health. Further studies in the 1970s by Rahe and colleagues suggested that high LCU scores were linked with heart disease (e.g. Theorell and Rahe, 1971). However, as the methodology has improved, and more longitudinal studies have been conducted, results have tended to be less consistent.

ACTIVITY BOX 3.2

Look at Table 3.1 and work out your own LCU score for the past year. Do you think this is a reasonable indication of the stress you have experienced in the last year? Before you read on, write down any problems you can see with this approach to measuring stress.

There have been a number of criticisms of the life events approach highlighting limitations which may account for the large number of positive findings in the early literature. Some critics have commented on the fact that where two people both have the same score their subjective experience may actually be very different. In one study, researchers interviewed people about their responses and found that, for some people, the death of a close friend involved the death of a childhood friend who they had not seen for a long time whereas for others it was a much more significant loss. This has been labelled the problem of 'intracategory variability' (Dohrenwend, 2006).

A further criticism, which you may have identified, is that the Social Readjustment Rating Scale does not discriminate between positive and negative events (Jones & Kinman, 2001). However, most people would assume that only negative events would be harmful for health, while positive events might even be beneficial. Because of this criticism many more recent approaches to life events measurement also take into account people's appraisals of each event.

Research on life events has also been criticized for the reliability and validity of measures (that is, do people produce the same scores if asked to complete the questionnaire after a time interval and do the measures actually measure what they are intended to measure). In the 1970s and 1980s researchers considered reliability over time (usually called test–retest reliability). One study found that, when people repeated the measure after 1–2 weeks, there was only 70% agreement (Steele et al., 1980), and other research has indicated that reliability declines dramatically over longer periods (Dohrenwend, 2006). Related to this, there are concerns that retrospective reports may not be valid when, as is often the case, they are reported by people who are already diagnosed with a disease. In these circumstances people may be inclined to want to find an explanation for their illness, leading them to report more life events than those who have no illness (Brown, 1974). This factor may account for some of the positive relationships found in the early studies. Nowadays limited credence is given to studies unless they use longitudinal approaches which assess life events prior to the development (or at least the diagnosis) of disease.

Over the years there have been improvements to life events methodology and many different measures of stressful life events have been developed. Some have been established that are relevant to particular subgroups. For example, there are a range of scales specifically for use with children and adolescents. Others have tried to overcome the methodological limitations of the checklist approach by using the much more time-consuming approach of semi-structured interviews where people describe events which are then rated by trained individuals. The most well-known example of this is the Life Events and Difficulties Schedule (LEDS) developed by Brown and Harris (1978). This was used in an important study of life events, social support and depression which is described in more detail in Chapter 5 (Brown & Harris, 1978).

Over the past 50 years researchers have studied the relationship between life events and disease. Yet there is still controversy concerning whether major life events do cause disease. The early studies showed strong links but have been subject to criticism. Literature on breast cancer provides a good example of how some well-publicized studies find links between life events and cancer (e.g. Chen et al., 1995) but other research fails to support the findings (e.g. Protheroe et al., 1999). Many studies have used what is known as a 'limited prospective design'. For example, Chen et al. (1995) studied 119 women who were referred for biopsies for suspected breast cancer. They were interviewed and their experience of life events was assessed before they received a definitive diagnosis. The researchers found that 19 out of 41 women who were subsequently diagnosed with cancer had experienced threatening life events during the five years before diagnosis compared with 15 out of the 78 controls. While isolated studies such as this often get media publicity and strengthen public perceptions that there is a link, literature reviews and meta-analyses of the overall associations tend to conclude that there is little evidence to link life events and breast cancer incidence (e.g. Nielsen & Brønbæk, 2006), though it is still unclear whether stress may effect progression of the disease. However, the search for possible links between stress and breast cancer continues to fascinate researchers (see Antoni & Dhabhar, 2019).

Stressful life events may be more strongly linked to psychological outcomes. Research into life events in extreme situations such as wars and natural disasters suggests that exposure to such events is likely to lead to serious psychopathology (Dohrenwend, 2006). There is also convincing evidence that stressful life events are linked to an increase in depression and suicide risk (e.g. Howarth et al., 2020). However, it is clear that there are considerable individual differences in people's susceptibility. The idea that some people are genetically more susceptible to stressors is known as the stress diathesis model (the term 'diathesis' meaning a predisposition to illness). A number of studies have suggested that some people are indeed more genetically vulnerable to stressful life events than others (e.g. Kendler et al., 1995). Advances in genetics have now enabled researchers to explore specific genes which may be associated with this susceptibility. For example, Lessard and Holman (2014) provide evidence that long-term health impacts of exposure to child abuse and stressful life events in adulthood are moderated by hypothalamic–pituitary–adrenal (HPA) axis polymorphism genotypes. More recently, O'Connor et al. (2018; 2020) found that childhood trauma was associated with dysregulation in the cortisol response to stressors and the amount of cortisol individuals released in the morning when they awaken – suggesting that the HPA axis was not functioning properly. There has also been the development of the important related area of behaviour genetics that explores how genetic differences in people leads to differences in their psychology and behaviour (Harden, 2021).

Overall, despite the many criticisms of life events research, it seems to be an approach that is here to stay with the number of studies increasing dramatically decade by decade (Dohrenwend, 2006). Furthermore, modifications in methodology have helped to improve reliability and validity of measurement.

Transactional theory and the daily hassles and uplifts approach

One of the most influential critics of life events research was Richard Lazarus who suggested that the focus on major life changes, which are comparatively rare, ignores the fact that a great deal of stress stems from recurrent day-to-day problems or chronic conditions which he describes as daily hassles. He also suggested that many of the other limitations of the approach (which are discussed above) stem from the fact that it is essentially atheoretical (Lazarus, 1999).

Lazarus (Lazarus & Folkman, 1984) suggested a new approach to stress based on his own transactional theory of stress. Central to this theory and to his definition of stress (see above) is the notion of appraisal. Lazarus takes the view that stress is not a property of the environment (as suggested by the life events approach), nor is it a property of the individual (as implied by research into physiological markers discussed in Chapter 2), rather it is a transaction between the individual and the environment (Lazarus, 1999). The focus is therefore on the process of appraisal and coping. In any potentially stressful transaction or encounter, a person may appraise the situation as involving harm or threat of harm, or alternatively they may see it in a positive, optimistic light and view it as a challenge. The type of appraisal will then determine the person's coping processes, which will in turn determine subsequent appraisals (see Chapter 5 for further discussion of the role of coping in this theory). Lazarus is therefore describing a constantly changing relationship between the person and the environment. Furthermore, he suggests that stress is a complex phenomenon which involves many variables in terms of inputs, outputs and mediating factors associated with appraisal and coping.

This approach clearly has implications for the way stress is measured. In particular, Lazarus (1999) suggests that the search for a single satisfactory measure is 'doomed to failure'. He argues that stress needs to be assessed by a series of different measures which each capture different aspects of the stress process. Relevant measures therefore might include environmental inputs (e.g. daily stressors as well as life events), measures of individual differences, coping, and physiological and psychological responses. A critical feature of this approach is that, because stress is a process, assessments should be repeated over time. This theory led to the development of a measure of daily stressors known as the Hassles Scale (e.g. Kanner et al., 1981) and subsequently a shorter Hassles and Uplifts Scale (DeLongis et al., 1982). In this measure 53 items are listed, for example 'your children', 'your fellow workers', 'your health', and respondents are asked to rate separately the extent to which each item is a hassle or an uplift. A number of studies have examined the extent to which both daily hassles and major life events predict ill health and these have tended to suggest that hassles are more predictive (e.g. Kanner et al., 1981; DeLongis et al., 1982). Research based on the transactional theory has been associated with a growth in daily assessment to tap the stress process. This typically uses 'daily diaries' which contain rating scales, such as the Hassles and Uplifts Scale. In addition, they may also offer scope to provide qualitative descriptions of daily events (see Research methods Box 3.2).

RESEARCH METHODS BOX 3.2

Using diaries in health psychology research

Approaches to studying stress differ in their focus. For example, compare the life events approach with the transactional approach. The life events approach has been criticized on methodological grounds and stress research, like other areas in health, social and clinical psychology, has been criticized for over-reliance on cross-sectional, 'snap-shot' methodologies (see Nezlek, 2001 for further discussion). For example, research into the impact of stress on eating behaviour has tended to use laboratory-based methods which employ single measures of stress (e.g. life events over the previous year) or one-off retrospective measurements of stress in the short term (e.g. perceptions of stress over the past two weeks). Such research ignores the substantial evidence showing that changes in within-person stressful daily hassles are important in understanding stress-outcome processes (see Bolger & Laurenceau, 2013).

We are often interested in investigating causal relationships between study variables and/or determining whether a particular psychological variable influences a later health outcome, e.g. on the following day or week (known as a lagged effect). Imagine we wanted to find out if negative mood was associated with the onset of pain episodes in arthritis patients or whether in psoriasis patients, stressful events on one day could trigger 'flare ups' the next day. Conventional cross-sectional or longitudinal study designs would not be very useful here because they miss the detailed daily variation driving the causal processes we are interested in. In these cases, and others in health psychology research, the dependent variable under investigation is a daily process, that is, it changes from day to day and/or frequently within days. Therefore, in order to assess it we need to measure it repeatedly during and over several days. A diary and/or an ecological momentary assessment approach (EMA) is ideally suited to such research (Junghaenel & Stone, 2020).

What are the advantages of using diary designs and measuring daily processes? Affleck and colleagues (1999: 747) argue that daily diary studies allow researchers '(a) to capture as closely as possible the "real-time" occurrences or moments of change (in study variables); (b) to reduce recall bias; (c) to mitigate some forms of confounding by using participants as their own controls, and (d) to establish temporal precedence to strengthen causal inferences'. In addition, using daily diaries permits researchers to use sophisticated statistical techniques (e.g. hierarchical linear modelling) to examine day-to-day within-person effects together with the impact of between-person factors such as personality or gender.

There are important procedural differences in the way daily diary studies are conducted. If we were designing a study, we would have to consider how frequently our participants completed their diaries. Three main methods exist:

1.   Interval-contingent: the participant completes diary at regular intervals (e.g. before going to bed).
2.   Event-contingent: the participant completes diary each time a specific event happens (e.g. every time they experience a daily hassle).

3. Signal-contingent: the patient completes diary in response to random 'alarms' or 'beeps' from a smartphone or similar device.

Crucially, researchers have to decide which method suits their study and best allows them to answer their research question(s). They also need to consider how many days the study should last and balance the number of study days against the burden placed on the participants.

Inevitably, Lazarus' approach has not been without critics. Criticisms have primarily focused upon the notion that by including appraisal of the stressful nature of transactions within measures of hassles, items may be inadvertently measuring psychological distress. If correct, this would inevitably lead to positive correlations between stressors and strains (Dohrenwend & Shrout, 1985). Dohrenwend and Shrout suggested that while life events measures may also sometimes include items which are symptoms rather than causes of distress, this is much more of a problem for Lazarus' measures. Here the mere instruction to rate severity of hassles implies a level of distress. Thus, all items are potentially confounded with psychological distress. Dohrenwend and Shrout (1985: 782) argue that environmental events should be measured 'uncontaminated by perceptions, appraisals or reactions'. While self-report measures are arguably always likely to be influenced by the individual's appraisal, the implication of this argument is that researchers should use items which ask about the existence of stressors (e.g. whether or not a particular event happened) rather than items which ask people to rate stress or hassles associated with the event. This more objective approach to stressors is commonly found in the work stress literature (see Chapter 4), where researchers (and employers) are primarily concerned with identifying the negative effects of work irrespective of individuals' idiosyncratic appraisal.

Within the current literature you may spot both relatively objective measures of stressors and measures which include elements of appraisal of distress. In your reading of research, it is important to look out for instances where there is overlap between stressors and strains. It is likely to be a particular problem where, for example, individuals' ratings of hassles are correlated with a rating of anxiety or depression. The findings may not be very meaningful if both measures are essentially measuring anxiety! However, subjective ratings may not be a problem if ratings of hassles are correlated with a more objective outcome such as a physiological measure or a rating of health behaviour (see Research Methods Box 3.3)

Nowadays, a range of different types of approach to measuring hassles and other daily stressors are used. For example, the study described in Research methods Box 3.3 asked people to describe their own hassles which were then categorized by independent raters. There have also been significant advances in the technologies available to collect and assess daily stressors, together with other health-related and psychological variables. For example, mobile phones, tablets, sensors and other ambulatory monitors are now widely used (Kaplan & Stone, 2013). Mobile technologies represent an exciting way forward to 'bring the laboratory and clinic to the community' (Kaplan & Stone, 2013).

RESEARCH METHODS BOX 3.3

Daily hassles and eating behaviour

Background

When under pressure we may be more likely to skip exercise sessions and replace nourishing meals with quick fast-food snacks or indulge in comfort eating of sweets and other high fat foods. Such negative health behaviours may be one of the ways in which stress indirectly contributes to both cardiovascular disease and cancer risk. A study by O'Connor et al. (2008) set out to explore the complex relationship between stress (assessed as daily hassles) and eating behaviour in a sample of employed men and women in a naturalistic setting using a multilevel prospective diary design.

The study also aimed to explore the different types of stressors that may affect changes in eating behaviour. A number of researchers have previously found that particular types of stress had different effects on eating. For example, in the laboratory, Heatherton and colleagues (1992) found stressors of an ego-threatening nature (e.g. where there is a fear of failure) were associated with an increase in eating whereas physical threats (e.g. fear of an electric shock) led to a decrease in eating. Therefore, the study described here looked at the effect of a range of different daily hassles, namely ego-threatening, interpersonal, physical and work-related stressors.

A final aim of the study was to investigate the influence of individual difference variables on the relationship between hassles and eating. Individual difference models of stress hypothesize that certain groups of individuals will show different responses to stress (e.g. the obese and non-obese; women and men; and those with certain eating styles such as emotional eating). In addition, at the time, few previous studies had explored multiple individual differences variables, therefore not allowing conclusions to be drawn about the relative importance of these different variables (e.g. Conner et al., 1999; O'Connor & O'Connor, 2004).

Design and methods

A total of 422 employees completed daily diaries over four weeks in which they recorded daily hassles and provided free response reports of between-meal snacking, fruit and vegetable consumption, and perceived variations in daily food intake. Eating styles were assessed using the Dutch Eating Behaviour Questionnaire and the Three Factor Eating Questionnaire. Each of the hassles reported was coded by independent raters as to whether or not it was ego-threatening (e.g. job interview, public talk, criticism), interpersonal (e.g. argument with partner, family problems, visiting relatives), work-related (e.g. difficult work task, late for meeting, deadline) or physical in nature (e.g. anxious/frightened, feeling ill). The data were analyzed using a technique known as hierarchical linear modelling which allowed the researchers to examine the day-to-day changes (in hassles and eating) together with the eating style variables.

Results

The results showed daily hassles were associated with increased consumption of high fat/sugar snacks and with a reduction in main meals and vegetable consumption. Ego-threatening, interpersonal and work-related hassles were associated with increased snacking, whereas physical stressors were associated with decreased snacking. In addition, an emotional eating style was found to be the most important moderator of the hassles–snacking relationship such that individuals who had higher levels of emotional eating consumed more snacks in response to daily stressors.

Conclusion

Daily hassles were associated with an increase in unhealthy eating behaviour, with most marked effects for those who were emotional eaters. These results highlight an important indirect pathway through which stress influences health risk. More recently, O'Connor, Armitage and Ferguson (2015) have developed a stress management support tool to help reduce stress-related unhealthy snacking and to promote stress-related healthy snacking.

Compared to life events research, less work has examined the relationship between hassles and health despite the fact that there are strong arguments in favour of examining the effect of day-to-day events and hassles in order to fully understand stress-outcome processes. Over 40 years ago, Kanner et al. (1981: 3) argued that it is 'day-to-day events that ultimately have proximal significance for health outcomes and whose accumulative impact . . . should be assessed'. Nevertheless, of the existing studies, a number have demonstrated that daily hassles can have a substantial cumulative effect on health and well-being (e.g. Chiang et al., 2018; Kaplan & Stone, 2013; Kong et al., 2021). The outcomes that are measured in this research are rather different to those in the life events literature. Thus, while researchers looking at major life events have looked at long-term effects on the likelihood of contracting serious diseases such as cancer, those looking at daily events have focused on much shorter time scales and linked hassles to much more proximal changes in physiological markers of stress, or the occurrence of minor diseases such as colds, as well as longer-term risk of chronic disease. As a result, this focus has also enabled them to shed more light on processes whereby stress may impact on disease. For example, Chiang et al. (2018) found that greater increases in negative affect in response to stress in everyday life were associated with the development of future chronic illnesses.

Nowadays, a range of different types of approach to measuring hassles and other daily stressors are used. For example, the study described in Research Methods 3.3 box asked people to describe their own hassles, which were then categorized by independent raters. There have also been significant advances in the technologies available to collect and assess daily stressors, together with other health-related and psychological variables. For example, mobile phones, tablets, sensors and other ambulatory monitors are now widely used (Kaplan & Stone, 2013; Keusch & Conrad, 2022). Mobile technologies represent an exciting way forward as they allow researchers to collect self-reports of stressors, mood, wellbeing together with passively measured behaviours and states including locations, movement and activity (Keusch & Conrad, 2022).

Researchers have found that hassles transmit their harmful effects directly through psycho-physiological pathways as well as indirectly via changes in health behaviours. In a two-year longitudinal study, Twisk and colleagues (1999) explored the effects of changes in daily hassles and life events on a number of biological and lifestyle variables associated with coronary heart disease risk. The main findings of this study showed that daily hassles were more important than life events and they predicted changes in lipoproteins (a combination of fats and proteins found in the blood), daily physical activity and smoking behaviour. In another study conducted by Newman, O'Connor and Conner (2007), daily hassles were associated with increased (high fat) snack intake over a two-week period. However, these effects were only observed in women who had previously been identified as high cortisol reactors following a laboratory stressor and not in low cortisol reactors. Moreover, a recent study in children also found that daily hassles were associated with unhealthy snacking, but only in children who had previously been found to release higher levels of cortisol in response to a laboratory stressor (Moss, Conner & O'Connor, 2020). These findings are noteworthy because they suggest that the impact of daily hassles on eating behaviour is moderated by individual differences in cortisol reactivity.

FOCUS BOX 3.1

Stress and health behaviours

As outlined earlier, stress is thought to influence health via two pathways; a direct, biological pathway and an indirect, behavioural pathway. So far in this chapter, we have outlined evidence on how stress can directly influence biological outcomes and health processes. Here we turn briefly to consider research that has explored the extent to which stress can change health behaviours. For example, previous research has shown that high levels of stress are associated with poorer sleep behaviours (Lo Martire et al., 2020), increased alcohol/drug use (Fonk et al., 2020) and reduced physical activity (Stults-Kolehmainen & Sinha, 2014). In terms of eating behaviours, a large number of studies have found that stress is associated with increased consumption of unhealthy foods, particularly those high in fat and sugar (Hill et al., 2022). In contrast, stress has been found to be negatively associated with consumption of healthy foods, particularly a reduction in fruit and vegetables (Hill et al., 2022). Moreover, a recent systematic review of studies investigating the effects of stress on eating behaviour in children and adolescents found clear evidence of associations between stress and eating in children as young as 8 or 9 years old (Hill et al., 2018). This is concerning as habits around eating behaviours may stay with children and adolescents as they progress into adulthood leading to increased health risks in the future. More broadly, all of these findings are important, because if stress-related disruptions to health behaviours are maintained over time, they are likely to be damaging for future health. Therefore, it is important to be 'stress aware' and recognise the different types of stressors that may change your own health behaviours.

Previous studies have demonstrated that daily hassles have the capacity to activate the HPA axis, as evidenced by increases in cortisol levels (e.g. Figueroa et al., 2021). In fact, hassles that produce negative emotional responses have been found to be most likely to activate the stress response. Jacobs et al. (2007) found daily hassles were associated with increased negative affect, decreased positive affect, agitation and raised cortisol levels. However, only negative affect accounted for the effects of daily hassles on cortisol. As you will recall from Chapter 2, frequent and excessive cortisol secretions over a prolonged period can cause wear and tear to the body's cardiovascular and immune systems leading to physical illness. In a recent seven-day diary study exploring the effects of daily stressors in sexual and gender minority young adults on cortisol levels, weeks with more daily minority stressors (i.e. stressors linked to being lesbian, gay, bisexual or transgender) were found to be associated with elevated cortisol levels in the morning (Figueroa et al., 2021). In addition, it has been suggested that increased cortisol secretion caused by daily hassles may contribute to several common psychological disorders such as depression (Sher, 2004). In other words, repeated minor daily hassles akin to having an argument with your partner or boss may lead to depression in vulnerable individuals.

Daily hassles have also been found to make some chronic illness conditions worse. In a study of irritable bowel syndrome sufferers, daily stress was shown to be associated with greater symptomatology (Dancey et al., 1998). Daily hassles can also impact on important self-care behaviours in people with chronic conditions. For example, Riazi, Pickup and Bradley (2004) found that daily hassles disrupted glycaemic control (i.e. regulation of blood glucose levels) in patients with type I diabetes who were prone to respond to stress. More recently, a study of adults with a binge-eating disorder found that moments with a greater build-up of stress (i.e. an accumulation of stress over the day) predicted greater subsequent binge-eating symptoms and food cravings (Smith et al., 2021). Another investigation demonstrated that yesterday's daily stressors influence the amount of cortisol that is released the following morning, and these (lower) levels of cortisol are associated with a greater frequency of physical symptoms on the same day (Gartland et al., 2014).

Taken together, these studies indicate that daily hassles are able to influence health and illness processes by disrupting habitual health behaviours, increasing the release of stress hormones as well as exacerbating symptomatology and disrupting self-care behaviours in a number of chronic illness conditions. This work suggests that stress management programmes may prove to be very beneficial for longer-term wellbeing (see Chapter 4 for more detail on approaches to stress management). Moreover, researchers have recently argued that using approaches that tap into daily processes (such as examining daily hassles) that include periods of in-depth and intensive sampling in real-life settings, will provide powerful insights into how stressors experienced in daily life may also forecast individual health and wellbeing (Ong & Leger, 2022).

Where is stress located?

Theorizing by Segerstrom and O'Connor (2012) has built upon each of the approaches outlined earlier and suggested that identifying where stress is located is important to improve its conceptualisation and assessment. Specifically, in keeping with Lazarus and Folkman, it is argued that stress can be located in the environment, in appraisal or in response (i.e. emotions or physiology), however, in order to fully understand the stress process, there is a need to investigate how each of these locales interact. For example, the experience of a major life event, such as unemployment or divorce, is likely to have a knock-on effect on the frequency and intensity of minor daily stressors such as being late for a meeting or having an argument with your partner, and conversely, minor daily stressors may reduce the ability to cope with a major life event; thus, the system is reciprocal (Segerstrom & O'Connor, 2012). Both types of stressor are located in the environment; however, the relationship between these events is dynamic, bi-directional and will change frequently overt time.

Therefore, a major challenge for stress research is to 'appropriately and explicitly locate stress and to understand the effects on other stress *locations*' (Segerstrom & O'Connor, 2012: 131). In order to do this, it is imperative that researchers adopt an integrated approach to measurement and ensure that the different locations of stress are assessed using a variety of longitudinal, panel, multi-level and daily research designs. For example, a major life stressor such as unemployment is likely to lead to an increased number of minor daily stressors (e.g. financial stressors), which are likely to influence appraisals of threat, challenge, and loss, which may generalise to other situations and stressors, thereby resulting in increased levels of psychological distress. However, importantly, such a cascade will also depend on personality (see Ferguson, 2013; Luo, Zhang & Roberts, 2021). For example, losing one's job, may result in reduced stress (assuming all else is equal in terms of financial constraints), in people who tend to be cautious, methodical and emotionally stable.

Conservation of resources theory – a resource-based model of stress

An approach to stress, which poses a challenge to the transactional model, is the conservation of resources model (COR; Hobfoll, 1989, 2001). This represents a shift away from the emphasis placed on appraisal in the transactional model back towards a more objective approach. This model suggests that resources (not demands) are the key variables of importance and that people strive to 'retain, protect and build resources' (Hobfoll, 1989: 516). Stress is defined as a reaction to loss, a threatened loss, or a failure to gain resources following an investment of resources. This may include personal resources (such as sense of mastery) and social resources (such as social support) which have been well-studied outside of the context of this theory (see Chapter 5). However, they also include a range of other factors such as financial/material resources. The model predicts that when faced with stress people will seek to minimize the potential loss of resources. In the absence of stress, Hobfoll suggests they will seek to build resources as a hedge against future stressors. He argues that the association of social resources with positive well-being is an example of the benefits of resource building.

A central principle of the theory is that 'resource loss is disproportionally more salient than resource gain' (Hobfoll, 2001: 343), so that in circumstances of equal resource loss and gain, the loss will have greater impact. Hobfoll suggests that this emphasis on resources differentiates this theory from transactional theory which emphasizes appraisals. In the COR approach, although stress processes may be assessed via people's appraisals, most are resources which are objectively observable. The model is also distinct from the transactional theory in its idea of building resources for prevention of, or protection against, future stressors. Thus, it highlights the importance of proactive coping (see Chapter 5). It also introduced the notion of 'resource caravans'. This is the idea that resources cluster together in groups so that if you have one major resource such as self-efficacy this is likely to be linked to a range of others such as social support and other positive coping styles. Over time these caravans travel with us such that resources at one time period tend to carry over into future times (Hobfoll, 2001). Hobfoll further suggests the notion of loss or gain spirals whereby initial resource gain leads to future gain, and loss leads to future loss. These principles seem intuitively sensible and Hobfoll supports them with examples, frequently drawing on studies of stress and coping in disaster areas. For example, Hobfoll has suggested that resources are an important predictor of resilience in the face of disasters (Hobfoll, 2011). Research based on data from the September 11, 2001, terrorist attack in New York, supports this theory. The presence of resources (such as social support) predicted resilience whereas those who experienced resource loss (in terms of income decline) were less than half as likely to be resilient as participants who did not experience this loss. Resilience was defined in terms of low levels of depression, substance abuse and post-traumatic stress disorder (Bonanno et al., 2007; for more on resilience see Chapter 5 and Troy et al., 2023).

The model has produced a certain amount of controversy, particularly as it can be seen as a challenge to Lazarus' highly influential theory. It was hotly debated in a series of articles in *Applied Psychology: An International Review* (2001). Here Hobfoll describes the theory and a number of other experts, including Lazarus himself, debate the issues in a series of subsequent articles. Lazarus (2001) attacks the theory in no uncertain terms and states that all the elements of the COR theory can already be found in his transactional theory. For example, there are plenty of references to resources within his theory and resource loss is central to the idea of loss appraisal, for example in the grief process (e.g. Lazarus & Folkman, 1984; Lazarus, 1999). His view is therefore that the COR approach is 'fundamentally unsound and fails to advance us beyond what we know' (Lazarus, 2001: 381). Others take a more moderate view. For example, Schwarzer (2001) suggests that Hobfoll's and Lazarus' views differ in emphasis rather than in fundamental principles. He argues that the difference lies in the centrality of either objective or subjective resources. Thus, Lazarus takes the view that objective resources are simply antecedents which lead to appraisals (subjective resources) which are the direct precursors of perceptions of stress. In contrast, Hobfoll examines both objective and subjective resources but emphasizes the former. Schwarzer further suggests that the inclusion of the notion of resource investment and proactive coping introduces a forward time perspective which opens up new research questions. Thus, he suggests that this theory represents an advance on the earlier theories rather than a major paradigm shift. This view is echoed in a more recent review by Hobfoll and his colleagues (2018). They argue that one of the major advantages of the COR theory is that it allows researchers to test a range of specific hypotheses unlike some of the more general theories of (work) stress that you will be introduced to in the next chapter.

Why do some people get ill in response to stress and others do not?

It is often claimed that stress can cause all sorts of diseases including cancer. In fact, consideration of the life events literature suggests that the evidence linking stress and many diseases is far from clear. Evidence is much clearer that experiencing certain stressors can have negative impacts in terms of increasing risk of coronary heart disease and can impact on immune functioning and day-to-day deterioration in health outcomes (e.g. Cohen, 2005; O'Connor, Thayer & Vedhara, 2021). However, not everyone who feels stressed becomes ill, distressed or experiences stress-related disruptions to their normal health behaviours. In fact, researchers now believe that certain individuals are more vulnerable to the effects of stress due to differences in their psychological as well as biological makeup. As you will see in Chapter 5, the effects of stress can be buffered by having a good social support network of friends and family and being well equipped to cope with different stressful situations. Personality also plays an important role in the stress process and will be covered in detail in Chapter 6. A number of personality traits have been found to predispose people to respond negatively to stress (e.g. type A personality, neuroticism, perfectionism). This is another example of the stress-diathesis paradigm. For example, individuals who have perfectionistic tendencies are more likely to experience serious psychological distress after each stressful encounter as it represents a chance for them to fail to meet their high standards (see O'Connor et al., 2007). Therefore, as you can imagine, people who are perfectionistic may be more vulnerable to suffering from the negative effects of stress in the future. Relatedly, a recent large-scale study of nearly 500,000 adults found that individuals with personalities that were mostly characterised by nervousness were at greater risk of having a heart attack (Dahlén et al., 2022).

As well as psychological differences, researchers have identified biological differences in the way people respond to and recover from stressful situations. It has been proposed that certain individuals generally may have a large physiological response to stress (this process is known as stress reactivity), while for others the body may take much longer to return to normal once the stressor has passed (this process is known as stress recovery). In both cases, over time, the body is likely to experience greater wear and tear. If such differences exist, then they may explain why some people are more likely to become ill as a result of stress and others do not. These exciting developments are considered in the next section.

Stress reactivity

The central idea linked to the 'stress reactivity hypothesis' is that individuals who have large emotional and physiological responses to stress may be more likely to develop health problems in the future (Kamarck & Lovallo, 2003). In particular, people who are prone to having dramatic increases in heart rate and/or blood pressure after stressful situations may be at greater risk of developing high blood pressure and cardiovascular disease. Over the last 25 years, evidence has accumulated in support of this hypothesis from animal as well as human studies. In a sample of monkeys, Manuck, Kaplan and Clarkson (1983) found greater evidence of heart disease in monkeys who were previously identified as being high reactors to stress compared to the low reactors. The high reactors were also found to be more aggressive than the low reactors. In a human study, the results from the Kuopio Heart Study in Finland showed that men who had a greater cardiovascular response to stress were more likely to develop hypertension (i.e. high blood pressure) and stroke (e.g. Everson et al., 2001). In another longitudinal study known as the Coronary Artery Risk Development in Young Adults (CARDIA) study, Matthews et al. (2004) found that cardiovascular reactivity to stress at the beginning of the study was associated with higher blood pressure levels 13 years later!

However, not all studies have been supportive with several researchers suggesting that the mixed findings may be associated with methodological inconsistencies (e.g. using different laboratory stress challenges; time of testing, Kamarck & Lovallo, 2003) and with individual differences (e.g. cynical hostility (see Chapter 6), morningness-eveningness; Kamarck & Lovallo, 2003; Willis et al., 2005) which may obscure the effects. For example, Willis et al. (2005) found that stress reactivity levels were moderated by morningness-eveningness (i.e. the extent to which you are a 'lark', who prefers doing tasks in the morning, or an 'owl' who prefers the evening). They found that 'owls' had a higher heart rate generally and in response to stress in the afternoon compared to the morning. Therefore, it seems that the research into the impact of stress reactivity is far from clear-cut. In addition, a number of researchers have begun to argue that low or blunted reactivity (and not just high!) may also be associated with negative health outcomes (e.g. Whittaker et al., 2021). These authors have suggested that departures from the norm in either direction may indicate that the bodily systems are operating in a biased state. Overall, it seems that there is fairly strong evidence showing that people who have large or small responses to stress may be at greater risk of becoming ill following the long-term effects of stress.

Stress recovery

More recently, researchers have turned their attention to exploring the impact on health outcomes of the amount of time it takes the body to return to normal after stress. This is known as stress recovery and it is proposed that people who take longer to recover may be more vulnerable to future ill health (e.g. Schneider et al., 2003). For example, in a study by Steptoe and Marmot (2005) in which the effects of stress reactivity and post-stress recovery on blood pressure three years later were investigated, they showed that increases in blood pressure levels three years later were most strongly associated with longer post-stress recovery. More impressively, these effects were independent of all the other risk factors measured (e.g. age, gender, body mass index, socio-economic status, smoking status, hypertension medication, etc.). Steptoe and Marmot (2005) also suggested that post-stress recovery may become more important as we get older. When we are young our recovery from stress tends to be swift and efficient, whereas, as we age, it may become less well controlled. One reason for this may be linked to McEwen's concept of allostatic load – longer post-stress recovery may develop as a result of wear and tear to the cardiovascular system caused by the body having to frequently respond to stress over several decades. This area remains relatively under researched, therefore we cannot draw firm conclusions about the importance of stress recovery; however, it is clear that there is room for much more investigation and inquiry (Whittaker et al., 2021).

Perseverative cognition

Important developments in stress theory have highlighted the importance of worry, rumination and repetitive thought in improving our understanding of stress-disease relationships. Brosschot et al. (2006), in their perseverative cognition hypothesis (PCH), suggested that worry or repetitive thinking may lead to disease by prolonging stress-related physiological activation by amplifying short-term responses, delaying recovery or reactivating responses after a stressor has been experienced. There is a growing body of evidence that has demonstrated that perseverative cognition is associated with somatic outcomes and negative physiological health outcomes both cross-sectionally and prospectively (see Ottaviani et al., 2016 for a review). For example, Brosschot and van der Doef (2006), in a worry intervention study, showed that reduction in worry was associated with a decrease in somatic complaints. In a more sophisticated design using electronic diaries, Verkuil and colleagues (2012) clearly demonstrated that worry intensity was predictive of the frequency of somatic complaints, and intensity mediated the effect of stressful events on these complaints. Building upon this work, another investigation found that stress-related thinking (triggered by the disclosure of traumatic thoughts) was associated with higher cortisol levels and upper respiratory infection symptoms at follow-up (O'Connor et al., 2013). More recently, the PCH has been extended to health behaviours with evidence now showing that worry and rumination also play a

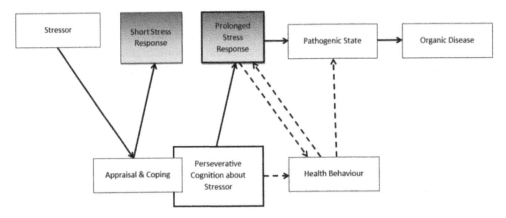

Figure 3.2 Brosschot et al.'s (2006) model of PC and health extended to include additional pathways to illness via health behaviours (represented by dashed lines). PC may mediate the
negative effects of stressors on health behaviours that will influence the pathogenic
state (pathway #1). PC may also influence health behaviours through its effects on
the prolonged stress response (pathway #2) and health behaviours may also have a
bi-directional influence on the prolonged stress response (pathway #3).

role in explaining the relationship between stress and negative health behaviours and sleep disruption (Clancy et al., 2016; 2020). Similar to stress recovery, research exploring the effects of perseverative cognition on health is an exciting avenue for future work.

Conclusions

We have presented a range of perspectives on stress and its relationship with health. These have
included research which has sought to establish links between the existence of objective stressors
(such as measures of major life events) and physical health outcomes, research which has focused
on the appraisal of stress (e.g. drawing on transactional theory), and research which has shed light
on physiological processes. Across this research gradually stronger links are emerging between
stressors, the processes whereby stressors lead to disease (e.g. impaired immune functioning) and
actual disease outcomes. However, we are still a long way from knowing for sure the extent to
which stress is implicated in most diseases.

At the start of this chapter we asked you to consider whether stress has increased in recent
years. It is of course not possible to give a definitive answer to this question. Clearly the types of
stressors we experience have changed over the last 50 years. For most in western society, standards
of living, working conditions, life expectancy and health have improved. Thus, it might seem we
have little to complain about. However, the pace of life seems to be ever increasing, the rate of
change in technology, employment (for example) and unexpected global pandemics impose new
stressors. It is certainly the case that people are more aware of stress due to the work of psychologists and social scientists and the publicity that this has generated. Some have even suggested that
stress is produced, or at least exacerbated, by the increased awareness and expectation of stress in
society (e.g. Pollock, 1988). While this may be a negative impact of our increased knowledge of

stress, information about the impacts of psychological (as well as physiological) processes is essential for improving individual health and wellbeing.

Summary

References to 'stress' are widespread in society but the term is used in different ways in different contexts. Lazarus suggested that stress is best regarded as a rubric or umbrella term which covers a wide range of variables (including stressors such as life events or hassles, and strain outcomes, such as physical symptoms or depression). Historically, stress has been variously viewed as a stimulus, a response or in terms of an interaction between the two. Selye's influential work on the general adaptation syndrome focused particularly on the physiological response. More recent approaches to research on allostatic load, which build on Selye's work, have helped to explain the ways in which stressors lead to disease.

Psychologists have developed a range of different perspectives on stress. Life events researchers claim that major life events are a key predictor of disease. Transactional researchers have focused on appraisals of stress and specifically the impacts of appraisals of minor day-to-day hassles and uplifts. Conservation of resource theorists focus on the impact of loss of resources as the main predictor of stressors. These approaches are sometimes seen as in conflict but can also be viewed as all contributing a useful perspective on a complex phenomenon. All have had some success in predicting negative health and psychological outcomes. However, links between stressors and major physical health outcomes such as breast cancer have not been robustly established.

People do clearly differ in their individual responses to stress, so some will get ill in response to stressors while others will not. For example, it is likely that some people are physiologically more reactive to stressors and/or take longer to recover and worry, rumination and repetitive thought appear to play an important role in stress-disease relationships.

Key concepts and terms

- Allostatic load
- Conservation of resources (COR) model
- Diseases of adaptation
- General adaptation syndrome (GAS)
- Hassles and uplifts scale
- Hierarchical linear modelling
- Life events
- Perseverative cognition
- Social Readjustment Rating Scale
- Stress
- Stress diathesis
- Stress reactivity
- Stress recovery
- Transactional theory

Sample essay titles

- 'Having a stressful life increases the likelihood of contracting disease.' Evaluate this statement with reference to examples from the psychological literature.
- Compare and contrast the transactional approach and the conservation of resources approach to stress.
- Why do some people get ill in response to stress and others do not? Discuss.
- Critically evaluate two approaches to measuring the effects of stress on health.

Further reading

Books

Cooper, C.L., & Quick, J. (2017). *The handbook of stress and health: A guide to research and practice*. Wiley & Sons.

Journal articles

Hobfoll, S.E., Halbesleben, J., Neveu, J-P., & Westman, M. (2018). Conservation of resources in the organizational context: The reality of resources and their consequences. *Annual Review of Organizational Psychology and Organizational Behavior*, *5*, 103–128. https://doi.org/10.1146/annurev-orgpsych-032117-104640

McEwen, B.S. (1998). Protective and damaging effects of stress mediators. *New England Journal of Medicine*, *338*, 171–179. https://doi.org/10.1056/nejm199801153380307

Ottaviani, C., Thayer, J.F., Verkuil, B., Lonigro, A., Medea, B., Couyoumdjian, A., & Brosschot, J.F. (2016). Physiological concomitants of perseverative cognition: A systematic review and meta-analysis. *Psychological Bulletin*, *142*, 231–259. https://doi.org/10.1037/bul0000036

Segerstrom, S.C., & O'Connor, D.B. (2012). Stress, health and illness: Four challenges for the future. *Psychology and Health*, 27, 128–140. https://doi.org/10.1080/08870446.2012.659516

Steptoe, A. & Kivimaki, M. (2013). Stress and cardiovascular disease: An update on current knowledge. *Annual Review of Public Health*, *34*, 337–354. https://doi.org/10.1146/annurev-publhealth-031912-114452

Whittaker, A.C., Ginty, A., Hughes, B., Steptoe, A., & Lovallo, W.R. (2021). Cardiovascular stress reactivity and health: Recent questions and future directions. *Psychosomatic Medicine*, *83*, 756–766. https://doi.org/10.1097/psy.0000000000000973

4 Stress and health in context

4. Stress and health in context

Chapter 3 examined a range of different approaches to stress and considered the links between stress and health. In this chapter we look at the effect of environmental or contextual factors on stress and their relationship to health.

In the first section, we consider the effect of socioeconomic status (SES) and social inequality on stress and health. It is well established worldwide that poverty and deprivation are associated with poor health and that even within affluent societies lower SES is linked to poorer health. We consider the role of stress in this relationship.

We then consider stress at work in a subsequent section. For most people, their job determines their income and therefore their SES. Indeed, researchers typically classify individuals into social classes based on their occupation using formal classification systems such as the UK National Statistics Socioeconomic Classification (NS-SEC; Office of National Statistics, 2022). Most people spend a significant proportion of their lives at work and evidence suggests that many people feel that it is a major source of stress (Health and Safety Executive, 2022). Work stress is also of great interest to employers who need to have healthy and productive workforces.

Work stress is also known to have implications beyond the work environment. If we feel stress at work this cannot always be easily switched off when we go home, and similarly major problems in our personal lives may affect our work. Work stressors may impact even more on our home lives if we work long hours and take work home with us. Increasingly, the barriers between work and home are being eroded by new technology and changing working patterns particularly as a result of the COVID-19 pandemic in the latter case (Major and Germano, 2006; O'Connor et al., 2020). Therefore, researchers have examined the relationships between work and home lives, looking at such concepts as work–family conflict, work–home spillover and work–life balance.

In the final section of the chapter we discuss ways to intervene to reduce stress, with a particular focus on work stress. This includes what governments, organizations and individuals themselves can do to reduce stress. Thus, there are four sections to this chapter:

1. Socioeconomic status, stress and health.
2. Work stress and occupational health psychology.
3. Stressors in work and home life.
4. Preventing and reducing stress at work.

DOI: 10.4324/9781003171096-6

Learning outcomes

When you have completed this chapter you should be able to:

1   Discuss the impact and the causes of social inequality on health.
2   Describe and evaluate key theories of work stress.
3   Describe the impacts on wellbeing of a range of different types of stressor, e.g. family stressors, conflict between home and family, etc.
4   Discuss the ways stress can be reduced in the workplace.

Socioeconomic status, stress and health

Poverty is linked to poorer health within most countries. It is easy to think of reasons why this might be the case. Poorer housing conditions, inadequate diet and reduced access to healthcare services are just a few potential explanations. However, there is a difference between the relationship found within each country and what we observe when we compare one country with another (i.e. comparisons between countries).

We might expect that, even in the western world, relatively more prosperous countries would have relatively lower mortality than poorer countries. However, comparing countries, we find that in poor countries increases in gross national product (and average income) over time are correlated with life expectancy but above a certain threshold this correlation disappears, that is, there is no further increase in longevity as people become richer. Wilkinson (1996: 29) calls this the 'epidemiological transition'. Yet within these countries there remains a strong link between income and mortality.

Wilkinson suggested that in affluent societies (beyond the epidemiological transition), health is affected less by changes in material standards and more by relative poverty (e.g. Wilkinson, 1996). Wilkinson argues that it is our position in this hierarchy, including our feelings of relative advantage/disadvantage within society, that causes stress and poorer health. He considered England and Japan to illustrate this phenomenon. In 1970, England and Japan had very similar life expectancies and similar income distribution. However, between 1970 and the 1990s Japan's income distribution shifted to become much narrower (that is, people had more similar incomes clustered around the mean), while in England the distribution became much wider (with increasing differences between the richest and poorest). At the same time, Japan's life expectancy increased dramatically while the UK moved down the international longevity league tables. Wilkinson argues that this phenomenon is not easily explained by factors such as health policies or nutrition.

Potential explanations of this effect include the role of psychological factors associated with the stress of relatively low social status in an affluent society. This explanation is bolstered by animal studies. For example, Wilkinson (1996) draws on Sapolsky's (1993) work showing that baboons lower in dominance hierarchies show higher levels of glucocorticoids indicating more frequent stress responses that could be detrimental to immunological functioning. In addition, these lower dominance animals have higher resting blood pressure and their blood pressure returns more slowly to resting levels following stressful encounters. High status animals also show changes in hormonal and cardiovascular functioning indicative of stress when their position in the hierarchy changes, for example, when a larger male is introduced into their group. Similar correspondence between such physiological indices of stress response and social position is observed in people, e.g. among civil servants working at different levels within government (Marmot et al., 1991; Wilkinson, 1996).

A further puzzling finding is that, while SES is strongly linked to mortality in men (when their SES is determined by their occupation) this is not the case for women. In fact, women's mortality is more strongly affected by socioeconomic class when they are classified according to their husband's job and not their own (Bartley et al., 2004). One explanation is that, traditionally, a husband has been the main breadwinner and his participation in the workforce was often more enduring. Thus, men's occupation has more influence on the overall living standards of the family and so determined family members' positions within the societal hierarchy.

Traditionally, it has been hypothesized that inequalities in health are due to material/structural and cultural/behavioural differences between socioeconomic groups. However, researchers debated whether social inequality causes ill health or ill health causes social inequality (Carroll et al., 1993). This has given rise to two opposing explanations. The first is known as the social causation hypothesis which states that low SES causes ill health. In other words, factors associated with occupying a low socioeconomic position has a negative impact on health. The alternative explanation is known as the social drift hypothesis which states that ill health causes low SES, that is, when an individual becomes ill, they drift down the socioeconomic hierarchy because they may be unable to hold down a job. In general, more evidence supports the former explanation. In longitudinal studies following large samples of individuals over time, baseline measures of SES have been found to be good predictors of subsequent health status, whereas health status has been found to be a weaker predictor of SES. Moreover, if ill health caused SES decline one might expect to see differences between fast-acting fatal illnesses (e.g. lung cancer) where there is usually little time to change SES and chronic illnesses (e.g. chronic bronchitis). Yet the SES gradient is seen equally strongly in both types of illness (Carroll et al., 1993).

More recently, a longitudinal study called the Whitehall II cohort study has been examining whether social inequalities are present before or after people become ill with a range of adverse health conditions (Dugravot et al., 2020). This study has been running for nearly 40 years and has included good indicators of socioeconomic status by collecting data on education, occupational position and literacy and as well as multiple health outcomes over many years. The main findings showed that socioeconomic status affects the risk of developing what is known as multimorbidity (i.e. having more than two chronic health conditions), frailty and disability but do not influence the risk of death after developing these adverse health conditions. These findings are important as they highlight that social inequalities exist in the transition from being healthy to becoming unhealthy but not the transition from being unwell to dying. Therefore, the authors argue that primary prevention strategies are urgently required before the development of multimorbidity, frailty and disability in order to help reduce the inequalities in mortality rates.

Stress and social inequality

Cardiovascular disease has been found to be associated with SES and this relationship is not eliminated after conventional risk factors such as smoking are taken into account. This has led researchers to search for additional factors that explain these social inequalities. Two hypotheses have been suggested relating to the role of stress in contributing to social inequality (e.g. Adler et al., 1994). First, the differential exposure hypothesis maintains that the higher prevalence of health problems in low socioeconomic groups may be associated with a greater exposure to psychological stressors in these groups. Second, the differential vulnerability hypothesis suggests that individuals in lower socioeconomic groups are less well equipped to cope with stressors due to having fewer resources (e.g. having less money to buy healthy foods, choosing less effective coping strategies, and having limited social support networks) and as such their impact is much greater in these groups. Evidence supporting both hypotheses has been found, although the most consistent findings relate to the differential vulnerability hypothesis. However, Stronks et al. (1998) have suggested that the importance of the differential exposure hypothesis has been underestimated. Nevertheless, recent theorising has highlighted the need for policy makers to set targets, priorities and prevention strategies that recognise both the vulnerability and exposure pathways and as such they should target high-risk individuals, whole populations and vulnerable groups (Diderichsen, Hallqvist & Whitchead, 2019).

Cohen, Doyle and Baum (2006) investigated the link between SES and a number of stress hormones. After controlling for race, age, gender and body mass index, the results showed that lower SES was associated with higher levels of cortisol, adrenaline and noradrenaline, mirroring Sapolsky's work with baboons. More impressively, Cohen et al. also showed that the effects of SES on these stress hormones were mediated via smoking status, not eating breakfast and having a less diverse social network. These findings emphasize the importance of psychological, biological and behavioural factors in understanding the effects of SES on health. They suggest that health behaviours and social resources, typifying lower SES, explain why those in lower SES positions suffer greater stress-related illness.

Work stress and occupational health psychology

Investigating and reducing work stress has become a major focus of the field of psychology known as occupational health psychology. The US National Institute of Occupational Safety and Health (NIOSH) states that 'Occupational Health Psychology concerns the application of psychology to improving the quality of working life and to protecting and promoting the safety, health and wellbeing of workers' (NIOSH, 2013). The emphasis here is on reducing occupational stress, injuries and illness and there are now a number of postgraduate courses which are concerned with psychosocial and organizational issues relevant to occupational health and safety. The research literature on stress is vast but some key models of work stress can be identified.

Theories and models of work stress

A number of writers have produced useful frameworks and models summarizing key variables that might cause stress for individuals at work (Warr, 1987; Cooper et al., 1988). For example, Warr (1987) listed nine key stressors which are like vitamins, in that a certain amount is essential for good mental health. Thus, to minimize stress, a job needs to have: 1) appropriate levels of personal control over activities and events, and 2) the right amount of opportunity to use existing skills and develop new skills. The job also needs to provide 3) opportunities to pursue goals or meet demands, and have the right amount of 4) variety, 5) clarity and 6) opportunity for interpersonal contact. Like some vitamins (e.g. vitamins A and D), either too much or too little of these variables may be bad for wellbeing. However, the final three factors (like vitamins C and E), are only thought to be stressful if there is a shortage. These are 7) money, 8) physical security (e.g. job security or working conditions) and holding a 9) valued social position. This framework simply focuses on external environmental stressors. However, as we noted in Chapter 3, people vary in their perceptions of stressors and in their ability to cope, so what is a reasonable demand for one person will overload another.

FOCUS BOX 4.1

What are theories and models? Why do we need them in health (and occupational health) psychology?

Theories are descriptions of how things, or people, are constructed and how they behave. Science is the process of generating theories and testing their capacity to account for observations of events. As scientists, psychologists use theory in their efforts to describe, explain, predict and change cognition, emotion and behaviour. In psychology, theory includes descriptions and categorizations that allow us to distinguish between types of people, for example in relation to cognition or personality, and between types of social situation, for example in terms of work demands or role relations. Identifying correlations between characterizations of people (e.g. personality) or jobs (e.g. work demands) and health or health-related outcomes is the first step in theory development which next proceeds to articulating processes which explain correlations. These causal explanations describe sequences of interconnected mechanisms underlying psychological responses and behavioural patterns. Once such processes are understood we can predict relationships between theorized variables and intervene to change such processes (Abraham, 2004). For example, see the development of psychological processes linking personality to coronary heart disease (as described in Chapter 6). Thus, developing and testing theory helps us explain why people behave differently and thereby facilitates prediction of the behaviour of particular types of people or people in particular roles and/or situations (Abraham, 2004).

The terms 'framework', 'model' and 'theory' are often used interchangeably in psychology and the distinctions are not clear-cut. However, generally speaking, a framework is a loose set of constructs that does not clearly specify linking mechanisms. Models may provide clearer links between constructs but theories should ideally specify interconnecting causal mechanisms which can be experimentally tested (see our discussion of testing social cognition models in Chapter 7).

In research in the area of occupational health psychology, many theoretical constructions are more accurately described by the term 'model' than 'theory' and we still have few theories to help us understand the processes whereby work stressors may damage health. Better theories would help us to design more effective interventions. Arguably, theoretical development is more advanced in other areas of health psychology such as predicting and changing motivation and health behaviour (see, e.g. Chapters 7–9).

The limitations of such frameworks have prompted some researchers to develop more complex models incorporating all possible stressors and influences (Beehr & Newman, 1978; Cooper et al., 1988). For example, the model developed by Beehr and Newman incorporated 150 variables. Unfortunately, such models are too complex to be easily testable or to provide practical guidance to those attempting to provide interventions to reduce stress. The breadth of the concept of stress, and the large number of variables involved has undoubtedly rendered it challenging to develop concise and comprehensive theories of work stress.

ACTIVITY BOX 4.1

Working in groups, make a list of all the things that you think are stressful about work (i.e. independent variables). Then note down individual characteristics that would allow some people to cope with these stressors better than others, for example, personality (see Chapter 6) or other resources they might have (i.e. moderators – see Research methods box 5.1). Then, finally, think of all the possible outcomes (i.e. physical, psychological and behavioural) that might result from high levels of stress (i.e. dependent variables).

Much has been written about the key elements of a good theory (e.g. Popper, 1963). Usually this includes that the theory should be falsifiable and concise (or parsimonious). Do you think it would be possible to produce a concise and falsifiable theory of the causes of work stress from your three lists of variables? Discuss why it might be difficult to produce a good theory of work stress.

Thus, most research has focused on more specific testable models focusing on a limited number of variables and potential interactions between them. Three such models have stimulated a great deal of research in recent years: the job demand–control (JDC) model (also known as the job strain model; Karasek, 1979), the job demand-resources (JD-R) model (Demerouti et al., 2001) and the effort–reward imbalance (ERI) model (Siegrist, 1996).

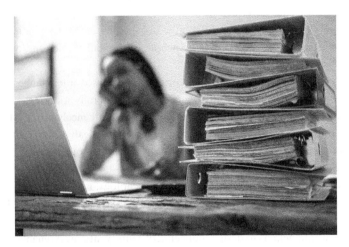

Figure 4.1 A high demand job is a job with heavy workload.
Copyright of Andrey_Popov/Shutterstock.

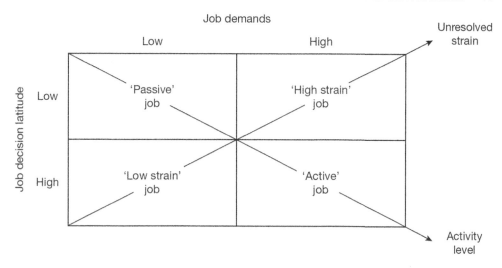

Figure 4.2 The job strain model. Adapted from Karasek, 1979.

Karasek's job demand–control model

In its original form this model focused on two key aspects of work – demands and control – as suggested by the name of the model (Karasek, 1979). A high demand job is a job with heavy workload, fast pace of work and conflicting demands (see Figure 4.1). A high control job means the employee has a say in decisions relating to their job. The model predicts that jobs that have a combination of high demand and low levels of control would result in high levels of psychological and physical strain for employees, i.e. they would be 'high strain' jobs (see Figure 4.2). Typical jobs of this type might include call centre work or being a junior doctor or nurse in a busy casualty department. The opposite combination, low levels of demand and high levels of control would result in low levels of strain. While there is a common view that it is senior executives in a company who are likely to experience stress, it is in fact the case that those lower down an organization suffer the most heart disease (e.g. Marmot et al., 1991). The JDC model suggests that this is because they have low levels of control and may therefore be unable to moderate their job demands.

The JDC model also describes two further job types. Active jobs are those with high levels of demand and high control. These are hypothesized to be less stressful than high strain jobs because they offer the individual opportunities to develop protective behaviours, encourage active learning and motivate engagement in new behaviours (Karasek, 1979). Thus, for example, a high-level manager or senior executive might have high job demands, but may also be in a position to delegate some of the work. By contrast, passive jobs, that is, those with low demands and low control (for example, an assistant in a seaside cafe out of season) are essentially boring and are suggested to result in learned helplessness and reduced activity. The original conceptualization of the model (Karasek, 1979) emphasized the importance of the interaction between the two variables in predicting strain. In a later publication, Karasek (1989) argued that this interaction is not of central importance. The model is, therefore, frequently considered supported if there is an additive effect of demands and control. However, van der

Doef and Maes (1999) make a clear distinction between two alternative hypotheses which are tested in different studies:

1. The strain hypothesis (the additive hypothesis) which states that greater psychological strain and physical illness will be suffered by those in the high strain quadrant of the model (see Figure 4.2).
2. The buffering hypothesis which states that there is an interaction between demand and control (i.e. control moderates, or buffers, the impact of demand). This can be tested by entering a multiplicative interaction term into a multiple regression equation predicting strain outcomes, after the main effects terms (of demand and control).

The model has subsequently been expanded by the addition of social support to form the job demand–control–support model (Johnson & Hall, 1988) and both forms of the model have stimulated considerable research looking at a wide range of physical and psychological outcomes (for reviews see van der Doef and Maes, 1998, 1999; de Lange et al., 2003; Hausser et al., 2010). This has been facilitated by the availability of measures of the core variables. The 'job content questionnaire' (Karasek, 1985) aims to measure demand and control as objectively as possible using a self-report questionnaire to tap the existence of particular stressors using items such as 'My job requires working very fast' or 'My job allows me to make a lot of decisions on my own'. People are asked to respond to these items by ticking one of four options ranging from 'strongly agree' to 'strongly disagree'.

The JDC model has been successful in predicting cardiovascular disease (Kivimaki et al., 2012) and associated risk factors (e.g. ambulatory blood pressure levels) as well as psychological wellbeing (van der Doef and Maes, 1998, 1999; O'Connor et al., 2000a) although there is less support for the buffering hypothesis. More recently, a systematic review and meta-analysis of prospective cohort studies found that job strain was associated with an increased risk of mortality and that these effects were more pronounced for men compared to women (Amiri & Behnezhad, 2020). Job strain has also been found to be associated with the development of common mental disorders such as depression and anxiety (Harvey et al., 2018). Using data from a large UK cohort study, this team of researchers found that high job strain was an independent risk factor for risk of developing a common mental disorder in midlife. There is also evidence that it predicts health behaviours such as physical activity and unhealthy eating (e.g. Heikkila et al., 2013). However, evidence relating to health behaviours is often complex and inconsistent (Jones et al., 2006). Indeed, a study of daily health behaviours suggested that, on a day-to-day basis, within-person fluctuations in mood and work hours were more important than the stable features of the work environment (Jones et al., 2007).

The model has been influential and it has inspired a number of successful interventions to increase control and reduce demand e.g. see Bambra et al. (2007), discussed later in this chapter and it has formed the basis of other more integrated approaches (e.g. Sara et al., 2018). However, job redesign attempts have not always been successful (van der Klink et al., 2001). Critics have suggested that the key variables are too broad and/or confounded with other work characteristics, leaving the precise nature of required interventions unclear (e.g. Jones et al., 1998; O'Connor et al., 2000b). The model has also been criticized for not including individual differences (e.g. coping characteristics), which have been found to buffer the relationship between work features and employee well-being (e.g. de Rijk et al., 1998). In these respects the next two models have some advantages.

The Job Demand-Resources Model

The Job Demand-Resources Model (JD-R) is one of the most recent approaches to work stress (Demerouti et al., 2001). It addresses some of the criticisms of the above model. It was originally proposed as a model of burnout. This is a syndrome consisting of exhaustion, depersonalization and lack of personal accomplishment (Maslach, 1982). Those working in human service occupations (social workers, teachers etc.) were assumed to be particularly vulnerable to burnout but more recently the concept has been extended to other occupations as the core dimensions of exhaustion and disengagement may be found in many occupations (Bakker & Demerouti, 2007). The model has since been used to predict other outcomes, such as depression, job satisfaction and, recently, to the perceived risk of being infected with COVID-19 at work (e.g. Falco et al., 2021; Nielsen et al., 2011).

Like the JDC and the ERI, the JD-R model suggests that stress results from a lack of equilibrium between sets of broadly positive and broadly negative variables. This model focuses on the equilibrium between *job demands* and *resources*. *Job demands* are defined as the 'physical, social, or organizational aspects of the job that require sustained physical and/or psychological (cognitive and emotional) effort or skills and are therefore associated with certain physiological and /or psychological costs' (Bakker & Demerouti, 2007: 312). *Job resources*, on the other hand consist of a broad range of aspects of the job that serve to either help the individual to achieve their work goals, help reduce their job demands or facilitate personal growth and development (Bakker & Demerouti, 2007). This may include control and rewards as well as social resources. The model has also been expanded to include personal resources such as optimism and self-efficacy (Xanthopoulou et al., 2007). It is consistent with the tenets of the Conservation of Resources theory (see Chapter 3).

The model suggests two processes, *the health impairment process* whereby excessive demands may lead to exhaustion and health problems, and the *motivational process* whereby job resources may lead to increased work engagement and performance (Bakker & Demerouti, 2007). A number of studies have now supported these two core processes in relation to psychological burnout and job engagement (e.g. Schaufeli et al., 2009; Xanthopoulou et al., 2007).

In addition to these main effects, the JD-R model, like the JDC model, proposes that interactions between the core variables are also important in predicting strain and motivation. Because of the large number of potential resources and demands, a range of interaction effects are possible whereby specific job resources (control, support, feedback, role clarity etc.) may buffer the impact of different types of demands (Bakker & Demerouti, 2007). Not only may the effects of job resources reduce the negative impact of high demands, but the model also proposes that resources may aid motivation when demands are high. Studies by the models' originators have found many significant interaction effects, though a large cross-national study has been unable to replicate these (Brough et al., 2013).

Unlike the JDC and the ERI model, the JD-R has primarily been tested on psychological outcomes such as burnout and work engagement, for which it was designed, rather than health outcomes. It has, however, been useful in predicting work-home interference (Bakker, ten Brummelhuis, Prins & van der Heijden, 2011) and organizational outcomes such as turnover intention and low organizational commitment (Hu, Schaufeli & Toon, 2011). Moreover, a recent review and meta-analysis of longitudinal studies found broad support for the model, however, it was noted that there was a mix of high- and low-quality studies and there was a need to investigate the reciprocal relationships between the job characteristics and employee outcomes (Lesener, Gusy & Wolter, 2019).

Effort–reward imbalance model

The effort–reward imbalance (ERI) model (Siegrist, 1996) assumes that people involved in social exchanges (such as the employer–employee relationship) expect reciprocity, i.e. mutual give and take. If these expectations are not met they experience the situation as stressful. Thus, the model proposes that an imbalance between the efforts that employees believe that they put into their work and the rewards they receive results in negative outcomes for health and wellbeing (see Figure 4.3). Efforts follow from work demands including time pressure, responsibilities or physical demands. Rewards stem from the nature of the social contract and include money (adequate salary), esteem (respect and support) and career opportunities (including security) (e.g. Siegrist, 2012). However, Siegrist (2012) suggests that the kind of person who is likely to suffer particularly from feeling that their work is associated with high costs and low gains is the individual who suffers from 'overcommitment', that is, they may overestimate the demands upon them or underestimate their ability to cope. Siegrist (2012) suggests that people remain in situations where efforts are high and rewards are low where there are no alternative job choices available or where they may have a strategic reason to do so (for example, because of long-term anticipated benefits) or where they are overcommitted to work.

Like the JDC model, the ERI has its own standardized questionnaire (Siegrist, 1996). While it has been less frequently tested than the JDC, the evidence is generally supportive. For example, the potential impact of lack of reciprocity (i.e. jobs that combine high effort and low rewards) has been highlighted in research conducted by van Vegchel et al. (2001). In this study, the risk of health symptoms was between six and nine times higher for employees who reported high efforts and low rewards than those with low efforts and high rewards. There is also evidence that an imbalance between efforts and rewards is associated with heart disease and recent findings have shown it is associated with higher incidence of suicidal ideation across ten European countries (e.g. Kivimaki et al., 2002; Lai-Bao et al., 2020).

Siegrist (2012) suggests that the model may be useful for designing worksite interventions. For example, improving leadership skills of supervisors and increasing their awareness of the need for recognition and constructive feedback may help increase perceptions of rewards among employees. He also suggests that structural interventions designed to increase non-monetary incentives, e.g. flexible working time, job security and increasing contractual fairness, may also reduce imbalance.

Some researchers have combined the JDC and ERI to predict psychological and physical health outcomes (e.g. Pena-Gralle et al., 2022; van Vegchel et al., 2005). Studies have typically indicated that variables from the ERI, i.e. effort–reward imbalance (and in some cases overcommitment), together with low job control (from the JDC model), predict negative health outcomes.

Overall, research based on all these models has told us a great deal about the range of factors that are stressful at work and how they impact on our health. They also suggest ways in which work can be structured and organized to reduce stress. A limitation of all these models is that they focus on work stressors in isolation, failing to take into account how work and other roles are interlinked. Stressors in home and family life cannot be clearly separated from those in work life.

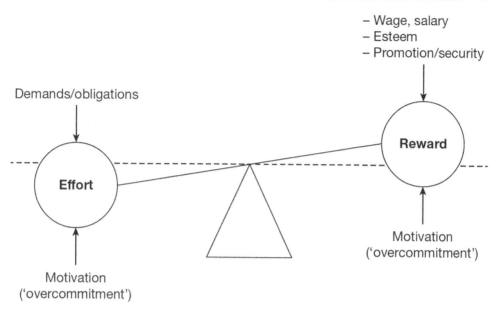

Figure 4.3 Effort-reward imbalance model. Adapted from Siegrist, 2012.

Stressors in work and home life

How does work life or university life affect you during your leisure time? If you are stressed during the day do you worry in the evening and feel low, or do you switch off and make sure you do something pleasant to compensate for the hard day you have had? These kinds of questions have interested researchers investigating the relationships between stressors in different domains of life and they are becoming increasingly important as the boundaries between work and home life are reduced. More women (including those with young children) are now working so both men and women occupy potentially conflicting roles. Furthermore, given that many jobs simply require access to laptop computers, emails and mobile phones a large number of employees can work anywhere. This is linked to a trend for work to be more flexible with more people working outside the traditional 9-to-5 day to cater for demands for 24-hour services (e.g. supermarkets, call centres) as well as to facilitate working in global organizations operating across different time zones. This has led to an increasing concern among employees about lack of work–life balance (Lee & Sirgy, 2019; Major & Germano, 2006). Moreover, the impact of the COVID-19 pandemic on how we work, live, socialise, shop, parent and function has significantly contributed to the further blurring of the work and home life balance (O'Connor et al., 2020).

   Three types of relationships between work and home life have been considered (Staines, 1980). First, the impact of work was hypothesized to spillover to affect the individual at home. For example, those experiencing negative emotions at work would take these to the home environment. However, this hypothesis has been extended beyond stressors and is assumed to also apply to activities and behaviour. So those with active and stimulating jobs would seek similar types of experience out of work. In contrast the compensation hypothesis, suggested that, for example, those with active stimulating jobs might seek calm and undemanding leisure activities and vice versa. A third hypothesis, the segmentation hypothesis, suggested no relationship, implying that work and non-work domains are independent (Staines, 1980). Early studies have tended to support the spillover hypothesis. For example, Meissner (1971) found that individuals who were isolated at work were also isolated at home. However, most studies were cross-sectional leaving the direction of causation unclear. Did work stressors spillover to the home or were home stressors affecting people at work, or was a third variable (such as personality) responsible for the link? Longitudinal studies have helped clarify these relationships. For example, Williams and Alliger (1994) showed that spillover occurs in both directions, with moods experienced in one environment influencing those in the other. However, in common with most other studies, they found that work seems to interfere more with family life than vice versa.

These findings have been extended by examining crossover of stress. This is the idea that stressors in one environment (usually work) not only affect the individual directly experiencing them when that person is at home but also affect others who share the home environment. Support for this phenomenon has now been found in numerous studies (Bakker et al., 2009). For example, a study of more than 2000 couples found striking evidence that workplace aggression experienced by one member of a couple was associated with an increase in psychological distress in their partner (Haines et al., 2006). Song et al. (2011), got couples to complete daily diaries and found crossover between unemployed and employed partners. Children have also been found to suffer from their parents' work stressors. Repetti and Wood (1997) studied working mothers and their pre-school children in a laboratory setting after work for five consecutive days. They found that on days when they reported heavier workloads, or where they had experienced interpersonal conflicts, the mothers were more withdrawn from their children. For men, the link between work stress and negative interaction with children seems to be moderated by neuroticism, that is, for men high in neuroticism job stress was linked to more negative emotional response to their children (Wang et al., 2011). Taken together, these findings are rather concerning, however, some recent theorising has suggested that the movement to more digital workplaces which allow for schedule flexibility and telecommuting (i.e. remote working) may have a positive influence on work–life balance and job satisfaction (Lee & Sirgy, 2019). This is an important area for future investigation.

Work–life conflict

Relationships between work and other aspects of life have been investigated in terms of role conflict, that is, when a person feels incompatible pressures from two separate roles. Most commonly this has focused on work–family conflict (Greenhaus & Beutell, 1985). For example, it may be that time spent at work prevents people from participating in family activities, or it may be that strain experienced at work affects people psychologically at home, or that particular behaviours found useful at work spill over and cause problems in the home environment. Thus, classic work by Greenhaus and Beutell introduced the concepts of time-based, strain-based and behaviour-based conflict. Like spillover, conflict can occur in two directions, work may affect family life (work-to-family interference) and family issues may impact on work (family-to-work interference: O'Driscoll et al., 2006). There has been some criticism of the emphasis on 'family' implied by the term 'work–family conflict', as increasing numbers of people live alone but nevertheless may experience conflicts with personal life and leisure activity. Many researchers now prefer to look at 'work–life' conflict (e.g. Siegel et al., 2005).

Research suggests that in the past work-to-family conflict was typically higher among men than women, while family-to-work conflict was higher in women. However, research suggests that these effects have levelled out to some extent (O'Driscoll et al., 2006). This is probably due to more equal roles in both work and home life. The negative effects of work–family conflict include increased work turnover and poorer work performance, reduced job satisfaction, increased distress and depression, poorer physical health and increased alcohol consumption.

Grandey and Cropanzano (1999) suggest that the effect of work and family stress can be explained by the conservation of resources theory (see Hobfoll et al., 2018 and Chapter 3). For example, conflict arising in the work role may result in fewer resources (such as time) being available to spend in the other role. However, those with additional resources such as marital partners may suffer less than those with fewer overall resources. Consistent with this, research has found that long work hours are linked to work–family conflict and that having a partner is linked to reduced conflict both from work to family and family to work (e.g. Brough & Kelling, 2002).

Recovery from work stress

Previously, interest in the work family interface has led to a focus on recovery from work stress. Jobs which are high in demand and low in control (i.e. high strain jobs), for example, have been found to linked to a high need for recovery (Sonnentag & Zijlstra, 2006). Sonnentag and Zjilstra define 'need for recovery' as 'a person's desire to be temporarily relieved from demands in order to restore his or her resources'. This in turn was linked to poorer wellbeing and fatigue (i.e. recovery mediates the relationship between demands and control and wellbeing outcomes). Psychological detachment, relaxation, mastery and control experiences in time off work have been shown to help recovery (e.g. Sonnentag et al., 2008). Engaging in pleasant activities is also related to greater recovery as is physical activity (e.g. van Hooff et al., 2011). The presence of children in the family, not surprisingly, helps detachment (Hahn & Dormann, 2013). Researchers are starting to look at whether training can help recovery. A recovery training programme with modules promoting psychological detachment, relaxation, mastery and control (Hahn et al., 2011) led to increased recovery experiences during off-work time and improved sleep quality and reduced perceptions of work stress. However, more commonly, interventions for work stress deal with reducing or managing the stress in the workplace. These are examined in the next section

Preventing and reducing stress in the workplace

A number of different types of intervention have been used in the work setting. Organizational change and job design interventions reduce stress by modifying the job to remove stressors. Other types of intervention aim at modifying the individual's ability to cope with stress, for example, by training, counselling or by changing the individual's physical fitness. These are described in further detail in the following sections.

Preventing or reducing stress by changing the work environment

Removing or reducing stressors at source wherever possible seems both sensible and ethically desirable. Furthermore, the focus of the work stress models discussed above is to determine sources of stressors with, by implication, a view to intervening to change the nature of jobs. This may be done by, for example, changing task characteristics such as job control as suggested by the JDC model.

This type of intervention has gained in importance with increased public and governmental pressure to reduce work stressors throughout Europe, Australia and North America. For example, in the UK, the Health and Safety at Work Act (1974: 2) states that employers have a duty 'to ensure as far as is reasonably practicable, the health, safety and welfare at work of all employees'. Since the 1990s this has been interpreted to include work demands, organization and work relationships (HSE, 1995). UK employers are now also required to assess the risk of stress-related ill health arising from work and to take steps to control such risks. This approach is now formalized within the Management Standards approach to work stress advocated by the UK Health and Safety Executive (see Table 4.1). For each of the standards listed there is the additional standard that 'systems are in place locally to respond to any individual concerns' (HSE, 2017). These standards are not legally enforced, rather they are recommendations to help employers meet legal obligations.

Interventions aimed at changing the workplace and thereby reducing or removing causes of stress are perhaps the most challenging type of stress management both to conduct and to evaluate rigorously and thus there is less research evidence in this area (Randall et al., 2005). For example, a meta-analysis (see Research methods box 8.1) by van der Klink et al. (2001) considered 48 experimental evaluations of stress reduction interventions to be of sufficient rigor to be included (see too discussion of intervention evaluation in Chapter 9). However, only five of these were organizational interventions aimed at reducing stressors (the rest being interventions targeting the individual). These researchers found no overall significant effect across the five studies. However, another review (Bambra et al., 2007) looked at 19 studies of interventions to restructure tasks and found that interventions which increased demand and reduced control (i.e. the opposite of the recommendations of the JDC), resulted in poorer health, as the JDC predicts. There were also health benefits where interventions increased control and reduced demands but these were less marked. A study by Bond and Bunce (2001) found that increases in job control were related not only to improved well-being but also to better self-rated performance and reduced sickness absenteeism. It is likely that the extent to which organizational interventions are of benefit to health will vary from person to person and researchers have started to consider the effects of individual differences. For example, those with greater psychological flexibility have been found to benefit more from an intervention to increase job control (Bond, Flaxman & Bunce, 2008).

Overall, organizational interventions face numerous challenges. For example, uncontrolled variables, such as changes in market conditions causing job insecurity, may undermine positive influences. Furthermore, organizational change may itself be stressful. Murphy (2003) suggests that simultaneous individual interventions may be needed to help people adjust to planned organizational change. A recent review of workplace-based organizational interventions aimed at promoting mental health and happiness among healthcare workers highlighted the importance of employee engagement in the intervention development and implementation process (Gray et al., 2019). Moreover, these authors argued that there is a need for more research in

Table 4.1   UK Health and Safety Executive Management Standards (HSE, 2017)

Stressor area	Description	The standard
Demands	Includes workload, work patterns and work environment	Employees indicate that they are able to cope with the demands of their jobs
Control	How much say the person has in the way they do their work	Employees indicate that they have a say about the way they do their work
Support	Includes the encouragement, sponsorship and resources provided by the organization, line management and colleagues	Employees indicate that they receive adequate information and support from their colleagues and superiors
Relationship	Includes promoting positive working to avoid conflict and dealing with unacceptable behaviour	Employees indicate that they are not subjected to unacceptable behaviours, e.g. bullying at work
Role	Whether people understand their role within the organization and whether the organization ensures that the person does not have conflicting roles	Employees indicate that they understand their role and responsibilities
Change	How organizational change (large or small) is managed and communicated in the organization	Employees indicate that the organization engages them frequently when undergoing an organizational change

low- and middle-income countries as well as for more studies investigating the longer-term effectiveness of organizational interventions. Nevertheless, while evidence concerning such interventions continues to develop, the pressure to reduce the causes of stress in the workplace remains high.

In recent years, the call for greater work–life balance has led to new organizational interventions aimed at helping people to manage the interface between home and work, for example the introduction of policies enabling employees to work more flexibly both in terms of working hours and work location (Lee & Sirgy, 2019). Such interventions might be expected to enhance employees' control and thereby reduce stress. While there is little evidence concerning the stress reducing effects of interventions to increase flexibility, studies indicate that perceptions of work flexibility are linked to improved wellbeing, health behaviours improved perceptions of health and work–life balance (Butler et al., 2009; Grzywacz et al., 2007; Lee & Sirgy, 2019).

Reducing stress by stress management training

A common approach to reducing stress in the workplace is to offer employees stress management training courses, a form of intervention which is not unique to the workplace. There is no set format for these courses and they are likely to include information about the nature of stress and a series of emotion-focused and problem-focused coping strategies (see also Chapter 5).

Emotion-focused techniques typically involve some form of relaxation training. This frequently involves a technique known as progressive muscle relaxation in which individuals are instructed to focus on specific groups of muscles in turn and progressively tense them and then release the tension (e.g. 'Clench your fist as tight as you can, then let it go'). Finally, they aim to tense and release all muscles together. Relaxation may be accompanied by the use of music or visualization techniques (e.g. 'Imagine you are lying on a beach, you can hear the waves in the distance and feel the gentle breeze'). Tapes are also available for people to use these techniques at home. Biofeedback is also sometimes used as an adjunct to relaxation. This gives individuals continuous feedback throughout a relaxation session about physiological processes such as muscle tension or blood pressure.

Problem-focused techniques can include techniques such as assertiveness or teaching time management skills (see Chapter 9). However, the most commonly used techniques are derived from cognitive behaviour therapy which seek to alter people's appraisals of stressful situations, inhibit automatic thoughts and enhance coping skills. Some people exacerbate the stress they experience by negative cognitions. Thus, for example, when faced with a disagreement with a work colleague about how to do a piece of work, a typical thought might be 'he obviously does not like me, maybe no-one likes me'. This irrational response illustrates personalizing and catastrophizing. This would be explored with the individual and different responses considered, e.g. 'We obviously do not see eye to eye on this task. How can we resolve this difference?' This response is much less likely to generate stress and depression and more likely to lead to constructive problem solving. Stress management techniques which draw on cognitive behaviour therapy involve people examining their reactions and developing skills to stop what for many are automatic negative thoughts and to replace them with more constructive cognitions. This then leads to rehearsal of different appraisals and new coping skills. These kinds of techniques have been demonstrated to be effective in therapeutic interventions (Holman et al., 2018).

Stress management training courses vary greatly in the length of the course and the components used within the course. In the workplace they may consist of very brief one-off sessions for participants who are not particularly stressed at the outset. It is not surprising if evaluations of such interventions show little improvement. However, rigorous evaluations of longer training interventions for individuals with high levels of anxiety show significant improvements in wellbeing (e.g. Ganster et al., 1982). Identifying which components are responsible for benefits has proved more difficult (see Chapter 9). Comparisons between different methods often show all techniques to be equally successful. However, meta-analytic reviews of workplace interventions have found those based on cognitive behavioural approaches to be most effective though other techniques such as relaxation also show benefits (e.g. van der Klink et al., 2001; Richardson & Rothstein, 2008). Moreover, a recent overview of stress management interventions (Holman et al., 2018) concluded that there remains a real need for more robust methodological designs (such as randomized controlled trials) and investigation of which components of the interventions are most effective (an issue we will come back to in Chapters 8 and 9). They also highlighted the need for further work to understand the precise work contexts and individuals who benefit most from the interventions in order to help improve the effectiveness.

A number of new developments in stress management training have been introduced in recent years (e.g. Prudenzi et al., 2021). The success of therapies based on the concept of mindfulness has meant this has inevitably had an influence on approaches to dealing with employees. 'Mindfulness' involves deliberate focus on an awareness of what is happening in the present moment (Kabat-Zinn, 2003). Mindfulness based therapies (such as Mindfulness Based Stress Reduction and Mindfulness-Based Cognitive therapy) aim to help people to cope more effectively with experiences, by accepting emotions and discomforts and paying attention to experiences without

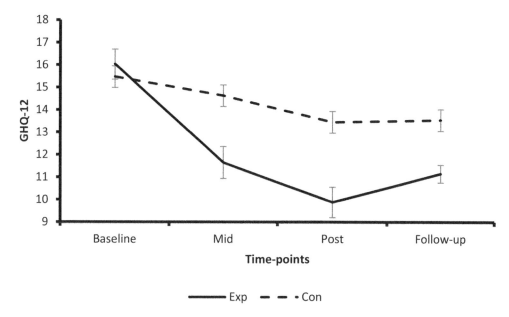

Figure 4.4 Psychological distress (GHQ-12) scores (and standard errors) at pre-intervention, mid-intervention, post-intervention, and follow-up for the ACT (Exp) and waitlist control (Con) groups (Prudenzi et al., 2022).

analytic or dysfunctional thought processes. Mindfulness exercises utilise meditation extensively to encourage focus on the present moment. Clinical trials have shown these approaches to be effective in reducing anxiety and depression (Piet et al., 2012). In the work environment, mindfulness-based approaches have successfully been used as stress management training for local government employees (e.g. Flaxman & Bond, 2010) and as part of an intervention to help people return to work after stress-related sickness absence (Netterstrom et al., 2013). A new stress management training approach has also emerged known as Acceptance and Commitment Therapy (ACT). This therapeutic approach is influenced by the earlier work on mindfulness, but has been modified for delivery and training in workplaces and in group settings. A review of the latest evidence of group-based ACT interventions for healthcare professionals has shown that the interventions are effective in improving general distress and work-related distress (Prudenzi et al., 2021). A good example of their effectiveness (see Figure 4.4) is shown in a recent randomized controlled trial in healthcare professionals (Prudenzi et al., 2022).

Counselling

The provision of counselling services for distressed employees is now a popular form of intervention which primarily aims to treat rather than prevent stress. This is now typically provided via Employee Assistance Programmes available to employees and (frequently) their families. Such services are provided by a specialist provider retained by companies. The level of service offered is variable and may range from telephone counselling and advice to the provision of a series of face-to-face counselling sessions. Typically, employees are provided with a card offering a 24-hour telephone service. The best services offer a range of help which may include specialist legal and financial advice, relationship support and trauma counselling. Some are also providing online support and support for health behaviour change. It has proved difficult to rigorously evaluate these schemes because random allocation to treatment and control groups is not possible when individuals refer themselves for services. Furthermore, withholding treatment from distressed employees would be unethical. However, studies do suggest that employees find such services useful and they report improved wellbeing and that they are cost effective for the organizations employing them (e.g. Csiernik, 2011).

Worksite lifestyle change interventions

Physical fitness is the main lifestyle intervention that has clear benefits in terms of stress reduction as well as its more obvious benefits for health (see Chapter 1). It can be seen as both an emotion-focused and a problem-focused strategy (Long & Flood, 1993). It can distract the individual from stressful emotions and invoke a relaxation response that is incompatible with stress. However, it can also increase people's confidence and self-esteem which may affect appraisal of their ability to cope with problems, that is, it may increase task-specific self-efficacy (see Chapter 8). Many workplaces now encourage physical activity by provision of sports facilities on site or negotiated rate reductions with local facilities. It is in an employer's interest to have a healthy workforce who will be less prone to sickness absence, and it may also have other organizational benefits in terms of employee relations. Exercise can be promoted at an individual or organizational level. While large-scale good quality evaluations of outcomes of worksite interventions are rare, indications are that such interventions can be effective for both improving physical health and reducing stress (e.g. Clemow et al., 2018; Holman et al., 2018).

ACTIVITY BOX 4.2

Chris is a qualified social worker with a good track record. He is one of the most experienced workers in his team. He therefore has one of the heaviest caseloads including a number of children who are at risk of child abuse. He frequently works long hours and faces aggressive clients alone. He is feeling increasingly overloaded and most days can do little more than respond to crises. He often has to cancel routine visits and is unable to make constructive plans to work towards improving his clients' situations. Because he does not have time to get round to all his clients, he is anxious that one of the children in his care may be harmed before he has the chance to intervene. He feels that he does not get adequate support from his manager and gets little feedback about how well he is doing. Recently the situation has become so bad that Chris feels perpetually anxious and unable to sleep. He is beginning to feel that he can no longer cope with the job and is considering looking for alternative employment.

What do you think Chris' managers should do to alleviate the problem? Consider the role of each of the types of interventions described in this chapter.

What type of intervention is most successful?

Removing stressors at source seems the most desirable and ethically acceptable approach but there have been relatively few successful interventions of this kind because job redesign operates in a complex context in which other factors can cancel out potential benefits. This relatively weak evidence base is not a justification to abandon this type of intervention. Indeed, in the UK, any company that did so would be likely to fall foul of the Health and Safety at Work Act (1974). Instead, Murphy (2003) advocates using a range of interventions. Many jobs are inherently stressful at times or include elements that will be stressful for some employees, while other employees will be suffering as a result of unavoidable stressors outside of work. The provision of a range of interventions which are based on the best possible evidence and which combine both organizational change and individual support would seem likely to offer the best chance of success.

Summary

Social inequality is linked to poorer health within countries around the world, even within affluent countries. In richer countries ill health and mortality are associated with relative poverty. Evidence suggests that it is low SES causing ill health rather than vice versa. Stress is implicated in this relationship. Those in lower SES positions are exposed to more stressors and tend to be more vulnerable to their effects.

The workplace has been a dominant focus of stress research and a number of models of work stress have been proposed. The JDC, JD-R and the ERI models have been particularly influential. Together these models highlight the importance of having a manageable level of work demands (or efforts) and the need for these to be balanced by appropriate rewards, including recognition and status, and the importance of adequate levels of control over your job as well as other resources such as adequate support from colleagues and management. There is evidence that a lack of these components is related to increased coronary heart disease.

Changes in the nature of work have led to an increase in concern about poor work–life balance. When work and family demands conflict or when work spills over into home life it can have negative impacts on individuals and on other family members. However, work can also bring psychological benefits that may have positive effects on home life.

There are a range of interventions to reduce stress which include removing stressors by organizational interventions such as job redesign, reducing the impacts of stressors by stress management training, treating stressed individuals by counselling and changing aspects of lifestyle to help people to be able to resist or cope with stress. All can play a useful part in reducing the effects of stress at work as well as in other environments.

Key concepts and terms

- Biofeedback
- Cognitive behaviour therapy
- Compensation
- Counselling
- Employee assistance programmes
- Job redesign
- Mindfulness

- Recovery
- Relative poverty
- Segmentation
- Social causation hypothesis
- Social drift hypothesis
- Social inequality
- Socioeconomic status
- Spillover
- Stress management training
- Work–family and family–work facilitation
- Work–family conflict
- Workplace counselling

Sample essay titles

- Does being poor make people less healthy? Discuss with reference to psychological research.
- Evaluate current theoretical approaches to work stress. How useful have they been for guiding interventions to improve the work environment?
- 'Work stress is unpleasant for employees but it has no real implications beyond the workplace.' Discuss.
- Imagine you have been asked by a company management team to advise on how they should reduce stress amongst their employees. What evidence-based advice would you offer?

Further reading

Books

Marmot, M. (2016). *The health gap: The challenge of an unequal world*. London: Bloomsbury.

Journal articles

Amiri, S., & Behnezhad, S. (2020). Job strain and mortality ratio: A systematic review and meta-analysis of cohort studies. *Public Health, 181*, 24–33. https://doi.org/10.1016/j.puhe.2019.10.030

Diderichsen, F., Hallqvist, J., & Whitehead, M. (2019). Differential vulnerability and susceptibility: How to make use of recent development in our understanding of mediation and interaction to tackle health inequalities. *International Journal of Epidemiology, 48*, 268–274. https://doi.org/10.1093/ije/dyy167

Gray, P, Senabe, S, Naicker, N, Kgalamono, S, Yassi, A, & Spiegel, J.M. (2019). Workplace-based organizational interventions promoting mental health and happiness among healthcare workers: A realist review. *International Journal of Environmental Research and Public Health, 16*, 4396. https://doi.org/10.3390/ijerph16224396

Lesener, T., Gusy, B., & Wolter, C. (2019). The job demands-resources model: A meta-analytic review of longitudinal studies. *Work & Stress, 33*, 76–103. https://doi.org/10.1080/02678373.2018.1529065

PART 3

Coping resources

Social Support and Individual Differences

5 Coping and social support

Coping and social support

Chapters 3 and 4 examined a range of theories relating stress to health outcomes. However, not everyone reacts in the same way to the pressures of life. This chapter explores ways in which different approaches to coping and the availability of social support can affect health.

In the course of normal life we are all faced with a range of stressors and challenges. When faced with a threat such as failing an important exam or having an argument with a friend, how do you cope? Do you try to think calmly about how you can address the problem, do you feel angry and distressed and express your feelings, do you talk to a friend or do you go for a drink or cigarette? Perhaps you use several of these strategies? These are just a few of the many ways of coping that have been identified by researchers in a range of different typologies of coping strategies. Does the way you cope depend on the circumstances or do you behave consistently across different situations? For example, do you tend to adopt a problem-solving approach or, alternatively, deny the threat? Consistent (or dispositional) coping tendencies are known as coping styles that are related to personality. How we cope affects the outcomes we experience. In this chapter we will consider a range of coping approaches and their implications for health.

Friends, family and work colleagues are, for most people, particularly important in times of stress. We may seek out our friends to listen to us express our feelings, distract us from insoluble problems or help us to find solutions. Thus, for many people, using social support is an important coping strategy and most measures of coping ask people about the extent to which they use social support. Of course, social support depends on having a friend or network of friends who we can call on. Thus, friends and family are regarded as coping resources. The availability of these resources seems to be important for our wellbeing regardless of whether they are providing social support in times of stress or whether we deliberately draw on them as a coping strategy. The chapter is divided into two sections:

1. Coping.
2. Social support.

DOI: 10.4324/9781003171096-8

Learning outcomes

When you have completed this chapter you should be able to:

1. Describe and critically evaluate studies of coping and social support, including strategies and styles of coping.
2. Discuss the implications of coping and social support for health.
3. Discuss the mechanisms by which coping and social support affect health.
4. Suggest ways to intervene to help individuals to cope with stressful situations.

Coping

Coping is a key element of Lazarus and Folkman's (1984) transactional theory of stress, described in Chapter 2. In this theory, coping is viewed as part of the stress process, defined as "constantly changing cognitive and behavioural efforts to manage specific external and/or internal demands that are appraised as taxing or exceeding the resources of the person" (Lazarus & Folkman, 1984: 141). You may recall the two types of appraisal. Primary appraisal involves the individual assessing the potential harm, loss, threat or challenge imposed by the stressor, that is, what's at stake. This leads to secondary appraisal in which the individual evaluates the coping options and resources available. In the case of potentially failing an exam, primary appraisals might range from "this does not matter too much, it's just a setback" to "this means I am hopeless and my future is bleak". Secondary appraisals will depend partially on the primary appraisal but also on the resources the individual feels they have (including their confidence, their intellectual resources, financial resources, etc.). In relation to the exam threat, secondary appraisals could include investigating the possibility of re-sitting the exam and planning how to do more work in future or eliciting the support of others to go out and "drown your sorrows". Thus, appraisal provides the basis for coping and so leads finally to the outcome that may involve emotional responses, behaviour and health. Arranging to re-sit the exam and/or planning to do more work would both be described as problem-focused strategies. These are strategies that involve trying to obtain information and formulate actions that will change the situation, e.g. to reduce or remove the impact of the stressor. However, "drowning your sorrows" would be an example of an emotion-focused strategy that simply aims to regulate the emotions generated by the stressor, in this case, by avoiding thinking about it. An alternative emotion-focused approach would be to think about the problem in a different light (i.e. appraising it more positively such as by thinking, "this has taught me a lesson I won't forget"). Thus, coping is a mediator between the stress appraisal and the final outcome (see Focus box 5.2 for a further discussion of mediation).

To assess how people cope, Folkman and Lazarus (1988) developed a measure called the Ways of Coping (WOC) Questionnaire. They used factor analysis of responses to a range of coping items to produce eight overall subscales. These are: 1) confrontive coping, 2) distancing, 3) self-controlling, 4) seeking social support, 5) accepting responsibility, 6) escape avoidance, 7) planful problem solving and 8) positive reappraisal. Some subsequent researchers have criticized these measures on the grounds that other studies have failed to replicate these eight subscales. For example, in a review of coping measures, Skinner et al. (2003) argue that eight studies that used the WOC produced eight different sets of categories based on factor analyses with the number of categories ranging from two to nine. Carver, Scheier and Weintraub (1989) also criticized the model for its lack of comprehensive coverage of coping methods.

To overcome this problem, Carver et al. (1989) produced an alternative, theory-based questionnaire called the COPE. This is based on both Lazarus' theory and their own model of behavioural self-regulation. The strategies measured by this questionnaire are shown in Research methods box 5.1. The measure includes more distinct types of strategies than the WOC questionnaire. However, there is considerable overlap between these two measures and both have proved popular and have been widely used in coping research over the last 30 years.

RESEARCH METHODS BOX 5.1

Measuring coping using the COPE (adapted from Carver et al., 1989)

The COPE questionnaire consists of subscales to assess each of the following types of coping. The response scale can be adjusted to apply to a particular situation or to assess dispositional coping. The measure (or sometimes specific subscales) is still frequently used in a wide range of research (e.g. Jonason et al., 2020; MacKay et al., 2021).

Primarily problem-focused coping

- Active coping, e.g. "I take direct action to get around the problem".
- Planning, e.g. "I make a plan of action".
- Suppression of competing activities, e.g. "I put aside other activities in order to concentrate on this".
- Restraint coping, e.g. "I hold off doing anything about it until the situation permits".
- Seeking instrumental social support, e.g. "I try to get advice from someone about what to do".

Primarily emotion-focused coping

- Seeking emotional social support, e.g. "I discuss my feelings with someone".
- Focus on and venting emotion, e.g. "I get upset and let my emotions out".
- Behavioural disengagement, e.g. "I give up the attempt to get what I want".
- Mental disengagement, e.g. "I go to the cinema or watch television, to think about it less".
- Positive reinterpretation and growth, e.g. "I learn something from the experience".
- Denial, e.g. "I act as though it hasn't even happened".
- Acceptance, e.g. "I learn to live with it".
- Turn to religion, e.g. "I try to find comfort in my religion".
- Alcohol/drug use, e.g. "I use alcohol and drugs to help me get through it".
- Humour, e.g. "I make jokes about it".

Lazarus (1999) argues that there is no universally effective (or ineffective) coping strategy. What works in one situation will not work in another. Furthermore, Lazarus suggests that the effectiveness of coping strategies will depend on the type of person and the outcome they are considering. Different coping strategies may also be useful at different stages of dealing with a stressor. Folkman and Lazarus (1985) found that just before an exam, problem-focused coping strategies are used most, whereas in the period waiting for results emotion-focused strategies predominate. Emotion-focused approaches, such as denial, are often unhelpful because they leave the threat unchanged. However, in some situations, they may be useful in the short term. For example, when experiencing the symptoms of a heart attack, denial is likely to be dangerous and even life-threatening because it may lead to delay in seeking treatment. However, once in hospital, denial may be helpful in reducing the anxiety that is likely to exacerbate the medical condition. Once the patient is discharged from hospital denial again may be dangerous as it may lead to resistance to modifying health behaviours.

Lazarus (1999) suggests that when there is nothing that can be done to alter the stressor or reduce the harm (i.e. when there is little control) then denial can be beneficial. Emotion-focused coping may also be important for people with high trait anxiety who are more likely to become anxious when faced with potential stressors. In a prospective study, Sultan et al. (2008) found that emotion-focused coping enhanced glycaemic control among diabetics high in trait anxiety (so that trait anxiety moderated the emotion-focused coping–health outcome relationship). However, problem-focused coping was also found to reduce trait anxiety, suggesting that for this highly anxious group of patients both coping strategies were important. Interestingly, recent theorizing has suggested that personality traits can be viewed as an emergent property of responses to the experience emotion (Segerstrom & Smith, 2019). In other words, how we cope – emotion-focused or problem-focused – may be underpinned by a diverse range of personality traits such as positive and negative urgency, emotional expressiveness and alexithymia (the latter is discussed later in this chapter). Further research is needs to understand the inter-relationships between personality and coping.

Critical evaluation of coping research

The literature on coping is extensive and complex and has been much criticized, not least because it has provided limited information on which to base interventions and because the factor structure of coping questionnaires is inconsistent (e.g. Jonason et al., 2020; Somerfield, 1997). The limitations of classification systems and the over-reliance on questionnaires are key problems.

In this chapter we have considered two well-established classification systems but many others have been proposed. In a review, Skinner et al. (2003) found over 100 different classification systems which, collectively, specified more than 400 ways of coping. Typically, these are classified into a range of higher order categories. The three most common higher-level categories were a) problem-focused coping versus emotion-focused coping, b) approach coping versus avoidance coping, c) cognitive coping versus behavioural coping. Skinner et al. suggest that this range of diverse classifications has made it difficult to make progress. They argue that many systems such as the two discussed above are based on exploratory factor analyses and, as a result, have a number of flaws. First, there is often a lack of clarity or distinctiveness in the different categories. Second, it is difficult to ensure that the categories are comprehensive and, finally, even where items do load onto a single category they may still represent more than one underlying category, which perhaps have a single underlying emotional tone. For example, both rumination and avoidance coping may load on to a single factor because worrying is common to both, even though the response is very different. Skinner et al. (2003: 248) suggest that there is a need for a comprehensive list of ways of coping that can then be classified into "conceptually clear and mutually exclusive action types". They identify 13 families of coping that fit this description. They are problem solving (e.g. direct action); support seeking; escape (e.g. avoidance, disengagement and denial); distraction; cognitive restructuring (e.g. positive thinking); rumination (e.g. worry and self-blame); helplessness (e.g. giving up); social withdrawal; emotional regulation (e.g. by emotional expression or self-calming); information seeking; negotiation (e.g. compromise or prioritizing); opposition (aggression or blaming others) and delegation (e.g. maladaptive help seeking). It is interesting to note that the debate around the factor structure of coping classifications is unlikely to end any time soon. For example, a recent review investigated studies that had tested the factor structure of the brief version of the COPE and found that studies had reported between two and 15 underlying factors with a two-factor solution being the most frequent (Solberg, Gridley & Peters, 2021).

Do we have consistent styles of coping across different situations?

When faced with a stressful situation, we do not all adopt the same coping strategy. Thus, we need to consider individual differences or the ways personality affects choice of coping strategy. However, the extent to which coping is determined by stable factors, rather than varying across situations, has been a source of debate among researchers (Segerstrom & Smith, 2019; Troy et al., 2023). Those such as Lazarus who are interested in the different strategies used in different circumstances take a situational view, while those who focus on consistency across different situations take a dispositional (or trait) approach to coping.

Carver and Scheier (1994) argue that there are dispositional tendencies to use emotion-focused or problem-focused coping. The COPE is designed to be used as either a dispositional or a situational measure depending on whether the individual is asked to complete it in relation to specific situations or in relation to general tendencies.

Some researchers are sceptical about the accuracy of people's reports of their general coping tendencies. Lazarus (1999) suggested that dispositional tendencies to use particular coping strategies are better obtained by looking at the individual in a range of different situations. One study that compared people's ratings of how they generally coped with their average coping across a number of specific episodes found that asking people how they generally coped was a poor predictor of what they did in a specific situation, although the tendency to use escape-avoidance or religious coping showed more consistency across situations (Schwartz et al., 1999). The tendency to use avoidance (versus approach) coping is a key feature of two coping trait classifications, namely, repressive coping and monitoring (versus blunting) coping. Recent approaches have started to move away from using checklists and questionnaires to measure coping styles and strategies (e.g. Somers & Casal, 2021). For example, an innovative study has used what is known as a person-centred model to study coping in combination with advances in machine learning (Somers & Casal, 2021). Specifically, in this study on work stress, participants are asked "How do you cope with or reduce the stress you experience at work?" The responses are then quantified using advanced analytics yielding coping profiles which, the authors argue, better represent the constellation of coping behaviours and how they are distributed across individuals. This is a promising new method that appears to bridge the trait-like, dispositional approaches and the more transactional, situational approaches.

Repressive coping

People who have a repressive coping style direct attention away from threatening information or stimuli or interpret such information in a non-threatening manner (Derakshan & Eysenck, 1997). This has clear links to the Freudian notion of repression and was originally contrasted with "sensitizing", a form of approach coping. A person high on repressive coping will avert attention from negative feelings to the extent of being unaware that they feel anxious or depressed. However, this is different from intentional suppression of disturbing thoughts or feelings (Myers et al., 2004). A characteristic of repressors is that, when faced with stressful tasks, there is a discrepancy between their self-reports of anxiety (which are low) and their scores on physiological indicators of anxiety (which tend to be high). This has been demonstrated in experimental studies where people have been asked to perform anxiety-provoking tasks such as public speaking (e.g. Newton & Contrada, 1992).

FOCUS BOX 5.1

The alexithymic personality

A personality trait often considered alongside repressive coping is alexithymia. The term alexithymia, when literally translated, means "lacking words for feelings" and relates explicitly to an individual's capacity to process and express emotion. Alexithymia can be assessed using the Toronto Alexithymia Scale which measures the extent to which respondents have difficulty in identifying, labelling and understanding emotions, thereby identifying individuals who show impaired capacity for emotional expression (Bagby et al., 1994). However, unlike people with a repressive coping style who are unconsciously motivated not to recognize negative emotions such as anger, fear and stress, individuals with an alexithymic personality experience negative emotional states but are unable to identify, label and understand the emotion. Interestingly, the term alexithymia was introduced in the 1970s by psychodynamically-oriented clinicians who noticed that many clients who presented with stress-related or psychosomatic illnesses exhibited little insight into the causes of their stressful experiences or negative moods (see Lumley et al., 1999). Typically, when an individual with an alexithymic personality is asked about a significant relationship or an emotionally charged situation, they will be unable to answer (e.g. "I don't know"), or they will provide simple and non-specific responses (e.g. "I felt bad").

It has been suggested that this emotional deficit may negatively impact on an individual's ability to cope with stressful and traumatic events. Evidence indicates that the alexithymic personality is associated with mortality and morbidity from all causes. In particular, research has shown a link between alexithymia and increased risk of developing cardiovascular disease (e.g. Aluja et al., 2020; Tolmunen et al., 2010). The alexithymic personality has been found to be associated with chronic pain and greater pain intensity (Aaron et al., 2019). These findings suggest that alexithymic individuals may be more likely to use maladaptive coping and engage in more health risk behaviours.

Measuring repression is problematic because repressive copers will, by definition, be unaware of their feelings of anxiety. In most cases they will not even know that they have tendencies to repress feelings. An early self-report measure of repression (the repression–sensitization scale, Byrne, 1961) was found to correlate so highly with measures of trait anxiety that repression was effectively equivalent to low anxiety (Eysenck & Matthews, 1987). However, for a measure of repression to be useful, repressors need to be distinguishable from those who are simply not anxious. Weinberger, Schwartz and Davidson (1979) have developed a method of measuring repression using a measure of anxiety together with a measure of defensiveness. This is the most frequently used approach. To be defined as a repressor a person must have a low score on anxiety and a high score on defensiveness. The measure of defensiveness often used is the Marlowe–Crowne measure of social desirability (Crowne and Marlowe, 1960).

Repression has been linked to poorer immune functioning, increased coronary heart disease risk factors such as high cholesterol and more recently to lower cortisol reactivity to stress (e.g. Esterling et al., 1993; Oskis et al., 2019). A recent study examining repressive coping in a sample of children with chronic pain revealed some interesting findings (Ruskin et al., 2022). These authors found that children who were classified as repressive copers reported lower levels of depressive and somatic symptoms but higher levels of pain intensity and pain unpleasantness compared to "true low anxious" children. Moreover, the caregivers of the repressive coper children reported that their children had higher levels of adaptability. However, the authors argue that this is concerning, because as a result these children may be less likely to present to primary healthcare teams, become overlooked and not receive appropriate treatments and support in the longer term. An influential meta-analysis (Mund & Mitte, 2012) looked at 22 studies of repressive coping and somatic illness and found that repressive coping was associated with cancer and heart disease. However, the findings for cancer suggest that repressive coping does not precede cancer diagnosis, but is likely to develop subsequently in order to cope with the diagnosis. Furthermore, it was not possible to draw any conclusions about the relationship between repression and cancer progression. Mund and Mitte also found that repressors were at increased risk of hypertension and cardiovascular disease, however this result was based on only a single study and remains to be confirmed. Thus, exact implications of this coping style for health remain unclear.

Monitoring and blunting

Monitoring and blunting coping styles refer to the information-processing style of people facing threats. It has typically been studied in medical situations with a view to ascertaining the appropriate type of information to give to patients to help them cope with impending medical or surgical interventions. Those with a monitoring style will tend to seek out information about the threat and amplify or worry about it (e.g. Miller et al., 1988) whereas those with a predominantly blunting style will actively avoid it. Typically, these two dimensions are treated as independent (rather than being opposite poles of a single dimension) so that individuals are divided into high and low monitors and high and low blunters.

Research suggests that monitors and blunters react differently to medical stressors. For example, high monitors go to the doctor with less severe medical problems and demand more tests and information than low monitors (Miller et al., 1988). Miller et al. suggests that this is not accompanied by any greater wish for control, rather it is to reduce uncertainty and lower arousal.

Miller and Mangan (1983) suggested that a patient's level of arousal was lower if the level of information given was matched to their coping style (i.e. monitors require much more detailed information). This theory has been used to inform the design of appropriate health messages (see also Chapter 8). Williams-Piehota et al. (2005) matched messages about mammography to women's coping styles. They hypothesized that matched messages would be more effective in persuading women to attend for mammography. The leaflet designed for those classified as blunters was short and to the point. It gave basic facts such as "the key to finding breast cancer is early detection and the key to early detection is getting regular screening mammograms". In contrast, the leaflet for monitors gave details of symptoms and risk factors for cancer and explanations of mammography procedures, e.g. "for some women early detection may prevent the need to remove the entire breast or to receive chemotherapy". Both leaflets included information to reassure and address anxiety. Messages which were matched to monitoring style were more effective in promoting uptake of mammography during the following six months. However, the difference was only significant for blunters, for whom it may be particularly important to provide messages that are appropriate. A similar approach was also useful in promoting fruit and vegetable consumption, though here the monitor message was particularly successful (Willliams-Piehota et al., 2009). Furthermore, Kola et al. (2013) found that matching information to suit the monitoring/blunting coping style of patients minimised the distress of patients undergoing colposcopy (an investigative procedure commonly used following abnormal cervical smears). Overall, these studies suggest tailoring messages to be appropriate to the coping styles of recipients is important for health psychologists and medical practitioners. More recently, during the COVID-19 pandemic, the importance of matching information coping style (monitor vs blunter) and strategy deployment in dealing with an infodemic (i.e. release of excessive amount of reliable and unreliable information that spreads rapidly) was found to make a difference to anxiety levels and sleep disruption (Cheng, Ebrahimi & Lau, 2021). In a study conducted during the early stages of the pandemic it was found that high blunters who sought COVID-19-related information online more frequently and high monitors who sought information less frequently both reported greater anxiety and more sleep disturbance.

Personality, coping dispositions and situational coping

We have discussed situational and dispositional approaches to coping, separately. However, coping styles and strategies are interrelated and function within the context of general personality. Many studies have examined links between personality and coping strategies, especially neuroticism and optimism. Hewitt and Flett (1996) suggest that the relationship between personality and coping can be conceptualized in terms of the three types of relationships between variables shown in Focus box 5.2. Thus, for the mediational model, personality would determine coping style or strategy which then determines adjustment. In the additive model, personality and coping have independent effects and in the interactive (or moderation) model coping may buffer the impact of personality on adjustment.

FOCUS BOX 5.2

Direct effects, mediation and moderation

Researchers examining coping and social support have investigated the mechanisms by which these factors influence relationships between stressors and outcomes such as health and wellbeing. There are three main types of mechanisms that are examined in this research and in other areas of health psychology (see Figure 5.1).

1. Direct effects. In this case coping or social support, for example, has a direct impact on the outcome. For example, having good social support or a positive approach to coping could lead to better health irrespective of the amount of stress the person is experiencing. Figure 5.1a) illustrates a situation where a high level of stress and poor coping strategies would both independently act to decrease wellbeing (and vice versa). This is sometimes also described as an additive effect.
2. Mediated effects. This occurs when one variable has its effect on another via an intervening variable. In Figure 5.1b) coping acts as an intervening variable through which the stressor exerts its effects on the level of strain. For example, the experience of stress could result in poor coping (e.g. use of alcohol or drugs) which leads to deteriorated wellbeing. Social support could be said to be a mediator in circumstances where, for example, a breast cancer diagnosis leads to someone joining a support group, which in turn reduces their anxiety or depression. Alternatively, a stressor such as marital breakdown may lead to a reduction in support (through loss of a previously supportive partner and perhaps the partner's family and friends) that may increase anxiety and depression.

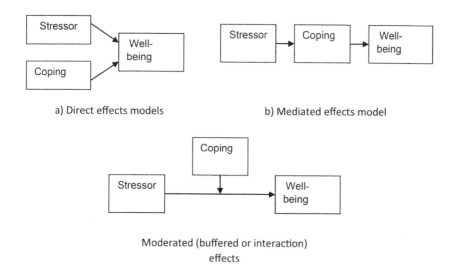

Figure 5.1 Direct effects, mediation and moderation: alternative models of mechanism.

3.   Moderated effects. Moderators, unlike mediators, change the nature of the relationship between two variables, e.g. the stressor–strain relationship. Moderators may alter either the strength or direction of this relationship. Thus, coping would be described as moderating the relationship between a stressor such as bereavement and an outcome such as wellbeing if, for example, bereavement led to poor health only for those who did not use social support or emotional expression as coping strategies. This kind of moderator is also referred to as a buffer because it reduces the impact of the stressor. This effect can be identified as an interaction effect (e.g. in a regression equation) because social support affects the association between stress and wellbeing. Other variables such as gender or personality may also act as moderators because, for example, some stressors may only result in strain for those scoring highly on a certain personality trait (e.g. neuroticism). Logically, however, fixed traits such as gender cannot act as mediators.

Bolger (1990) found that coping strategies mediated the relationship between personality and anxiety in the face of medical school entrance exams such that the personality trait of neuroticism led to ineffective coping. Specifically, they found that two ineffective coping strategies (wishful thinking and self-blame) mediated over half of the effect of neuroticism on anxiety. Fortunately, they found no effect of neuroticism on exam mark! Coping styles may also moderate the effects of personality. For example, O'Connor and O'Connor (2003) found that the negative effects of trait perfectionism on psychological wellbeing were moderated by coping styles. Specifically, the maladaptive effect of self-oriented perfectionism (i.e. having unrealistically high expectations for one's self) was reduced by the adaptive effects of positive reappraisal, while the harmful effect of socially prescribed perfectionism (i.e. the belief that others hold unrealistically high standards for one's behaviour) was exacerbated by the presence of an avoidance coping style.

Optimists and pessimists have also been shown to adopt markedly different coping styles and strategies (for a review see Carver, Scheier & Segerstrom, 2010). For example, pessimists tend to be more avoidant copers, whereas optimists are more likely to use approach styles and strategies such as problem-focused coping, cognitive restructuring and acceptance (Solberg Nes & Segerstrom, 2006). Optimism is generally linked to more positive approaches to coping that are considered in the next sections. Interestingly, there has been recent theoretical advances that challenge the traditional view that optimism is a bipolar construct with pessimism at the other end of the construct (Scheier et al., 2021). Michael Scheier, one of the most influential thinkers in this area, and his colleagues have argued that optimism and pessimism should be considered independent but related constructs. Indeed, in a recent reanalysis of earlier data, they conclude that pessimism is more strongly related to physical health outcomes than optimism. Moreover, this new conceptualisation ought to be incorporated into future research investigating the relationship between optimism, pessimism and coping styles.

Positive approaches to coping

It has been argued that coping research has focused unduly on the causes and consequences of stress and negative affect (e.g. Folkman & Moskowitz, 2000). In recent years there has been a move towards considering the role of positive affect and cognitions which may help prevent potentially negative events being appraised as stressful. Three such approaches are considered below.

Positive affect

Research has highlighted the importance of positive affect in the midst of threatening events. This work is in line with the positive psychology movement, which is a branch of psychology interested in positive human functioning (see Seligman, 2019 for a personal history of positive psychology). For example, Folkman (1997) studied care-giving partners of men dying of AIDS. They interviewed the carers at intervals before and, in many cases, after bereavement and reported that, even in these most distressing of circumstances, both positive and negative affect co-occurred. While participants reported higher levels of negative affect than is found in community samples, positive affect was experienced with at least as much frequency as negative affect among those whose partners did not die. Even after bereavement people still report positive affect. During difficult circumstances such as bereavement people may feel guilty that they still manage to enjoy a joke or feel quite cheerful. Yet this capacity may enhance adaptation and coping. Lazarus, Kanner and Folkman (1980) suggested that it might provide a respite or a breathing space in which people replenish resources. Being miserable all the time may simply become too tiring. Folkman and Moskowitz (2000) summarize other potential functions. These include: a) helping us to build social, intellectual and physical resources, b) helping to provide a buffer against physiological consequences of stress, c) helping prevent clinical depression by interrupting negative rumination spirals. They further point out that when people report more negative events they tend to also report more positive events. It may be that in bad times we create more positive events, or we may interpret neutral events more positively, to offset our negative experiences and induce positive affect.

Positive affect has been related to three particular types of coping (Folkman, 1997; Folkman & Moskowitz, 2000). First, it has been linked to positive reappraisal that is defined by Folkman and Moskowitz (2000: 650) as "coping strategies for reframing a situation to see it in a positive light (seeing a glass half full as opposed to half empty)". This coping strategy is incorporated in the COPE questionnaire (see above) as positive reinterpretation and growth. Second, positive affect is associated with problem-focused coping that involves direct efforts to solve or manage the stressor, i.e. by gathering information, planning, decision making. Third, positive affect is associated with the tendency to "infuse ordinary events with positive meaning" thereby generating good feeling about oneself or one's life.

Research attention has also focused on the possible health benefits of positive affect. At the daily level, positive affect has been shown to have a beneficial influence on physiological processes such as cortisol levels and ambulatory blood pressure (Steptoe & Wardle, 2005). Earlier research reviews suggest that positive affect can have significant effects on health both at the daily level *and* in the longer term with an effect size comparable to negative affect (e.g. Steptoe et al., 2009). For example, Ong, Bergeman, Bisconti and Wallace (2006) have suggested that the ability to maintain positive emotions in the face of stress is one pathway through which people can successfully adapt to stress and experience better health outcomes. A comprehensive review by Pressman and colleagues (2019) of research on positive affect and health concluded by arguing that there is compelling evidence for a robust relationship and there is a great potential to develop positive affect-related interventions to help improve future health and wellbeing and to protect against the negative effects of stress. For example, Moskowitz et al. (2019) developed a positive affect intervention called the Life Enhancing Activities for Family Caregivers (LEAF) intervention which incorporated a number of well-established positive affect techniques (such as noticing positive events, capitalizing on them, gratitude, positive reappraisal). In this study, caregivers were taught remotely the positive emotional regulation skills and then compared against a control group who did not receive the training (but were taught them after the study – known as a waitlist control group). The results found significant improvements in depression, anxiety and physical health symptoms after six weeks compared to the control participants. The authors note that these results show great promise for remotely delivered intervention to improve psychological wellbeing in caregivers of people with dementia and other chronic illnesses.

Benefit finding

Most people, faced with even the most serious of stressors, try to identify some benefit. For example, when faced with a stressor such as breast cancer a patient might identify benefits such as improvements in relationships or a greater appreciation of day-to-day experiences. Finding such benefits has been related to improved mental health (see Helgeson et al., 2006, for a meta-analysis). In addition, longitudinal research has suggested benefits in terms of objective measures of physical health. For example, Affleck et al. (1987) found that men who found more benefits seven weeks after a heart attack had lower incidence of further heart attacks during the next eight years. There is also evidence suggesting that benefit finding is related to improved immune functioning and a range of objective indicators of health in HIV and cancer patients (for a review see Bower et al., 2009). More recently, a review confirmed across 21 studies in cancer patients that higher levels of benefit finding were associated with lower anxiety, depression and distress (Zhu et al., 2022).

Benefit finding is linked to optimism and positive affect, i.e. those with higher optimism scores and positive affect are more likely to find benefit in adversity. It is also linked to positive reappraisal, though these are all distinct constructs (Sears, Stanton & Danoff-Burg, 2003). The mechanism whereby benefit finding affects health remains unclear. However, Bower et al. (2009), suggest a model whereby benefit finding is linked to changes in appraisal and coping processes, social relationships and/or priorities and goals. Changes in these factors in turn leads to more adaptive responses to future stressors thus minimizing the stress experienced and the harmful physiological effects of stress hormones. They further suggest that effects on health may also be mediated by positive affect.

Benefit finding is sometimes examined within the context of emotional writing interventions (see Focus box 5.3).

FOCUS BOX 5.3

Written emotional disclosure interventions

In 1986, James Pennebaker developed the "emotional writing paradigm" in which he explored the effects of writing for 15–20 minutes on three consecutive days about stressful or traumatic events on a range of health outcomes. Typically, individuals in the experimental group are asked to write about their deepest emotions and thoughts about the most upsetting experience(s) in their life. They are encouraged to really let go and to link their writing to other aspects of their life such as relationships, their childhood, their careers and who they would like to become, who they were in the past and who they are now. In the control group, individuals are asked to write about what they have done the previous day and to describe their plans for the following day.

Research has found that emotional disclosure through expressive writing can produce clinically significant changes on a number of physiological and psychological health outcomes such as enhanced responses to hepatitis B vaccination in healthy adults, improvement in lung function in asthmatic patients, increased lymphocyte counts in HIV patients and on wound healing (e.g. Petrie et al., 2004; Robinson et al., 2017). Emotional disclosure through writing has also been found to reduce physician visits at follow-up, increase exam performance, reduce psychological distress and increase re-employment following job loss (see Pennebaker, 1997).

Support for the benefits of emotional writing has also been found in meta-analyses (e.g. Frisina et al., 2004). However, two more recent reviews have shown that the effects of emotional disclosure are likely to be smaller than previously hoped and its impact is moderated by individual differences variables (e.g. personality and previous experience of trauma) and by the characteristics of the writing task (e.g. time spent writing, instructions received) (Frattaroli, 2006; Merz, Fox & Malcarne, 2014). In addition, in some cases, the beneficial effects of writing may only be observed when using more sensitive and subtle outcome measures such as implicit measures that are not contaminated by self-report bias or expectations (O'Connor et al., 2011).

How does emotional writing influence health? Several mechanisms have been suggested. For example, writing may reduce the cumulative physiological drain of not confronting upsetting experiences or facilitate cognitive processing of traumatic memories which in turn leads to affective and physiological change. One of the current mechanisms proposed to account for the positive effects of emotional disclosure involves exposure and cognitive processing (Sloan & Marx, 2004). By accessing the emotions, feelings and cognitions linked to a stressful or traumatic event, memory begins to be restructured. Through such restructuring the individual assimilates the stressor into their own self-schema and beliefs system, becomes aware of the associated feelings and considers methods of coping with the traumatic or stressful encounter.

An important line of work has concentrated on understanding the psychological processes associated with the beneficial effects of emotional disclosure. For example, Creswell and colleagues (2007) content analyzed the essays of early-stage cancer survivors and showed that essays that included self-affirmation writing (i.e. evidence that an important personal value was affirmed as a result of their cancer) were associated with fewer physical symptoms at three months' follow-up. In other work, O'Connor and Ashley (2008) have explored the importance of the emotional characteristics of disclosure essays together with the alexithymic personality trait. Using the computer programme, Linguistic Inquiry and Word Count (LIWC), they found that alexithymic participants who disclosed more negative emotion words compared to positive emotion words exhibited reduced blood pressure responses to stress two weeks after writing. Yet non-alexithymic participants who disclosed more positive and less negative emotion words displayed reduced blood pressure responses to stress.

Resilience

The term "Resilience" as a psychological construct was first used in the developmental literature to describe the ability to overcome negative childhood experiences. In recent years it has gained popularity in adult psychology in the context of loss and other traumatic events (Bonanno et al., 2012; Bonanno, 2021) and like the other approaches discussed above is linked to the growth in more positive approaches in psychology and the move away from an emphasis on negative wellbeing outcomes. It has spawned a complex literature on what factors contribute to resilience. Bonanno (2012) defines resilience as a "stable trajectory of healthy functioning in response to a clearly defined event" (p. 753). Typically, resilience is defined by this successful outcome. It is not a personality construct though personality traits (e.g. optimism) are predictors of the outcome (Carver et al., 2005; Zautra & Reich, 2011). Other factors seen as contributing to resilience include resources such as social networks, income and education.

However, in addition to these variables, processes of coping with stressful events are central to achieving successful outcomes. Researchers have investigated the links between coping strategies and resilience. For example, Bonanno et al. (2012) investigated the coping strategies (using the COPE scale) that predicted resilience (i.e. a stable pattern over time of low symptoms of anxiety and depression) in the face of spinal cord injury. They found that resilient patients were more likely to appraise the spinal cord injury as a challenge rather than a threat, and were more likely to cope using strategies of acceptance and fighting spirit and less likely to use behavioural disengagement. A study of child caregivers also showed that resilience is associated with higher levels of benefit finding (see above; Cassidy et al., 2014).

Nevertheless, it has been recently suggested that there is a resilience paradox (Bonanno, 2021). There is an abundance of evidence showing that the most common outcome following a trauma is a stable trajectory of healthy functioning, known as resilience. However, predicting resilience or who is likely to be resilient has proved very difficult and when predictors are identified, they turn out to make a small and modest contribution. Therefore, it seems, much more work is required in order to understand the characteristics and related factors that predict resilience.

FOCUS BOX 5.4

Building resilience

The American Psychological Association (APA, 2014) has produced a list of ten ways to build resilience

1. *Make connections.* Building relationships, accepting and giving help and support.
2. *Avoid seeing crises as insurmountable problems.* Change how you interpret and respond to difficult events.
3. *Accept that change is part of living.* This includes accepting circumstances that cannot be changed.
4. *Move toward your goals.* Develop realistic goals and take steps to move towards them.
5. *Take decisive actions.* Act on difficult situations rather than detaching from them or wishing they will go away.
6. *Look for opportunities for self-discovery.* Try to learn from difficult experiences.
7. *Nurture a positive view of yourself.* Develop confidence in your abilities to solve problems and trust your instincts.
8. *Keep things in perspective.* Avoid blowing problems out of proportion.
9. *Maintain a hopeful outlook.* Be optimistic. Visualize what you want rather than worrying about what you fear.
10. *Take care of yourself.* For example, engage in activities you enjoy, exercise etc.

Adapted from (APA, 2014).

ACTIVITY BOX 5.1

Consider each of the 10 ways of building resilience listed in Focus box 5.4. How do each of these relate to the coping strategies discussed earlier in this chapter.

Throughout this section on coping, we have seen that drawing on social support resources can make a positive contribution to coping. The role of strong social networks and other types of social supports are explored in further detail in the next section.

Social support

What do we mean by social support? What should researchers be measuring when they look at social support? Is it important to be part of community networks with large numbers of social contacts, or is it more important to have one close relationship perhaps with a spouse, cohabiting partner or close friend? Maybe the crucial issue is not the nature of the relationship but whether people perform behaviours that help out in a stressful situation. These are key questions addressed by social support research.

Types of social support

Various classifications of social support exist. Researchers have distinguished between structural and functional approaches to support (e.g. Uchino, 2009). Structural approaches examine the simple existence of networks and friendships, whereas functional approaches look at the actual function that such social contacts serve (e.g. providing practical help versus emotional support). Supports have further been categorized into perceived and received supports, with perceived support tending to show stronger relationships with health than received support (Uchino, 2009). In this section we examine research demonstrating the importance of being part of a social network followed by some studies examining the importance of having a small number of quality relationships. We then examine studies examining a range of different functions of social support.

Social networks

In 1979, Berkman and Syme published what is now regarded as a classic study demonstrating the value of social networks for health. The study, conducted in the USA, followed up a random sample of almost 5000 adults (aged 30–69) for nine years from 1965. At the start of the study the researchers recorded the presence and the extent of four types of social ties – marriage, contact with the extended family and friends, church membership and other formal and informal group affiliations. These were combined to form a social network index. They found that both the individual ties and the combined index predicted mortality over the next nine years. Those with low scores on the index were about twice as likely to die as those with high scores, even after controlling for self-reports of social class, smoking, obesity and health at the outset. One limitation of this study was the use of self-reports of health in the initial measurements but findings were later replicated using physical examinations. In a review of a range of such studies, House, Landis and Umberson (1988) concluded that evidence consistently supports the view that there is an increased risk associated with having few social relationships even after adjusting for other risk factors. However, there are gender differences. In particular, marriage has more health benefits for men than for women, and bereavement is more harmful for men. Poor social networks, or social isolation (as it is now more frequently called), have been linked to strokes, decline in cognitive functioning and depression. An influential key review paper has recently described social isolation as an underappreciated determinant of physical health (Holt-Lunstad & Steptoe, 2022).

Quality of relationships

Being part of a large social network does not guarantee that people will receive greater help when they need it. The correlation between the number of connections people have and the actual support they receive tends to be quite low, perhaps because one good relationship may provide better support than a large number of more superficial contacts (Cohen & Wills, 1985). The importance of quality rather than quantity of relationships is demonstrated by a well-known sociological study conducted by Brown and Harris (1978), who studied the origins of depression in women. They interviewed 400 women about the life events they had experienced in the past year. They also asked the participants to name the people they were able to confide in about their worries. Women were classified into one of the four following categories: a) those who had a close relationship with someone in the same household, b) those without such a relationship who had a friend or relative they saw at least weekly, c) those with a close friend or relative they saw less than weekly and d) those with none of these relationships. The study found that having a confiding relationship protected the women from depression following major life events. Among the women who experienced a stressful life event, only one in ten of those in category a developed depression, compared to one in four of those in category b and one in 2.5 of those in categories c or d. This suggests that having confiding social support buffered the impact of life stressors.

Functional social support

None of the above measures taps specific supportive behaviours. However, it is important to consider what types of behaviour may be most helpful if we wish to develop effective social support interventions. For example, what type of support would be most helpful when an individual received a diagnosis of cancer? Various types of specific social support have been assessed, including emotional support (helping the person to feel accepted or valued), instrumental support (i.e. practical support) and informational support (e.g. Cohen & Wills, 1985; Uchino et al., 2018a). The match between support provided and an individual's need may be crucial to effectiveness. For example, a study of support from family and friends provided for breast cancer sufferers (Reynolds & Perrin, 2004) compared a range of provided support with the support desired by the women. The study found that two behaviours which were intended to be supportive were unwelcomed by over 90% of the women. These both related to trying to find causes or explanations for the cancer. However, reactions to other types of support varied greatly between women. Using cluster analysis, a statistical technique which classifies people into groupings according to specified characteristics, they found four different patterns. Group 1 wanted many types of support which focused on reassurance that everything would be OK; group 2 wanted people to act normally and did not want to talk about cancer; group 3 wanted facts, information and general advice; group 4 wanted to talk but did not want advice. The four groups did not differ on measures of adjustment to breast cancer. However a mismatch of support was associated with poorer adjustment, particularly where people received support they had not wanted.

Health impact of social support

There is strong evidence for positive effects of social support such that it has been shown to be related to beneficial effects on cardiovascular, endocrine and immune functioning (e.g. Uchino et al., 2018a; 2018b). A recent meta-analysis clearly demonstrated that social support and social integration were related to lower levels of inflammation as measured by inflammatory cytokines (Uchino et al., 2018b). These researchers also found that interventions to improve social support had beneficial impacts on heart disease risk factors such as blood pressure.

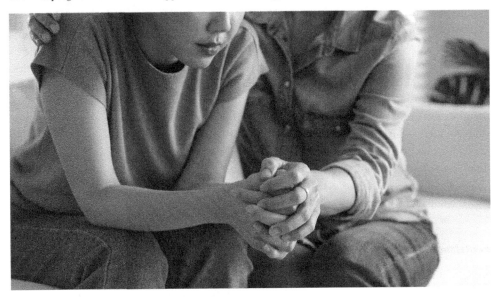

Figure 5.2 Greater social support is associated with better health.
Copyright of Chay_Tee/Shutterstock.

The mechanisms whereby social support impacts on health have been discussed at length. Cohen and Wills (1985) suggested two alternative pathways. First, social support may have a direct effect on wellbeing and health, i.e. it is beneficial regardless of the presence of stressors. Second, social support may buffer or moderate the impact of stressors on health so that it only benefits those facing threats (see Focus box 5.2). In a review of early literature, Cohen and Wills found evidence of direct effects for structural supports (e.g. when measures of social networks are used), but buffering was sometimes found when studies focused on close relationships. Studies tend to find buffering effects when measures of enacted supports are used. It is perhaps not surprising that, when close family or friends provide specific supports in response to a particular stressful situation, this buffers the stress, while simply having a large social network may not have the same effect. Social support may also have a positive impact on health through its effect on health behaviour (i.e. the social support–health relationship is mediated by health behaviours). Finally, it is also possible that the level of social support available to an individual is a stable individual difference that is linked to personality traits (e.g. agreeableness or lack of hostility, see Chapter 6).

FOCUS BOX 5.5

Can social support ever be bad for you?

In some situations social support can be unhelpful. We have seen that this is the case where there is a mismatch between our needs and the support provided. It is also not unusual for researchers to find that social support provided in the work situation is not beneficial. Support at work, especially from a supervisor, may make the recipient feel incompetent and so is not experienced as helpful. This idea was tested in an experimental study by Deelstra et al. (2003) which imposed instrumental support and found that negative affect was higher and self-esteem was lower when support was given, except when the problem could not have been solved without it. These effects were confirmed by physiological indicators (e.g. pulse rate).

Similarly, social networks may not always be supportive. For example, in a study of widowed women (aged 60–69), Rook (1984) found a stronger relationship between problematic relationships and reduced wellbeing than between positive relationships and improved wellbeing. Furthermore, most of those relationships identified as "problematic" were friends or relatives. The researchers suggested that many of these unhelpful relationships were not seen to be egalitarian, i.e. others were making decisions for them. There is also evidence from a meta-analysis that negative aspects of social relationships may have a negative impact on the immune system (Herbert & Cohen, 1993).

Finally, it is also worth considering the impact of social support on the provider of the support. We saw in Chapter 2 that carers of Alzheimer's patients showed slower wound-healing than matched controls (Kiecolt-Glaser et al., 1995), a clear instance of negative impact of offering social support. This may be an extreme example where giving support is damaging because it is extremely stressful. Generally, social psychologists researching reciprocity in social support have suggested that the feeling of giving more support than you receive is beneficial for health (e.g. Liang et al., 2001). However, there do seem to be gender differences. Vaananen et al. (2005) examined the long-term effects of perceived reciprocity in intimate relationships on sickness absence and found that women who gave more support than they received were healthier (compared to those who received more than they gave), whereas men who received more than they gave were healthier. They suggested that giving support was associated with enhanced self-esteem for women.

In summary, many of the findings in studies discussed in this section emphasize the importance of providing social support in a way that does not undermine individuals' self-esteem and feelings of competence.

Developments in social support research.

Loneliness and social isolation

Research has focused on the effects of social isolation and loneliness. Social isolation refers to a lack of social networks. For example, those living alone with few friends and family and limited contact with others are regarded as isolated (Shankar et al., 2011). As we have seen earlier in this chapter it is well established that such isolation is associated with a range of cognitive and health problems and with increased mortality.

Loneliness is the perception of social isolation and is not necessarily the same as objective isolation. Feelings of loneliness may occur in those who have considerable social contacts while some quite isolated people do not feel lonely. Social isolation is a particular risk for older people as they frequently live alone and may have lost partners or suffer deteriorating mobility. Loneliness in this group is also a matter of concern. A survey of older people (over age 65) in the UK found that 7% reported being often or always lonely (Victor et al., 2005). Loneliness is found to show a U-shaped relationship with age, being higher among those aged under 25 and those aged over 65 years (Victor & Yang, 2012)

Loneliness, like social isolation, has been linked to an increase in physical illness and mortality (e.g. Hawkley & Cacioppo, 2010, Smith & Victor, 2022). Hawkley and Cacioppo also report evidence of devastating effects of loneliness on mental wellbeing and cognitive functioning. It has been associated with increased risk of depression, cognitive decline and Alzheimer's disease. So serious are these effects that Hawkley and Cacioppo conclude that "A perceived sense of social connectedness serves as a scaffold for the self – damage the scaffold and the self starts to crumble". (p. 219).

Recent research has investigated the mechanisms whereby both loneliness and social isolation are linked to illness and mortality. It is unclear whether they have independent effects or whether loneliness mediates the relationship between social isolation and health (see Focus box 5.2) and few studies examine both variables in conjunction. Cornwell and Waite (2009) found that loneliness and isolation have independent effects on self-rated health, but loneliness appeared to mediate the association between isolation and mental health. Both have been linked to physical inactivity, smoking and other health behaviours (Shankar et al., 2011). However, Shankar et al. found that social isolation was linked to blood pressure and a number of inflammatory markers. This suggests that both loneliness and social isolation may affect health through their effects on health behaviour but that social isolation may have direct effects on biological processes implicated in heart disease development. Steptoe et al. (2013) also found that loneliness was not independently associated with mortality among older adults and also did not appear to mediate the link between social isolation and mortality suggesting social isolation is associated with ill health and mortality regardless of whether a person experiences loneliness. Steptoe et al. suggest that while reducing both social isolation and loneliness would benefit individuals' wellbeing, interventions to reduce isolation would be more important for reducing mortality. Interestingly, a recent large-scale study conducted in Germany found that loneliness and social isolation interacted synergistically to predict mortality with a follow-up period of up to 20 years (Beller & Wagner, 2018). These authors showed that the higher the social isolation, the larger the effect of loneliness on mortality, and the higher the loneliness, the larger the effect of social isolation.

Social isolation and social support in cyberspace

Over the last century the nature of social networks has gradually changed for many people. Greater social mobility means that many people work away from home and families are often dispersed around the world. At the same time new technologies have made it possible for people to maintain contact, at first by phone and more recently via the Internet (e.g. by email, social networking, instant messaging and use of Zoom, Skype, Teams). Opportunities to build new networks, often based on specific interests, are also offered via Internet chat rooms, discussion forums and social media platforms such as X (formerly Twitter) and Mastodon. In recent years there has been a rapid growth in studies examining the impact of the Internet for social networks and social support.

Whether the Internet has a positive or negative impact on social networks and individuals' wellbeing has proved controversial. Early research by Kraut et al. (1998) studied 179 people in 73 households over the first year or two of their Internet use. They found that greater use of the

Internet was linked to reductions in communication with others in their household, a decline in the size of their social circle and increases in feelings of depression and loneliness. This was true even though they used the Internet predominantly for communication purposes. They labelled this phenomenon the "Internet paradox". They followed up the same sample three years later (Kraut et al., 2002) and found that the negative effects had generally been replaced by positive effects in that more use of the Internet was associated with improved psychological wellbeing and more social involvement, although, on the negative side, there was also an increase in stress. However, there were important individual differences in the long-term effects of Internet use with better outcomes for extroverts and those who already had good social support but poorer outcomes for introverts and those lacking social support. Overall, they suggest that the Internet may have improved in the three years of the study, offering better information and communication services (e.g. instant messaging) that help maintain social contacts. There were also gender differences in Internet use such that women were more likely to use e-mail to keep in touch with family and friends who live far away (Boneva et al., 2001). It is clearly likely that the effects on social contacts are very dependent on type of use made of the Internet and whether it is a replacement for social contact or for other individual activities. The Internet also played a crucial role during the COVID-19 pandemic in ways that were not always positive. For example, Wilding et al. (2022), in a longitudinal study conducted during the first year of the pandemic, found that individuals who engaged in high levels of COVID-related information seeking reported poorer mental health outcomes, particularly clinically significant levels of anxiety.

ACTIVITY BOX 5.2

It has been suggested that excessive Internet use makes people isolated and withdrawn. Discuss whether you think this is the case. Do you think it is possible to improve your social support via the Internet?

For people who are perhaps isolated by illness or disability, the Internet can provide a unique and invaluable source of support. It can provide informational support and can also put people in touch with others experiencing similar circumstances who may be able to provide emotional support. Researchers have examined Internet social support for a range of illnesses, including breast cancer or HIV/AIDS, as well as sites offering support for behaviour change such as quitting smoking or losing weight. For example, Fogel et al. (2002) found that women with breast cancer who used the Internet for information on breast health issues reported greater social support and less loneliness. This was true even when the use of the Internet was less than one hour a week. Similarly, Kalichman et al. (2003) reported greater perceptions of social support, as well as greater active coping, among HIV-positive people who used the Internet for health-related information. Mo and Coulson (2012) suggest that participating in online support groups help individuals living with HIV/AIDS by four empowering processes, i.e. receiving useful information, receiving social support, finding positive meaning and helping others. More recently, Coulson and Buchanan (2022) reviewed the existing evidence base and found promising evidence that online support groups do yield benefits for individuals affected by HIV and AIDS (Coulson & Buchanan, 2022).

Researchers using qualitative methods to content analyze communications in Internet social support groups have shed light on the types of social support available. For example, Coulson, Buchanan and Aubeeluck (2007) analyzed communications online in a support group for people affected by Huntington's disease (an inherited degenerative neurological disorder). They found that informational and emotional supports were most commonly offered. Just less than 10% offered tangible help and this included indirect help such as advising someone of sources of direct help. Other studies confirm the finding that informational and emotional supports are the dominant forms of support in online communications.

Further research by Coulson (2013), using qualitative methods, has shown the value of membership of a web-based community for those with inflammatory bowel disease. The majority accessed the site daily and to obtain information and emotional support. They reported that it helped them to accept their illness and learn to manage it. It also helped them view their disease more positively and improved their subjective wellbeing. However, some disadvantages were also reported. For example, a focus on the negative side of the disease could be demoralizing.

In some cases there may be more worrying disadvantages to Internet use. For example, there has been considerable concern in the media and medical profession about pro-anorexia websites that provide support for life-threatening behaviour. In an experimental study of exposure to such websites, Bardone-Cone and Cass (2007) found evidence of negative effects on viewers' affect, self-esteem and perceived weight. Similarly, Whitlock et al. (2006) analyzed self-injury message boards for adolescents and suggested that while they may provide valuable support they may also normalize and so encourage damaging behaviour.

ACTIVITY BOX 5.3

Search for support groups online (e.g. type "support group" into Google). Pick three support groups for physical or psychological disorders and evaluate them. What kind of support do they offer? How likely is it to fit the needs of the target group?

Summary

Coping can be viewed both as a situational and dispositional variable. Researchers have identified a wide range of coping strategies that are typically measured using standard coping questionnaires. These have been used to explore coping in response to particular situations and to examine dispositional tendencies to use particular coping strategies. These strategies are often further grouped into overarching categories, e.g. emotion-focused or problem-focused coping.

Repressive coping is a form of avoidant coping style that is linked to health outcomes. The distinction between monitoring and blunting coping styles addresses people's information processing preferences and is useful in helping to design strategies to communicate medical information to patients. General personality styles are also linked to coping strategies. Coping strategies can be seen as mediators of the relationship between personality and wellbeing outcomes.

A positive or optimistic approach to the experience of threat has coping benefits. People typically report feeling positive affect (as well as negative affect) even in the most stressful times. This is thought to provide respite and help build resources. Positive affect and looking for benefits in stressful situations also benefits health. Positive approaches to coping are also central to developing resilience.

Social support has been classified into functional and structural forms of support and a distinction has also been made between perceived and received support. Types of functional support have also been identified e.g. emotional, instrumental and informational supports. Most types of support have been linked to positive health outcomes. Having good social networks has been shown to be beneficial for health and mortality but having one or two close confiding relationships may be more important in a crisis. Both direct and stress buffering effects have been found depending on the type of support considered. However, there are also some instances when social support may not be helpful. This may be particularly the case where social support is damaging to the self-esteem of the recipient. In some circumstances it may also be harmful to the support giver.

Recent developments in social support research discussed in this chapter include research on loneliness and isolation and on the role of new technologies for the provision of social support.

Key concepts and terms

- Benefit finding
- Blunter
- Coping resources
- Coping strategies
- Coping style
- Emotional writing
- Emotion-focused
- Monitor
- Primary appraisal
- Proactive coping
- Problem-focused
- Repressive coping
- Secondary appraisal
- Social networks
- Social support
- Loneliness
- Social isolation
- Resilience

Sample essay titles

- Moving house is generally considered to be a stressful experience. How does psychological theory and research help to explain why one person may cope with this experience better than another?
- "Coping is personality in action under stress". Evaluate this statement with reference to situational and dispositional approaches to coping.

- Are personal relationships helpful in reducing stress? Discuss with reference to the psychological evidence.
- Is the Internet a valuable resource in the provision of social support to isolated individuals? Discuss giving examples from the research literature.

Further reading

Books

Skinner, E.A., & Zimmer-Gemback (Eds). (2023). *The Cambridge handbook of the development of coping.* Cambridge University Press.

Journal articles

Carver, C.S., Scheier, M.F., & Weintraub, J.K. (1989). Assessing coping strategies: A theoretically based approach. *Journal of Personality and Social Psychology, 56,* 267–283. https://doi.org/10.1037//0022-3514.56.2.267

Holt-Lunstad, J., & Steptoe, A. (2022). Social isolation: An underappreciated determinant of physical health. *Current Opinion in Psychology, 43,* 232–237. https://doi.org/10.1016/j.copsyc.2021.07.012

Pressman, S.D., Jenkins, B.N., & Moskowitz, J.T. (2019). Positive affect and health: What do we know and where next should we go? *Annual Review of Psychology, 70,* 627–650. https://doi.org/10.1146/annurev-psych-010418-102955

Seligman, M.E.P. (2019). Positive psychology: A personal history. *Annual Review of Clinical Psychology, 15,* 1–23. https://doi.org/10.1146/annurev-clinpsy-050718-095653

Uchino, B.N., Trettevik, R., Kent de Grey, R.G., Cronan, S., Hogan, J., & Baucom, B.R.W. (2018). Social support, social integration and inflammatory cytokines: A meta-analysis. *Health Psychology, 37,* 462–471. https://doi.org/10.1037/hea0000594

6 Personality and health

Personality and health

Personality variables or traits refer to stable individual differences in thinking, feeling and behaving across a range of different situations. Much of the research on personality traits and health has focused on specific traits (e.g. optimism, type A behaviour, hostility, self-control). These specific traits can be considered as "blends" of five broader personality dimensions (openness, conscientiousness, extraversion, agreeableness, neuroticism). Research in the health domain has found that some personality variables are associated with poor health and reduced longevity, while others are linked to good health and increased length of life. The magnitude of these effects for personality variables can be similar to those of known biological risk factors such as cholesterol (Caspi et al., 2005). The aspects of personality associated with poor health outcomes include neuroticism (or negative affect), type A behaviour, and hostility. The aspects associated with good health outcomes include optimism, extraversion and conscientiousness.

In this chapter we review the evidence linking these personality variables to health outcomes and some of the mechanisms by which personality affects health. For example, personality variables might lead to greater exposure to stressful events, to a reduction in the effectiveness of coping strategies, or a change in coping resources such as social support. These explanations of the personality–health link build on the discussion of the impact of personality on coping in Chapter 5. Other personality variables such as hostility may affect health through changing the intensity and duration of physiological reactions to stress, linking personality to the biopsychosocial pathways considered in Chapter 2.

In this chapter we consider:

1. Optimism and health.
2. Type A behaviour and coronary heart disease.
3. Hostility and coronary heart disease.
4. Big five personality dimensions (openness, conscientiousness, extraversion, agreeableness, neuroticism) and health.

Introduction

This chapter reviews evidence suggesting that stable individual differences in the way people think, feel and behave (i.e. personality variables) are predictive of various health outcomes. We explore

DOI: 10.4324/9781003171096-9

how these stable individual differences can predispose individuals to respond to life challenges in a manner which, over time, damages or protects their health. Much research on personality in recent years has focused on five broad personality dimensions: openness to experience (or intellect), conscientiousness, extraversion, agreeableness and neuroticism (or emotional stability) (McCrae & Costa, 1987; Digman, 1990). This is often referred to as the Big Five Taxonomy or the OCEAN model of personality. A growing body of research now relates traits from the Big Five Taxonomy to various health behaviours and health outcomes. For example, Booth-Kewley and Vickers (1994) suggest that the Big Five personality traits may determine the extent to which people engage in general clusters of health-related behaviours such as substance use risk behaviours (e.g. smoking). It should be noted that research in relation to health has focused less on openness and agreeableness and more on extraversion, neuroticism and conscientiousness – a bias that our review reflects. The Big Five model is based on the assumption that a range of more specific personality traits can be understood as blends of the different Big Five traits. Some of the best evidence for the impacts of personality on health outcomes arises from work looking at more specific personality traits. So, for example, work has examined the impact of optimism or positive affect on health. We will consider work on optimism, type A behaviour pattern, and hostility as important areas of research relating personality variables to health outcomes. Some research has also suggested a cancer or type C personality type (see Focus box 6.1) and a distressed or type D personality type (see Focus box 6.3).

Learning outcomes

When you have completed this chapter you should be able to:

1. Explain how optimism is related to positive health outcomes and the role of attributional styles in this relationship.
2. Discuss the effects of type A personality and hostility on coronary heart disease and potential mediation of these effects through physiological reactions.
3. Describe the role of neuroticism (or negative affect) on poor health and the explanations of this effect through perceptions of stress, ability to cope and social support.
4. Describe the impact of extraversion on positive and negative health outcomes through effects on mood and health risk behaviours.
5. Describe the relationship between conscientiousness and positive health outcomes and the mediating effects of health behaviours.
6. Evaluate the different mechanisms through which personality variables affect health outcomes.

Since the magnitude of personality effects on health outcomes can be comparable to known biological factors, these effects must be taken seriously by health psychologists (Ferguson, 2013; Friedman & Hampson, 2021; Hampson et al., 2006; Hampson, 2012). In the western world the leading causes of morbidity and mortality in middle and later life are now various chronic diseases such as coronary heart disease, cancer, and diabetes; while in children, adolescents and young adults unintentional injuries are the leading causes of death. Personality variables may have important roles to play in both these periods of life. In relation to the development of chronic diseases, personality variables may play an important role in the maintenance of behaviours that are health-promoting (e.g. physical activity; fruit and vegetable consumption) or health-damaging (e.g. smoking and unhealthy eating) when engaged in over time. Similarly, accidents and unintentional injuries are usually a consequence of repeated exposure to risky situations rather than a single chance event. Personality variables may also influence health through a variety of other mechanisms such as increasing perceptions of stress. A key theme in this chapter is the different mechanisms by which personality variables affect health outcomes. In considering each personality variable and its impact on health we discuss potential explanations and then in a final section consider these explanations collectively. Table 6.3 (below) provides a summary of key explanations of the relationships between personality variables and health.

FOCUS BOX 6.1

Type C personality

This chapter reviews work on the "type A" or coronary prone behaviour pattern. The type A individual appears to be hostile, easily angered, competitive and hard-driving. Research by oncologists interested in the behavioural causes of cancer has suggested a "type C" or cancer risk pattern (Temoshok et al., 1985). Type C individuals are characterized by high levels of denial and suppression of various emotions, in particular anger. Type C includes a number of other features including "pathological niceness", conflict avoidance, high social desirability, harmonizing behaviour, over-compliance, over-patience, as well as high rationality and a rigid control of emotional expression. It is suggested that the excessive denial, avoidance, suppression and repression of emotions that characterize type C can, over time, weaken the individual's natural resistance to carcinogenic influences. Support for the link between type C personality and cancer is found in studies relating different immune parameters (e.g. natural killer cell activity, lymphocytes, serotonin uptake, mean platelet volume) to mood states, coping styles and personality traits (Cunningham, 1985). Recent research has suggested that there may be two facets of type C personality: submissiveness and restricted affectivity (Rymarczyk et al., 2020). It will be interesting to see if these two facets are replicated in additional studies and whether the two facets show differential relationships to cancer outcomes.

Alexithymia is a related personality type (a literal translation is the lack of words for emotions), characterized by difficulty identifying, labelling and understanding emotions, which is also found to be associated with negative health outcomes. Evidence exists to suggest that alexithymia is linked to an increased risk of developing cardiovascular disease (Waldstein et al., 2002). It has also been found to be associated with blood pressure reactivity following written emotional disclosure (O'Connor & Ashley, 2008; see also Focus box 5.1).

Optimism and health

Optimism refers to the expectation that in the future good things will happen to you and bad things will not. While we all may be optimistic in some areas of our lives and pessimistic in others, optimism taps the extent to which an individual is optimistic in general across a range of domains and over time. A number of measures of optimism have been developed. Scheier and Carver (1992) developed a measure that focuses on optimistic expectations. This includes items such as "In uncertain times, I usually expect the best" and "I always look on the bright side of life". Optimism has also been assessed using indices of an individual's sense of hope. A measure developed by Snyder et al. (1996) focuses on the extent to which individuals pursue their goals and their beliefs that their goals can be realised. Items include "I energetically pursue my goals" and "There are lots of ways around any problem". Other researchers have focused on how people explain the causes of bad events (Peterson, 2000). Such explanations or "attributions" can be classified along a number of dimensions such as whether they are internal or external to the individual (e.g. whether the cause is something about the individual versus their environment), whether they are likely to be stable or unstable over time (e.g. the extent to which the cause will affect most/all similar future outcomes or just this specific one), and whether they are general or specific causes (e.g. will the cause affect a range of life events for that individual or just this particular event). Optimists tend to attribute bad events to external, unstable and specific causes while pessimists see the same events as resulting from internal, stable and global causes (Peterson et al., 1988). For example, an optimist might believe that they got a minor illness because they were "run down" after an unusually busy time at work. In contrast, a pessimist might believe they contracted a minor illness because they are always susceptible to such things no matter what they do.

The outcomes of optimism include increased psychological wellbeing, better physical health and even greater longevity. For example, in relation to psychological wellbeing, Litt et al. (1992) found that optimistic individuals were less depressed after unsuccessful in vitro fertilization. Similarly, Carver et al. (1993) reported that optimism in women with breast cancer was associated with less distress following surgery and that this effect persisted one year later. Alloy, Abrahamson and Francis (1999) found that students with a pessimistic explanatory style were more likely to subsequently experience depression.

Research also demonstrates that high levels of optimism are associated with better physical health. Those with high levels of optimism have fewer infectious illnesses and report fewer physical symptoms even during periods of stress (Peterson & Seligman, 1987). They are also more likely to recover from surgery more quickly and less likely to be re-hospitalized (Scheier et al., 1999). Peterson and colleagues provide an impressive demonstration of the effects of optimism on physical health. In a sample of men, an attributional style measure of optimism assessed at age 25 was found to predict health status 35 years later as judged by doctors; the optimists were more likely to be in better health even when initial physical and mental health were statistically controlled for (Peterson et al., 1988).

Most impressively, those with high levels of optimism may even live longer. Danner, Snowdon and Friesen (2001) coded pieces of text that a sample of 180 Catholic nuns had written about themselves on entering the church as young women, for emotional content. The research then examined the survival rates of these same women when they were 75–95 years of age. Those who wrote sentences containing self-descriptions with the most positive emotions (e.g. happiness, pride, love) were more likely to live longer than those containing the fewest positive emotions. Comparison of the top and bottom 25% (quartiles) indicated that 24% of those in the top quartile had died compared to 54% of those in the bottom quartile. Similar results have been reported for men. Everson et al. (1996) examined the relationship between hopelessness and health outcomes in a large sample of men. Comparing the top and bottom 33% (tertiles) showed that those in the top tertile compared to the bottom tertile for hopelessness were 3.5 times more likely to die from all causes of death, 4 times more likely to die from cardiovascular disease, and 2.5 times more likely to die from cancer. Similarly, men with AIDS who are optimistic live twice as long as men who are pessimistic (Reed et al., 1994). More generally, among older individuals, those with positive attitudes towards ageing live an average of 7.5 years longer than those with more negative attitudes (Levy et al., 2002).

Recent research has suggested that optimism and pessimism may not be simple opposites and may have distinct effects on physical health outcomes. A quantitative review or meta-analysis has shown that both optimism and lack of pessimism may be associated with more positive health outcomes (Scheier et al., 2021). Interestingly the lack of pessimism was more strongly related to positive health outcomes than the presence of optimism.

These studies on health outcomes highlight an important but subtle distinction between optimism and positive affect. Whereas optimism refers to positive beliefs and feelings about the future, positive affect reflects a level of pleasurable engagement with the environment such as happiness, joy, excitement, enthusiasm and contentment. These two tendencies may overlap substantially as is shown in the Danner et al. (2001) study. However, research has begun to examine the effects of positive affect independently of optimism (see Pressman & Cohen, 2005, for a review of positive affect and health; see also Chapter 5). One important issue here is the extent to which positive affect is the opposite of, or alternatively distinct from, negative affect, a personality trait we consider below. Currently there is evidence supporting each view as we discuss below.

The explanation for the relationship between optimism and various health outcomes is still unclear. One interesting suggestion is that those high in optimism may be more likely to avoid certain high-risk situations. Some supporting evidence for this view comes from Peterson and colleagues (1988) who showed that those with an optimistic attributional style were less likely to die from accidental or violent causes than those with a pessimistic style, while the two groups did not differ in respect of mortality from cancer or cardiovascular disease. A further explanation for the relationship between optimism and health is through the effects of optimism on coping strategies. Those high in optimism are more likely to use adaptive and functional strategies for coping with problems such as acceptance, rational thinking, social support and positive reframing. For example, Scheier, Weintraub and Carver (1986) conducted a study in which students had to write about coping with stressful situations. Optimists were found to be more likely to use strategies such as making a plan and sticking to it, focusing intently on the problem, and seeking social support. Optimists were also less likely to distract themselves from thinking about the problem. Scheier et al. (1989) reported similar differences between optimists and pessimists in the way they coped with recovery from surgery that resulted in faster recovery among the optimists. The use of more constructive coping strategies may lead to better health outcomes, partly by helping individuals to avoid negative life events and also by helping them to confront and deal with problems earlier and more effectively. A further explanation focuses on the effect of pessimism on physiological reactions to stress in terms of immune functioning and cardiovascular response (Scheier & Carver, 1987). Some support of this explanation can be found in studies that have shown immune responses to be lower in pessimists (Segerstrom et al., 1998).

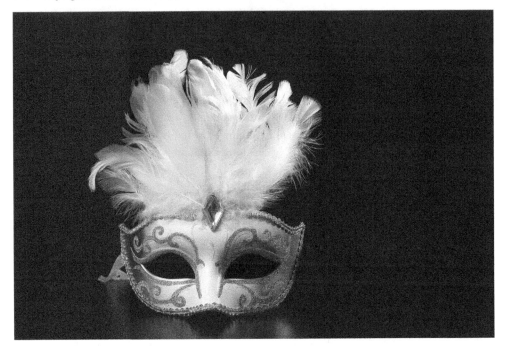

Figure 6.1 We can all show different "faces" to the world. Personality traits tap consistencies in
how we respond and behave. Such consistencies have been found to be important to the
maintenance of health and the development of illness.
Copyright of MirasWonderland/Shutterstock.

Type A behaviour and health

Type A behaviour pattern is typified by a competitive drive, aggression, chronic impatience and a
sense of time urgency (Rosenman et al., 1976). This type of behaviour is contrasted with the
opposite cluster of characteristics, type B behaviour pattern, which leads to a more relaxed, laid-
back approach to life. The concept of type A behaviour originated from the work of two cardiol-
ogists, Meyer Friedman and Ray Rosenman, who realized that their patients' disease was not
fully explained by conventional risk factors such as dietary cholesterol and smoking. For years
they failed to look beyond the physical symptoms and to consider the signs of stress in their
patients, even though patients tended to sit on the edge of waiting room chairs to the extent that
an upholsterer commented that the front edges of the waiting room chairs were unusually worn
(Friedman & Rosenman, 1974). Eventually, however, they sent out a questionnaire asking 150
businessmen what they believed had precipitated a heart attack in a friend. Few thought it was
due to diet or smoking and most felt it was due to "excessive competitive drive and meeting
deadlines" (Rosenman et al., 1964: 17). A subsequent study suggested that physicians agreed even
though this was not a recognized cause in the medical literature of the time. This and subsequent
research ultimately led to the identification of the constellation of characteristics described
above, and its long-term investigation in a large prospective study known as the Western
Collaborative Group Study. This examined risk factors for coronary heart disease (CHD) in a
sample of over 3000 healthy middle-aged men. The study started in 1960 and followed participants for more than 27 years. Rosenman and colleagues assessed the participants in the study

using a structured interview, in which the interviewer asked questions in a confrontational manner (including interrupting the participant) with the aim of provoking the participant in order to assess aggression and time urgency (Chesney et al., 1980). The men were then followed up at 8.5 and 22 years. The researchers found after 8.5 years that those men who were classified as type A had around twice the risk of developing CHD as those who were type B, even after controlling for other risk factors. At this stage it appeared that type A was a risk factor that was as important as smoking or high blood pressure for the development of CHD. However, on follow-up after 22 years, the researchers found that type A behaviour no longer showed a significant relationship with CHD (Ragland & Brand, 1985). Thus, after the initial enthusiasm about the importance of this risk factor, doubts were raised.

Many other research teams around the world were also conducting studies of type A behaviour during the 1960s and 1970s and in the early years (pre-1978) these tended to support the idea that type A was linked to CHD (Miller et al., 1991). However, after this time, the majority of subsequent studies, like that of the Western Collaborative Group itself, failed to support the original findings. As a result, the role of type A in causing heart disease became a controversial issue. A number of meta-analyses have been conducted over the years (e.g. Booth-Kewley & Friedman, 1987; Miller et al., 1996; Myrtek, 2001). For example, Miller et al. suggested that the null findings were due to a range of methodological differences between the early studies and those conducted later. First, the more recent studies often looked at samples that were already at high risk of heart disease. Second, over time, questionnaire measures (e.g. the Jenkins Activity Survey; Jenkins et al., 1971) have been used rather than the structured interview which allows assessment of behaviour in interaction. Compared to the interview, questionnaire items have limitations in terms of assessing behaviour and tend to be less effective in predicting CHD. Overall, Miller et al. (1996) concluded that type A behaviour was a risk factor for heart disease as, across studies based on structured interviews, about 70% of middle-aged males with CHD were type As, as opposed to 46% of healthy males.

Myrtek (2001) reviewed all prospective studies (a total of 25) published up to 1998 investigating coronary heart disease and type A behaviour. They concluded that taking all studies together there was no significant association between type A behaviour and heart disease and hence that type A is not a risk factor for heart disease. Since that time there seems no further evidence to support a link. Perhaps most damning of all for the type A construct has been a paper by Petticrew et al. (2012) which suggests that the initial positive results were due to the fact that much of the early research was funded by the tobacco industry and "selected results used to counter concerns about tobacco and health" (p. 2018). Evidence that type A caused disease could be used to suggest that smoking was merely a result of type A and not itself a risk factor.

However, interest in at least one aspect of type A continues as number of meta-analytic reviews (e.g. Booth-Kewley & Friedman, 1987; Matthews; 1988) raised the possibility that one component of type A behaviour (hostility) is predictive of heart disease. While a certain amount of research continues into the type A behaviour pattern the emphasis has now shifted towards investigating hostility.

Hostility and health

Hostility, like type A, is a complex and multidimensional construct. It has been defined as "a negative attitude towards others, consisting of enmity, denigration and ill will" (Smith, 1994: 26). Components of this characteristic are cynicism about others' motives, mistrust and hostile attributional style, i.e. a tendency to interpret other people's actions as aggressive (Smith et al., 2004). While this definition is primarily cognitive, the associated emotional and behavioural constructs of anger and aggression are often incorporated within the construct (Miller et al., 1996). The construct is measured using items such as "Some of my family have habits that bother and annoy me very much" and "It is safer to trust no-one"; with a response of 'true' indicating higher levels of hostility. These items are taken from the Cook–Medley hostility scale which is a commonly used measure (Cook & Medley, 1954). Hostility has been found to be correlated quite highly with the hard-driving component of type A behaviour (r = .44). It is also positively correlated with a range of measures of neuroticism (r = .27 to .54) and negatively with measures of extraversion (r = −.48) (Carmody et al., 1989). Some authors discuss hostility as one (negative) expression of the Big Five personality trait agreeableness (Ozer & Benet-Martinez, 2006), i.e. hostility is low agreeableness.

Following on from the tradition of research in type A behaviour, most research in this area has focused on the role of hostility in CHD. As for the research on type A, meta-analyses have assessed the strength of effects (Miller et al., 1996). Miller et al. included 45 studies in their review and concluded that hostility was an independent risk factor for CHD. As was the case with the research into type A, they found that the strongest relationships were found using structured interviews to assess hostility which emphasize the expressive component of hostility (i.e. verbally and physically aggressive behaviour). These studies suggested that the effects were at least of similar magnitude to those reported for traditional risk factors such as smoking, high blood pressure and cholesterol. Even among studies using self-report measures (the Cook–Medley scale: Cook & Medley, 1954), the review found small but consistent relationships with heart disease. It should be noted, however, that a more recent meta-analysis offers a less positive interpretation based on a smaller subset of papers (Myrtek, 2001), i.e. they suggest that while the effects are significant they are very small indeed. Furthermore, Petticrew et al. (2012) suggests that large amounts of tobacco industry funding also supported early research into hostility. In the main however, studies and reviews continue to suggest that hostility plays a role in causing CHD (e.g. Gallo & Matthews, 2003) and hypertension (Rutledge & Hogan, 2002). Most recently, Chida and Steptoe, (2010) reviewed prospective studies of the role of anger and hostility in heart disease including a number of studies published since the previous reviews. They conclude that both anger and hostility are associated with an increase in CHD events in those who were initially healthy, but also poorer prognosis for CHD patients. They suggest that interventions to reduce anger and hostility may help prevent and treat CHD. Focus box 6.2 considers one such intervention.

The possible mechanisms underlying the effects of hostility have also been discussed in some detail. Smith et al. (2004) discuss five possible models:

1. Psychophysiological reactivity model. This suggests that hostile individuals show exaggerated cardiovascular and neuroendocrine responses to stressors.
2. Psychosocial vulnerability model. This model suggests that hostile individuals experience more interpersonal conflict. Hostility may lead to more stress and also be associated with less social support.
3. Transactional model. This combines the above two models and suggests that hostile individuals experience more interpersonal conflict and also have greater physiological reactivity – a "double whammy" effect.

4. Health behaviour model. This suggests that hostility affects health because hostile individuals engage in health-risk behaviour patterns which mediate the effects of hostility on health. For example, hostile people may be cynical about health warnings or resistant to medical advice.
5. Constitutional vulnerability model. This model raises the possibility that individual differences (which might be genetic) are associated with both the personality tendency and the disease risk, i.e. the association between hostility and CHD is due to a third variable.

Overall, Smith et al. (2004) conclude that there is considerable support for a number of these models. Hostile people do display heightened physiological responses; they also experience increased levels of conflict and less social support. However, research has not yet established whether these tendencies mediate the relationship between hostility and health. There is some evidence that hostile people do display poorer health behaviour patterns but it is also clear that this does not wholly account for the relationship between hostility and health. Finally, the development of molecular genetics offers opportunities to explore the constitutional vulnerability model. Further research is awaited on these mechanisms. However, it is possible that each of several mechanisms play a part in explaining the association between hostility and health.

An interesting possibility in relation to the development of hostility is suggested by the work of Matthews et al. (1996). In this work, negative behaviours during parent–son discussions aimed at resolving disagreements were observed in 51 Caucasian adolescent (12–13 years of age) boys. Results showed that the frequency of negative behaviours in the family discussions predicted hostility and expressed anger assessed three years later even after controlling for baseline hostility. This would suggest that hostility may be nurtured within particular family backgrounds that are characterized by negative behaviours during interactions. In contrast, work by Caspi et al. (1997) shows that measures of temperament taken at three years old predict later health-related risk behaviour in early adulthood and that this effect is mediated by personality measures taken in late adolescence. This would appear to be good evidence that personality traits are something we are born with or at least develop very early in life and remain stable throughout our lives. Together, however, these studies suggest that, while certain aspects of personality may be stable from a very young age, other aspects change and develop over time as a result of our interaction with our environment. Thus both "nature" and "nurture" explanations may be needed to account for personality trait development.

FOCUS BOX 6.2

Interventions to reduce hostility

There is evidence suggesting that a hostility-reduction intervention aimed at CHD patients with high levels of hostility may reduce risks for heart disease. Gidron, Davidson and Bata (1999) conducted a randomized controlled trial in which 22 hostile male patients were assigned to either a treatment or control group. Hostility was assessed by observation during a structured interview and by self-ratings. The hostility-reduction intervention involved eight 90-minute weekly group meetings using cognitive behaviour techniques. Participants were taught skills to reduce antagonism, cynicism and anger. They were also asked to rate their hostility in a daily log and to record their use of the skills they had learnt. The control group had a one-session group meeting giving information about the risks of hostility and about basic hostility-reduction skills. The participants were followed up immediately after the trial and again after two months. Those in the intervention group were observed to be, and rated themselves to be, less hostile at follow-up than the controls. They also had lower diastolic blood pressure. Furthermore, reductions in hostility were correlated with reductions in blood pressure.

In a subsequent paper, Davidson et al. (2007) conducted secondary analysis of the data from the above study. They found that patients who received the intervention tended to have fewer hospital admissions in the six months following the intervention, and, importantly, had significantly fewer days in hospital (a mean of 0.38 days compared with a mean of 2.15 days for the control group). Consequently, their hospitalization costs were less. While more studies are needed with larger and more diverse groups, these findings suggest there may be potential to design efficacious and cost-effective hostility-reduction treatments.

FOCUS BOX 6.3

Type D personality

Similar to type A, type D personality is a risk factor for coronary heart disease. The type D, or distressed, personality describes individuals who experience high levels of negative emotions (negative affectivity) and inhibit the expression of these negative emotions in social interactions (social inhibition). The concept was introduced by Johan Denollet, of Tilburg University in the Netherlands.

Type D personality can be assessed by a self-report questionnaire containing items that tap negative affectivity (e.g. "I often make a fuss about unimportant things" or "I often feel unhappy") and social inhibition (e.g. "I often feel inhibited in social interactions" or "I find it hard to start a conversation"). The type D individual would be someone who scores highly on both of these dimensions. This is important because previous research has shown negative affectivity or neuroticism to be related to various negative health outcomes.

Denollet and colleagues have shown the type D personality to be a risk factor for adverse health outcomes in cardiac patients. So, for example, Denollet et al. (1996) assessed type D in a sample of 286 cardiac patients who were receiving treatment. Approximately one-third of the sample were classified as type D. Approximately eight years later, the patients were followed up. Among those classified as type D a total of 27% had died compared with a total of 7% of the rest of the sample. A majority of the deaths were due to heart disease or stroke. This translated into an odds ratio of almost four (i.e. being four times more likely to die if classified as type D compared to those not classified as type D). These effects were replicated in several studies. However, a meta-analysis including more recent studies suggested this was an overestimate and gave an odds ratio of 2.28 (Grande et al., 2012). More recent studies have often found smaller effects, a pattern seen in research in other areas discussed above, and have questioned the definition of the construct (see Ferguson et al., 2009).

The explanation for the relationship between type D and risk of death is not entirely clear. Those with type D personalities appear to have more highly activated immune systems and more inflammation (perhaps indicating more damage to blood vessels in the heart and throughout the body). They also show greater increases in blood pressure in reactions to stress. Recent research has suggested that type D individuals engage in fewer health behaviours and experience lower levels of social support and that these effects remain after controlling for neuroticism (Williams et al., 2008). Kupper and Denollet (2018) provide a recent review of evidence for type D personality as a risk factor for coronary heart disease.

FOCUS BOX 6.4

Personality and COVID-19 behaviours

Personality variables have been recently tested as potential predictors of engagement in behaviours that protect against the spread of the COVID-19 virus. For example, Zajenkowski et al. (2020) tested if any of the big five personality variables were associated with compliance with government guidelines to reduce the spread of COVID-19. Only low levels of agreeableness were significantly associated with being less likely to comply with guidelines.

Big Five personality dimensions and health

As noted earlier a significant proportion of personality research in the last few years has focused on five broad personality dimensions: openness to experience (or intellect), conscientiousness, extraversion, agreeableness and neuroticism (or emotional stability) (OCEAN; McCrae & Costa, 1987; Digman, 1990). In this section we consider how each of these five dimensions relate to health. Considerably more research has focused neuroticism, extraversion, and conscientiousness compared to openness and agreeableness and this is reflected here.

Neuroticism and health

Neuroticism refers to the tendency to commonly experience negative emotions such as distress, anxiety, fear, anger and guilt (Watson & Clark, 1984). Because of the focus on negative emotions it is sometimes referred to as negative affect. Those high in neuroticism or negative affect worry about the future, dwell on failures and shortcomings, and have less favourable views of themselves and others. There are a number of well-established measures of neuroticism. For example, the International Personality Item Pool (website: www.ipip.ori.org/ipip), which contains a set of public domain measures of the Big Five personality traits, includes statements such as "Worry a lot", and "Get upset easily"; those high in neuroticism are more likely to consider these statements as good self-descriptions. A variety of studies show that those high in neuroticism report themselves as experiencing more physical symptoms and that these symptoms are more intense (Affleck et al., 1992). For example, Costa and McCrae (1987) reported neuroticism to be related to frequency of illness, cardiovascular problems, digestive problems and fatigue across a sample of women with a wide variety of ages. These effects have been demonstrated in various cross-sectional and longitudinal studies.

Similar to the case for hostility, a number of mechanisms by which neuroticism might influence health outcomes have been suggested. One potential mechanism relating neuroticism to health outcomes might be through perceived or actual stress experienced. For example, those high in negative affect tend to perceive events as more stressful and difficult to cope with than those who are low in negative affect (Watson, 1988). In addition, those high in negative affect may experience more prolonged psychological distress after a negative event (Ormell & Wohlfarth, 1991). However, an important alternative suggestion in relation to neuroticism is that the reported impact on health symptoms may be attributable to the use of self-report measures of health. The hypothesis is that high levels of neuroticism lead to an individual noticing or complaining more about symptoms without this influencing the symptoms he or she experiences. Work that has objectively assessed physical health has indeed tended to report little association between such measures and neuroticism (Watson & Pennebaker, 1989). This importantly suggests the need to measure and control for the effects of neuroticism in any studies using symptom reports as outcome measures.

A further mechanism by which neuroticism may lead to negative health outcomes is through impact on coping mechanisms. Neuroticism might be related to maladaptive coping strategies in a similar way to pessimism. For example, Costa and McCrae (1990) showed that those high in neuroticism were more likely to engage in self-blame and less likely to engage in problem-solving in response to a scenario describing a nuclear accident. Another mechanism by which neuroticism influences health outcomes is through social support. It has been suggested that those high in neuroticism may have greater difficulties in forming and maintaining close relationships and may experience higher levels of interpersonal conflict. In support of this view, those high in negative affect have been shown to have lower marital satisfaction (Burke et al., 1980). These effects of neuroticism may have the result that those high in neuroticism experience less social support and so are less likely to experience the health protective effects associated with social support (see Chapter 5).

Neuroticism may also influence an individual's health behaviour patterns and, thereby, their health outcomes. Neuroticism is associated with more smoking and alcohol abuse, and less healthy eating and exercise (Booth-Kewley & Vickers, 1994). For example, in relation to smoking, longitudinal studies have found that those with higher neuroticism scores are more likely to take up smoking and maintain the habit (e.g. Canals et al., 1997). Thus, negative health outcomes associated with higher levels of neuroticism might be due, in part, to those with higher levels of neuroticism being more likely to smoke. Therefore, smoking may mediate the neuroticism-health relationship. Shipley et al. (2007) reported the impact of neuroticism on mortality in a sample of over 5000 UK adults over a period of 21 years. High neuroticism was associated with mortality from all causes and with mortality from cardiovascular diseases. However, these effects became non-significant after controlling for age, gender, social class, education, smoking, alcohol consumption and physical activity. This would suggest that the effects of neuroticism on mortality may be explained by sociodemographic factors and health behaviours. A final mechanism by which neuroticism may impact on health is through physiological changes. Research has highlighted the impact of high levels of neuroticism on reduced immune function (Kiecolt-Glaser et al., 2002) suggesting another potential mechanism through which neuroticism impacts on various health outcomes.

Extraversion and health

Extraversion is a Big Five personality trait where those with high levels of the trait are referred to as extraverts and those with low levels referred to as introverts. Extraverts tend to be outgoing, social, assertive and show high levels of energy; they also tend to seek stimulation and so enjoy new challenges but get easily bored. In contrast, introverts tend to be more cautious, serious and avoid over-stimulating environments and activities (Eysenck, 1967; Costa & McCrae, 1992). There are a number of well-established measures of extraversion–introversion. For example, Eysenck and Eysenck's (1964) measure contains items such as "Are you usually carefree?" and "Do you enjoy wild parties?" with extraverts more likely to agree with these items (see Figure 6.2). Extraversion has been found to be associated with positive psychological wellbeing and better physical health. For example, extraverts report more positive moods and higher levels of pleasure and excitement. Costa and McCrae (1980) showed that extraversion measured at one time point significantly predicted happiness ten years later. Extraverts tend to report lower rates of coronary heart disease, ulcers, asthma and arthritis (Friedman & Booth-Kewley, 1987). Some research has reported effects for extraversion

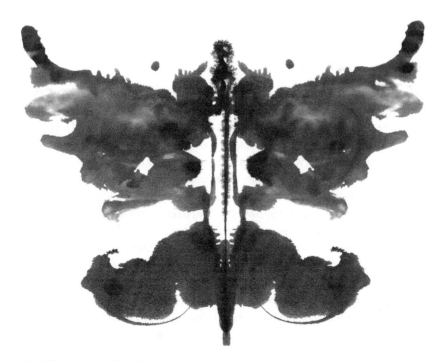

Figure 6.2 TheRorschach ink blot test for personality.
Copyright of xpixel/Shutterstock.

on mortality. For example, Shipley et al. (2007), in addition to examining the impact of neuroticism on mortality, also examined the impact of extraversion. In their sample of over 5000 UK adults examined over a 21-year period, extraversion was found to be significantly associated with a reduced risk of respiratory disease.

The explanation for the relationship between extraversion and health is not entirely clear. It is possible that this relationship is attributable to extraverts experiencing lower levels of stress, better coping strategies or more social support compared to introverts but there is as yet no strong evidence to support these explanations. Similarly, in relation to health behaviour patterns, extraversion appears to be associated with both health-protective behaviours like exercise (Rhodes et al., 2002) and health-risk behaviours like smoking (Booth-Kewley & Vickers, 1994)!

ACTIVITY BOX 6.1

The accident-prone personality?

Some research has addressed the idea that certain personality traits are precursors of accidents or unintentional injuries, i.e. the accident-prone personality. The best evidence supporting such a personality type comes from studies focusing on impulsivity. This research shows that childhood impulsivity predicts injuries both during childhood and later life (Caspi et al., 1997; Cooper et al., 2003).

What mechanisms might explain how impulsivity is related to injuries? Try reading these two articles and coming up with a list of potential mechanisms.

Conscientiousness and health

Conscientiousness refers to the ability to control one's behaviour and to complete tasks. Highly conscientious individuals are more organized, careful, dependable, self-disciplined and achievement-oriented than those low in conscientiousness (McCrae & Costa, 1987). High conscientiousness has also been associated with a greater use of problem-focused, positive reappraisal and support-seeking coping strategies (Watson & Hubbard, 1996), and a less frequent use of escape-avoidance and self-blame coping strategies (O'Brien & Delongis, 1996; see Chapter 5). In addition, conscientiousness is associated with a propensity to follow socially prescribed norms for impulse control (John & Srivastava, 1999; Bogg & Roberts, 2004; 2013). Recently, measures of conscientiousness with good levels of reliability and validity have become available. For example, the International Personality Item Pool contains statements such as "Am always prepared", and "Am exacting in my work" in order to tap conscientiousness. Those high in conscientiousness are more likely to consider these statements as accurate self-descriptions. A growing body of research shows conscientiousness to be positively associated with health-promoting behaviour patterns, health outcomes and even longevity prompting much recently research into the relationships between conscientiousness and health.

Some key evidence for an effect of conscientiousness on longevity comes from the Terman Life-Cycle personality cohort study. In this highly regarded study, a sample of over 1000 children born around 1910 completed various measures every five to ten years from the age of 11. The original sample of children were selected to have above average IQ and were drawn from the area around the Californian cities of San Francisco and Los Angeles. The personality assessments included measures of conscientiousness, optimism, self-esteem, sociability, stability of mood and energy level. Friedman et al. (1993) reported that of these variables only conscientiousness was significantly associated with lower mortality over time. The degree of association was such that those high in conscientiousness were more likely to live longer (by about two years) compared to those low in conscientiousness. Comparing the top and bottom 25% (quartiles) on conscientiousness indicated that those in the bottom quartile were one-and-one-half times more likely to die in any one year compared to those in the top quartile. Figure 6.3 shows the survival curves for participants in the Terman sample separately for males and females and for those with and without divorced parents among those with high and low levels of conscientiousness. Hampson et al. (2013) using a different cohort showed that childhood conscientiousness predicted objectively measured health when members of the cohort were in their 50s. Those with lower childhood conscientiousness were observed to have higher levels of obesity and worse blood lipids. Reviews have shown low conscientiousness to be a consistent risk factor for developing obesity across populations (Jokela et al., 2013a). Most recently, in the largest study of its kind, conscientiousness has been shown to be the only higher-order personality trait to be related to mortality risk across populations (Jokela et al., 2013b; see also Kern & Friedman, 2008).

An important mechanism by which conscientiousness may influence health is through health behaviour patterns. Howard Friedman et al. (1995) showed that the impact of conscientiousness on longevity in the Terman sample was partly accounted for by its effect on smoking and alcohol use, that is, conscientious children were less likely to become heavy smokers and

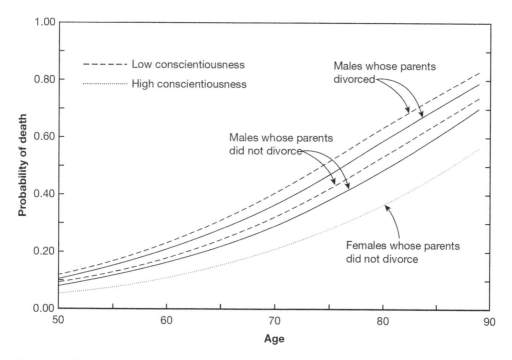

Figure 6.3 Survival curves for individuals from the Terman study.
Copyright Howard S. Friedman and Joseph Schwartz

drinkers. Consistent with these findings, Booth-Kewley and Vickers (1994) found that conscientiousness was more strongly correlated with clusters of health-related behaviours than the other Big Five traits, and was particularly strongly associated with health protection and accident control behaviours. Similarly, Courneya and Hellsten (1998) reported that, of the Big Five traits, conscientiousness was most strongly related to engaging in exercise behaviours, while Siegler, Feaganes and Rimer (1995) showed that regular mammography attendance was predicted by conscientiousness and extraversion. A comprehensive meta-analysis of work on the relationship between conscientiousness and behaviours (Bogg & Roberts, 2004) showed conscientiousness to be positively related to a range of protective health behaviours (e.g. exercise) and negatively related to a range of health-risk behaviours (e.g. smoking). In recent cohort study, school-related conscientiousness was found to be predictive of alcohol consumption and cigarette smoking in adolescents confirming its importance early in the life-course (Hagger-Johnson et al., 2013). Table 6.1 shows the size of these effects for a range of different health behaviours (the impact of health behaviours on health is further considered in Chapter 7). A further way in which conscientiousness may impact on health outcomes is through modifying behaviour following illness. So, for example, some studies have demonstrated that individuals high in conscientiousness are more likely to follow healthcare advice and that this difference is particularly apparent when the advice is difficult or time consuming to follow (Christiansen & Smith, 1995; Schwartz J.E. et al., 1999). A study (Booth et al., 2014) has shown that lower conscientiousness was associated with increased brain ageing (e.g. objectively measured brain tissue loss) using the Lothian Birth Cohort Study 1936 when the participants were in their 70s. Importantly this effect of conscientiousness on brain ageing appeared to be partly explained (i.e. mediated) by differences in health behaviours such as smoking, alcohol use, physical activity and diet.

Research has begun to examine how personality traits may produce changes in health behaviours through shaping the way in which individuals think about these behaviours. This work

Table 6.1   *Relationship between conscientiousness and various health behaviours based on a meta-analysis of available studies (from Bogg & Roberts, 2004).*

Behaviour	Effect size (r)	Total sample size
Physical activity	.05	24,259
Excessive alcohol use	−.25	32,137
Drug use	−.28	36,573
Unhealthy eating	−.13	6,356
Risky driving	−.25	10,171
Risky sex	−.13	12,410
Suicide	−.12	6,087
Tobacco use	−.14	46,725
Violence	−.25	10,277

Note. Cohen (1992) suggests that r = 0.1 equates to a small effect size, 0.3 to a medium effect size, and 0.5 to a large effect size; so these effect sizes for conscientiousness are mostly in the small to medium range.

suggests that our thoughts and feelings about performing a particular health behaviour (e.g. exercising) are a primary determinant of whether we perform that behaviour. That is, we tend to engage in behaviours that we have positive thoughts and feelings about (see Chapter 7). Consequently, conscientiousness may influence the amount of exercise we do by shaping our thoughts and feelings about exercising (i.e. thoughts and feelings mediate the impact of conscientiousness on exercise). Such mediation effects have been demonstrated by Siegler et al. (1995) who found that the effect of conscientiousness on mammography attendance was mediated by knowledge of breast cancer and the perceived costs of seeking mammography. Similarly, the impact of conscientiousness on the self-care activities of patients with type 1 diabetes has been found to be mediated by treatment beliefs (e.g. Christensen et al., 1999). However, other research has found both mediated and direct effects for conscientiousness when predicting health behaviour (Conner & Abraham, 2001; O'Connor et al., 2009; Vollrath et al., 1999).

In addition to mediation effects, conscientiousness might also operate as a moderator changing the relationship between health beliefs and health behaviour patterns. A few studies have examined the moderating role of conscientiousness. For example, in a retrospective study, Schwartz M.D. et al. (1999) found that conscientiousness moderated the relationship between breast-cancer-related distress and mammography uptake such that, among those with high levels of distress, those with high conscientiousness scores were more likely to have attended mammography screening than those with low conscientiousness scores. Conscientiousness scores had no effect on attendance among those with low levels of distress. Hampson et al. (2000) reported a similar significant interaction between conscientiousness and perceived risk in relation to changes in indoor smoking behaviour in response to the threat from radon gas, with greater response to risk among the more conscientious. In relation to exercise, Rhodes et al. (2002) reported conscientiousness to significantly moderate the intention–behaviour relationship, with higher levels of conscientiousness associated with stronger intention–behaviour relationships (see also Conner et al., 2007). Conner et al. (2009) showed intentions to be stronger predictors of resisting initiating smoking for an adolescent sample with high rather than low levels of conscientiousness.

Openness and agreeableness and the combined effects of the Big Five on health

Openness to experience is related to being intellectually curious and being creative and imaginative. Agreeableness is related to trust, altruism, kindness, affection and various prosocial behaviours. Those high in agreeableness tend to be more cooperative, while those low in agreeableness tend to be more competitive. Neither of these big five dimensions of personality has received the attention that neuroticism, extraversion and conscientiousness have in relation to health. Nevertheless, more recent work has suggested that agreeableness in particular may show similar sized effects on health as conscientiousness, extraversion and neuroticism. Strickhouser and colleagues (2017) reported a metasynthesis of the relationship between the big five personality dimensions and health and wellbeing. A metasynthesis combines the effects from different meta-analyses on a topic. The Strickhouser et al. (2017) metasynthesis combined 36 such meta-analyses including over half a million participants. The metasynthesis indicated that each of the big five personality dimensions were on average significantly related to health outcomes with neuroticism, conscientiousness and agreeableness being mostly strongly related to overall health, and extraversion and openness least strongly related to overall health. These relationships were positive (higher level of big five dimension associated with more positive overall health) for each dimension except neuroticism. These relationships were strongest for mental health and then health behaviours but were generally small and non-significant for physical health (see Table 6.2). Together the big five dimensions were moderately associated with overall health (R = .35; this equates to explaining about 10% of the variability in overall health). Future research could usefully follow this lead in further examining the combinations of the big five personality dimensions in predicting overall health.

Table 6.2   Relationship (correlations) between the big five personality dimensions and different outcomes based on a metasynthesis of available studies meta-analyses (from Strickhouser et al., 2017).

Big Five Dimension	Mental health	Health behaviour	Physical health
Extraversion	.11	−.02	−.02
Agreeableness	.21	.10	−.01
Conscientiousness	.22	.12	.03
Neuroticism	−.27	−.07	.00
Opennesss	.06	.00	.01

Note. Cohen (1992) suggests that a correlation of r = 0.1 equates to a small effect size, 0.3 to a medium effect size, and 0.5 to a large effect size; so, these effect sizes for conscientiousness are mostly in the small to medium range.

FOCUS BOX 6.5

Changing personality dimensions

The idea that changes in personality variables over time (either naturally occurring or as the result of intervention) may be associated with changes in health outcomes has received attention over the last few years. Socially desirable changes in personality dimensions (e.g. increasing agreeableness, conscientiousness and extraversion and decreasing neuroticism) may be beneficial for health. For example, Magee et al. (2013) showed that such socially desirable personality change was associated with self-reported health improvements over a period of four years. The improvement in health was particularly associated with increases in extraversion and conscientiousness and decreases in neuroticism. Takahashi et al. (2012) provided data to suggest that, at least in relation to increases in conscientiousness, it was effects on health-enhancing behaviours that explained the effects on self-reported health.

Recent studies have tested interventions to change different personality dimensions (e.g. Javaras et al., 2019; Stieger et al., 2021) with a particular focus on conscientiousness. The evidence would appear to suggest that such interventions can produce change that persists at least in the short-term (e.g. Stieger et al., 2021 report effects over three months). Future studies will hopefully address longer term changes and effects on different health outcomes. Such evidence would more directly address the causal effects of personality variables on health.

Conclusions

We have reviewed relationships between key personality variables and health outcomes and considered some of the explanations of this relationship. Out of the Big Five personality framework we noted that although there is as yet less evidence linking openness to health outcomes, there was more evidence in relation to conscientiousness, extraversion, neuroticism and agreeableness, with better health outcomes associated with high conscientiousness, high extraversion, low neuroticism and high agreeableness (or low hostility). We also noted that a body of research supports a link between optimism and positive health outcomes. The negative impacts of type A behaviour pattern and hostility on health were also noted, particularly in relation to the risk of coronary heart disease.

While discussing the effects of individual personality traits on health outcomes we also noted a number of important explanations for the relationship between the two. Table 6.3 provides a summary of these explanations and is worth reviewing now. Not all these explanations constitute true causal mechanisms. Indeed, part of the problem in interpreting any relationship between personality and health is that the data obtained is usually correlational (see Research methods box 6.1).

A further explanation of the relationship between personality traits and health outcomes is a measurement artefact explanation. Here the suggestion is that the personality variable may cause differences in the way certain health outcomes (e.g. symptoms) are reported. For example, we noted that, at least in relation to neuroticism, some of the relationship between this personality variable and health outcomes may be artefactual, caused by a reliance on self-report measures of symptoms (see Chapter 4). This would account for the stronger relationship between neuroticism and symptom reports compared to the relationship between neuroticism and non-self-report health outcomes (e.g. illness).

The remaining explanations of the relationship between personality variables and health outcomes are more easily interpreted as causal relationships. A key explanation may be that personality traits can lead to health outcomes through physiological mechanisms. So, for example, hostility might cause damage to arteries which in turn leads to a greater likelihood of heart disease. Another explanation focuses on the idea that certain personality traits may be associated with approaching certain risky situations. Friedman (2000) has referred to this idea as tropisms. Drawing on the analogy of phototropic plants that move towards sources of light, the suggestion is that certain personality types are drawn to particular situations which then pose a risk to the individual's health. For example, extraverts might be more likely to seek out situations where the risk of accidental injury is higher or where health risk behaviours such as smoking or drug use are common. Relatedly, personality variables may lead to negative health outcomes through changing engagement in health-related behaviours. We noted that conscientious individuals appear to be less likely to engage in health-risking behaviours such as smoking and more likely to engage in health-protective behaviours such as exercise. As we have already suggested, this might be through exposure to such behaviours in situations individuals are drawn to. Alternatively, personality variables like conscientiousness might make some health behaviours more likely by changing the way conscientious individuals think about behaviours such as exercise (Conner & Abraham, 2001). Thus, conscientious individuals might value health-protective behaviours more or might just be better at planning how best to engage in such behaviours. These cognitions about health behaviours are the focus of Chapter 7. Focus box 6.6 looks at recent research on mechanisms by which the personality trait of self-control might impact on engagement with health behaviours).

A final set of explanations for the relationship between personality traits and health outcomes relates to stress and the variables that protect against the effects of stress. So, for example, individuals high in neuroticism may perceive themselves as experiencing more stress. Such individuals may also be less likely to employ appropriate coping mechanisms or have access to coping resources such as social support to deal with this stress. In this case it may be the stress that causes the negative health outcomes, but it is high levels of neuroticism that cause the stress and the inability to cope appropriately with the stress. Penley and Tomaka (2002) provide an interesting discussion of the relationship between all of the Big Five personality traits and both stress and coping. While Ferguson (2013) has proposed a theoretical model explaining the role of personality in the illness process and identified six routes through which personality can have an influence on health (see also Bogg & Roberts, 2013 for a discussion of conscientiousness and health). Finally we should note that although personality variables have tended to be treated as relatively fixed from childhood/adolescence onwards more recently attention has focused on interventions to change personality variables as a means to change health outcomes (see Focus box 6.5).

FOCUS BOX 6.6

Mechanisms explaining the effects of self-control on health behaviours

Self-control is the capacity to override impulses and is known to predict engagement in health behaviours (de Ridder et al., 2012). Recent research has focused on *how* (i.e. the mechanisms) self-control drives health actions (Conner et al., 2023). Evidence for a number of mediation and moderation pathways by which self-control influences engagement with health behaviours is provided. In particular, Conner et al. (2023) show that high self-control helps individuals override negative impulses (feelings and habits) and how favourable are people's thoughts, feelings, and intentions about health behaviours. High self-control also leads to people giving higher priority to the perceived healthiness of the behaviour and how much control they have over its performance in forming their intention to act. High self-control also helps people translate their "good" intentions into health behaviours and form good habits. These different pathways were shown in a correlational study and need confirming in experimental studies that try to manipulate these pathways. Nevertheless, such a detailed approach to considering various mechanisms by which personality leads to health behaviour and health outcomes offers to provide important insights.

RESEARCH METHODS 6.1

Correlation and inferences of causation

When an independent (or predictor) variable (e.g. social support or attitude) is measured at the same time as a dependent (or outcome) variable (e.g. immune functioning or condom use) this is known as a cross-sectional study. When the dependent variable is measured at a later time then this is known as a longitudinal or prospective study. For example, if we measure job stress and then follow up our participants a year later this is a prospective study. Prospective studies offer more reassurance regarding the direction of causation because we know that the independent variable measure preceded the dependent variable measure in time. Prospective studies also allow us to control for levels of a dependent variable at time 1 so that we can predict change in the dependent variable from an independent variable. For example, we might find that lower reported social support (at time 1) predicts increases in stress over the following year (i.e. changes from time 1 to time 2). Thus, while we might use analysis of variance (ANOVA) to test whether an association between an independent and dependent variable is likely to be replicable, we can use analysis of covariance (ANCOVA) to assess the degree to which an independent variable can predict change in a dependent variable over time by including a baseline measure of the dependent variable as a covariate.

The direction of causation is ideally assessed in an experimental study in which we manipulate (rather than measure) the independent variable. In health psychology, interventions such as behaviour change interventions provide good examples of experimental methodology. For example, one group may receive an intervention to change attitudes or reduce work stress while another (control) group receives no intervention. If participants are randomly allocated to these two groups (to try to evenly distribute confounding factors across groups) or matched (to balance confounding factors) then any difference in the dependent variable following the manipulation (that is, the intervention) can be reasonably attributed to that manipulation. The classic use of experimental methodology in health psychology is the randomized controlled trial (RCT). It is of course worth noting that such experimental methods merely establish one causal determinant of the dependent variable, they do not necessarily demonstrate that this is the one and only causal determinant.

Unfortunately, we often cannot manipulate independent variables in health psychology and so must infer underlying causal mechanisms from correlational data. For example, in relation to smoking, the majority of the evidence supporting an impact of smoking on cancer and cardiovascular disease outcomes is correlational, at least for studies in humans. Similarly, the relationship between personality and health is based on correlational data.

There are well-known dangers in drawing causal inferences from correlational data. Two key issues are causal direction and the third variable problem. Causal direction refers to the issue of the direction of effect being unknown when two variables are correlated: did A cause B or B cause A? For example, in relation to personality and health this issue becomes one of whether a personality trait resulted in a health outcome or the health outcome produced the personality trait. So, for example, some patients with serious illnesses such as cancer may become anxious and neurotic. This might lead us to the erroneous conclusion that neuroticism played a role in causing the cancer when in fact the cancer had produced increased neuroticism.

Third variable problems refer to the possibility that a correlation between two variables might be due to both variables being caused by a third variable. So, for example, there is some evidence that a hyper-responsive nervous system is an underlying factor in both the development of an anxious personality (high neuroticism) and the development of heart disease. Here an anxious, reactive personality would be related to (that is, correlated with) heart disease without being a causal determinant of heart disease (McCabe et al., 2000). Similarly, Eysenck (1967) argued that extraversion relates to differences in the sensitivity of the nervous system that influences emotional reactions and reactions to socialization. Extraverts may also be more likely to seek stimulation through behaviours such as smoking. In both these cases it is not the personality trait itself which causes the health outcomes but an underlying biological mechanism that causes both the personality trait and the health outcome.

Table 6.3   Explanations of the relationship between personality traits and health outcomes.

Non-causal explanations	
Causal direction problem	Health outcome causes personality change (e.g. illness affects perceptions and behaviour)
Third variable problem	Both the personality trait and health outcome are caused by another underlying variable (e.g. disease)
Measurement artefact	The measurement of the health outcome is contaminated by the personality trait
Causal explanations	
Physiological changes	The personality trait causes physiological changes that in turn influences health outcomes
Tropisms	The personality trait means the individual is more likely to be exposed to risky situations
Health behaviours	The personality trait makes the individual more likely to engage in health-risk behaviours and less likely to engage in health-promoting behaviours
Stress impacts	The personality trait makes the individual more likely to experience stress and/or less likely to be protected from the effects of stress through coping mechanisms or social support

Summary

A number of personality variables or traits show significant relationships with various health outcomes such as morbidity and mortality. Indeed some of these relationships are of a similar size to those reported for more well-known risk factors like blood cholesterol levels. Of the Big Five personality traits that form much of the focus in modern-day personality research there is good evidence relating low levels of neuroticism and high levels of extraversion and conscientiousness to health outcomes (e.g. lower levels of illness and greater longevity). Evidence also suggests that optimism is positively related to health outcomes, while type A behaviour and hostility (low agreeableness) tend to be negatively related to health outcomes. In some cases (such as type A and type D) recent studies have shown declining effects and the importance of such variables remains a controversial issue.

The explanations of these relationships between personality and health are many and varied. They range from artefactual explanations, through mediating mechanisms, to direct biological or physiological effects. So, for example, much of the observed impact of neuroticism on self-reported illness is probably attributable to those higher in neuroticism being more likely to report symptoms. In relation to conscientiousness and health, for example, there is evidence of a mediating mechanism through greater engagement in health-protective behaviours and less engagement in health-risking behaviours, whereas in relation to hostility there is evidence of a direct effect through damage to arteries cause by over-reactivity to stress among those high in hostility. Detailing the range of effects that different personality dimensions can have on health and assessing the explanations of these effects is an exciting area of current research in health psychology.

Key concepts and terms

- Achievement-striving
- Agreeableness
- Big Five personality traits
- Conscientiousness
- Cynicism
- Direction of causation
- Extraversion
- Hope/Hopelessness
- Hostile attributional style
- Hostility
- Impatience/Irritability
- International Personality Item Pool
- Measurement artefact
- Mistrust
- Negative affect
- Neuroticism
- Openness to experience
- Optimism
- Optimistic attributional style
- Positive affect
- Psychophysiological reactivity model
- Psychosocial vulnerability model
- Third variable problem
- Tropisms
- Type A behaviour pattern

Sample essay titles

- Describe the evidence relating key personality traits to different kinds of health outcomes.
- Critically evaluate the mechanisms by which personality traits might have impacts on health.
- Do personality differences predict health? Discuss relevant findings and mechanisms.

Further reading

Journal articles

Bogg, T., & Roberts, B.W. (2013). The case for conscientiousness: Evidence and implications for a personality trait marker of health and longevity. *Annals of Behavioral Medicine, 45*, 278–288. https://doi.org/10.1007/s12160-012-9454-6

Ferguson, E. (2013) Personality is of central concern to understand health: Towards a theoretical model for health psychology. *Health Psychology Review*, 7, S32–S70. https://doi.org/10.1080/17437199.2010.547985

Hampson, S.E. (2012). Personality processes: Mechanisms by which personality traits "Get Outside the Skin". *Annual Review of Psychology, 63*, 315–339. https://doi.org/10.1146/annurev-psych-120710-100419

Pressman, S.D., & Cohen, S. (2005). Does positive affect influence health? *Psychological Bulletin, 131*, 925–971. https://doi.org/10.1037/0033-2909.131.6.925

Smith, T.W., Glazer, K., Ruiz, J.M., & Gallo, L.C. (2004). Hostility, anger, aggressiveness, and coronary heart disease: An interpersonal perspective on personality, emotion, and health. *Journal of Personality, 72*, 1217–1270. https://doi.org/10.1111/j.1467–6494.2004.00296.x

Book chapter

Friedman, H.S., & Hampson, S.E. (2021). Personality and health: A lifespan perspective. In O.P. John & R.W. Robins (Eds.), *Handbook of personality: Theory and research* (pp. 773–790). The Guilford Press.

PART 4

Motivation and behaviour

7 Health cognitions and health behaviours

Health cognitions and health behaviours

The prevalence of health-related behaviours varies across social groups. For example, smoking is more prevalent among those from more economically deprived backgrounds. This would suggest that these factors might be the focus of interventions to change health-related behaviours. However, socio-demographic factors may be impossible to change or may require political intervention at national or international levels (such as changes in income distribution or taxation). For that reason a considerable body of research has examined more modifiable factors that may mediate (or explain) the relationship between socio-demographic factors and health-related behaviours. A particularly promising set of factors are the thoughts and feelings the individual associates with the particular health-related behaviour. These are known as *health cognitions* and are the focus of this chapter. We consider:

1. Predicting health behaviours.
2. Social cognition models.
3. A critical appraisal of social cognition models.
4. The intention–behaviour gap.

Learning outcomes

When you have completed this chapter you should be able to:

1 Describe the key health cognitions associated with performing health behaviours.
2 Explain what the cognitive determinants of health behaviours are according to: a) the health belief model; b) protection motivation theory; c) theory of planned behaviour; and d) social cognitive theory.
3 Evaluate the contribution of stage models to the understanding of change in health behaviours.
4 Critically evaluate the contribution of social cognition models to understanding the determinants of health behaviours.
5 Describe the intention–behaviour gap in relation to health behaviours.

DOI: 10.4324/9781003171096-11

Predicting health behaviours

Can we predict who will perform health behaviours? Such knowledge might help us understand variations in the distribution of health behaviours and outcomes across society and suggest targets for interventions designed to improve health through changing health behaviours. As you might expect, a range of differences exist between those who do and do not engage in health behaviours such as smoking or physical activity. These include demographic factors, social factors, personality factors and cognitive factors (Conner & Norman, 2015).

Demographic variables show reliable associations with the performance of various health behaviours. Age, for example, shows a curvilinear relationship with many health behaviours, with higher incidences of health-risk behaviours such as smoking in young adults and much lower incidences in children and older adults (Blaxter, 1990). Health behaviours also vary between genders, with women being generally less likely to smoke, consume large amounts of alcohol or engage in regular exercise, and more likely to monitor their diet, take vitamins and engage in dental care, although such patterns can change over time (Waldron, 1988). Differences predicted by economic and ethnic status are also apparent for behaviours such as diet, exercise, alcohol consumption and smoking (e.g. Blaxter, 1990). Generally, younger, wealthier, better educated individuals are more likely to practise health-enhancing behaviours and less likely to engage in health-risking behaviours. Socioeconomic status (SES) differences are particularly apparent with "social class gradients" (i.e. increased longevity, better health and improved health behaviours as we move from lower to higher SES groups) apparent in most western countries (Mackenbach, 2006). Social factors, such as parental models, are important in instilling health behaviours early in life. Peer influences are also important, for example, in the initiation of smoking (e.g. McNeil et al., 1988). Cultural values also appear to be influential, for instance in determining the exercise behaviour of women across cultural groups (e.g. Wardle & Steptoe, 1991). We noted in Chapter 6 that personality traits are fundamental determinants of behaviour and that there is now considerable evidence linking personality and health behaviours (see Vollrath, 2006). For example, H.S. Friedman and colleagues (1993, 1995) found that childhood conscientiousness predicted longevity and that this was partly accounted for by conscientious individuals being less likely to engage in smoking and alcohol use.

In general, the correlates of health behaviours mentioned above cannot be easily modified (although see Focus box 6.5 on changing personality variables) and, therefore, they do not represent useful targets for interventions designed to change health behaviours. This is not the case for the cognitive antecedents of behaviour. A variety of cognitive factors distinguish between those who do and do not perform various health behaviours. Indeed recent research commonly refers to these cognitive factors as 'mechanisms of action' because they are often used to explain how an intervention to change a health behaviour exerts its effects. For example, knowledge about behaviour–health links (or risk awareness) is an essential factor in an informed choice concerning a healthy lifestyle (see Chapter 8). The reduction of smoking over the past 20–30 years in the western world can be largely attributed to a growing awareness of the serious health risks posed by tobacco use brought about by widespread publicity. However, the fact that tobacco continues to be widely used among lower socioeconomic status groups, and the continuing uptake of smoking among adolescent girls in some countries, illustrate that knowledge of health risks is not a sufficient condition for avoidance of smoking by all individuals.

Knowledge is just one of a number of cognitive correlates of health behaviours. Others include perceptions of health risk, potential efficacy of behaviours in reducing this risk, perceived social pressures to perform a behaviour and control over performance of the behaviour. The relative importance of individual cognitive factors in predicting performance of health behaviours has been the focus of numerous studies. For example, Cummings, Becker and Maile (1980) had experts sort 109 variables associated with performing health behaviours and derived six distinguishable factors:

1. Accessibility of healthcare services.
2. Attitudes to healthcare (beliefs about quality and benefits of treatment).
3. Perceptions of disease threat.
4. Knowledge about disease.
5. Social network characteristics.
6. Demographic factors.

These six groups of correlates may not be independent. For example, there may be considerable overlap between perceptions of disease threat and knowledge of the disease. In order to account for such overlaps and describe the relationships between different influences on health behaviours a number of models have been developed. Such models have been labelled "social cognition models" because of their use of a number of cognitive variables to predict and understand individual behaviours, including health behaviours. It is important to note at the outset that these models focus on behaviour-specific cognitions as determinants of the relevant behaviour. For example, on this view healthy eating is best understood in terms of cognitions about healthy eating rather than more general thoughts and feelings about health. In the health psychology area these are usually referred to as health cognitions.

FOCUS BOX 7.1

What are health behaviours?

The range of behaviours influencing health is extremely varied, from health-enhancing behaviours such as exercise participation and healthy eating, to health-protective behaviours such as health screening clinic attendance, vaccination against disease, and condom use in response to the threat of AIDS, through to avoidance of health-harming behaviours such as smoking and excessive alcohol consumption, and sick role behaviours such as compliance with medical regimens. A unifying theme across these behaviours has been that they each have immediate or longer-term effects upon the individual's health and are at least partially within the individual's control.

A number of definitions of health behaviours have been suggested (e.g. Kasl & Cobb, 1966). Conner and Norman (2005: 2) define health behaviours as "any activity undertaken for the purpose of preventing or detecting disease or for improving health and well-being". Behaviours encompassed in such a definition include medical service usage (e.g. physician visits, vaccination, screening), compliance with medical regimens (e.g. dietary, diabetic, antihypertensive regimens) and self-directed health behaviours (e.g. diet, exercise, breast or testicular self-examination, brushing and flossing teeth, smoking, alcohol consumption and contraceptive use). One useful distinction is between protection (e.g. physical activity), risk (e.g. smoking) and detection (e.g. breast or testicular self-examination) health behaviours.

The COVID-19 pandemic brought us a whole range of new health behaviours that were recommended to help prevent its' spread to our attention (e.g. hand washing, face mask wearing, social distancing; see Norman et al., 2020). Similarly concerns over global heating have drawn attention to various health behaviours (e.g. reducing red meat consumption) that may also reduce individual's impact on global heating.

FOCUS BOX 7.2

How do health behaviours impact on health outcomes?

A great many studies have now looked at the relationship between the performance of health behaviours and a variety of health outcomes (e.g. Doll et al., 1994). Large scale epidemiological studies have demonstrated the importance of a variety of health behaviours for both morbidity and mortality. For example, the Alameda County study, which followed nearly 7000 people over ten years, found that seven key behaviours were associated with lower morbidity and longer life: not smoking, moderate alcohol intake, sleeping seven to eight hours per night, exercising regularly, maintaining a desirable body weight, avoiding snacks and eating breakfast regularly (Belloc & Breslow, 1972; Breslow & Enstrom, 1980).

Health behaviours are assumed to influence health through three major pathways (Baum & Posluszny, 1999): first, by generating direct biological changes such as when excessive alcohol consumption damages the liver; second, by changing exposure to health risks, as when the use of a condom protects against the spread of HIV; and third, by ensuring early detection and treatment of disease, as when testicular or breast self-examination leads to early detection of a cancer that can more easily be treated.

Can you think of further examples for each of the pathways through which health behaviours might exert their effects on health?

FOCUS BOX 7.3

General models or behaviour-specific mModels?

The social cognition models considered here can be considered general models that could be applied to a broad range of behaviours. For example, the Theory of Planned Behaviour and Social Cognitive Theory were developed to apply to a broad range of social behaviours. The Health Belief Model and Protection Motivation Theory were developed to apply particularly in the health domain. Such models are useful because they help us understand a broad range of behaviours (see Conner & Norman, 2023 for a discussion). However, in relation to specific health behaviours then it may be useful to consider additional predictors not included in these models. For example, in relation to understanding blood donation the moral nature of the behaviour may be an important additional predictor (e.g. through measuring moral norms). We noted above the distinction between protection, risk and detection health behaviours. Some researchers have noted systematic differences in the power of predictors within models such as the Theory of Planned Behaviour and Reasoned Action Approach when explaining these different health behaviours. For example, Conner et al. (2017) showed differences for predicting intentions and behaviour for protection and risk health behaviours using the Reason Action Approach.

This links to a general difference in the way health psychologists work towards understanding and changing health behaviours. Some health psychologists focus across health behaviours aiming to form a general understanding of specific predictors and interventions. Other health psychologists focus on specific health behaviours and aim to develop a thorough understanding of that behaviour. These two approaches can form useful counterpoints in relation to health behaviours.

The journal *Psychology & Health* has over the last few years published a series of state-of-the-art reviews on specific health behaviours including smoking (West, 2017), physical activity (Rhodes et al., 2017), healthy eating (de Ridder et al., 2017), cancer screening (Sarma et al., 2019), sexual behaviours (de Wit et al., 2023), sun protection behaviours (Stewart et al., 2023) and medication adherence (Stewart et al., 2023). These can provide a useful resource to those interested in what is currently known about a specific health behaviour from a health psychology perspective.

Social cognition models

Social cognition models describe the important cognitions (i.e. thoughts and feelings) that distinguish between those who do and do not perform health behaviours. This approach focuses on the cognitions or thought processes that intervene between observable stimuli and behaviour in real world situations (Fiske & Taylor, 1991). This "social cognition" approach has been central to social psychology over the past quarter of a century. Unlike behaviourism, it is founded on the assumption that behaviour is best understood as a function of people's perceptions of reality, rather than objective characterizations of environmental stimuli.

Research into social cognition models can be seen as one part of what has been called "self-regulation" research. Self-regulation processes are defined as those ". . . mental and behavioral processes by which people enact their self-conceptions, revise their behavior, or alter the environment so as to bring about outcomes in it in line with their self-perceptions and personal goals" (Fiske & Taylor, 1991: 181). Self-regulation research has emerged from a clinical tradition in psychology which views the individual as striving to eliminate dysfunctional patterns of thinking or behaviour and engage in adaptive patterns of thinking or behaviour (Bandura, 1982; Turk & Salovey, 1986). Self-regulation involves cognitive re-evaluation of beliefs, goal-setting and ongoing monitoring and evaluating of goal-directed behaviour. Two phases of self-regulation activities have been defined: motivational and volitional (Gollwitzer, 1990). In the motivational phase costs and benefits are considered in order to choose between goals and behaviours. This phase is assumed to conclude with a decision or intention concerning which goals and actions to pursue at a particular time. In the subsequent volitional phase, planning and action directed towards achieving the set goal predominate.

Much of the research with health behaviours has focused on the important cognitions in the motivational phase, although recent research has begun to focus on the volitional phase. The key social cognition models in this area are:

1.   The health belief model (HBM; e.g. Janz & Becker, 1984; Abraham & Sheeran, 2015).
2.   Protection motivation theory (PMT; e.g. Maddux & Rogers, 1983; Norman et al., 2015).
3.   The theory of reasoned action/theory of planned behaviour (TRA/TPB; e.g. Ajzen, 1991; Conner & Sparks, 2015) and related Reasoned Action Approach (RAA; Fishbein & Ajzen, 2010).
4.   Social cognitive theory (SCT; e.g. Bandura, 2000; Luszczynska & Schwarzer, 2015).

A distinct set of models focus on the idea that behaviour change occurs through a series of qualitatively different stages. These so-called "stage" models (Sutton, 2015) importantly include the transtheoretical model of change (Prochaska & DiClemente, 1984; Prochaska et al., 1992) and the Health Action Process Approach (Schwarzer & Luszczynska, 2015). In the following sections we consider these different models and what they say about how cognitions help direct health behaviours. These social cognition models (SCMs) provide a basis for understanding the determinants of behaviour and also provide important targets (or mechanisms of action) which interventions designed to change behaviour should focus on if they are to change motivation (see Chapter 8) and, thereby, behaviour (see Chapter 9).

The health belief model

The health belief model (HBM) is the earliest and most widely used SCM in health psychology (see Abraham & Sheeran, 2015 for a review). For example, Hochbaum (1958) found that perceived susceptibility to tuberculosis and the belief that people with the disease could be asymptomatic (so that screening would be beneficial) distinguished between those who had and had not attended for chest X-rays. Haefner and Kirscht (1970) took this research further by demonstrating that health education interventions designed to increase participants' perceived susceptibility, perceived severity and anticipated benefits resulted in a greater number of check-up visits to the doctor compared to controls over the following eight months.

The HBM suggests that health behaviours are determined mainly by two aspects of individuals' representations of health behaviour: perceptions of illness threat and evaluation of behaviours to counteract this threat (see Figure 7.1). Threat perceptions are based on two beliefs: the perceived susceptibility of the individual to the illness ("Am I likely to get it?"); and the perceived severity of the consequences of the illness for the individual ("How bad would it be?"). Similarly, evaluation of possible responses involves consideration of both the potential benefits of, and barriers to action. Together these four beliefs are believed to determine the likelihood of the individual undertaking to perform a health behaviour. The particular action taken is determined by the evaluation of the available alternatives, focusing on the benefits or efficacy of the health behaviour and the perceived costs or barriers of performing the behaviour. Hence individuals are more likely to follow a particular health action if they believe themselves to be susceptible to a particular condition which they also consider to be serious, and believe that the benefits of the action taken to counteract the health threat outweigh the costs. For example, an individual is likely to quit smoking if he or she: believes him or herself to be susceptible to smoking-related illnesses; considers the illnesses to be serious; and that, of the alternative behaviours open to him/her, considers quitting smoking to be the most effective way to tackle his/her susceptibility to smoking-related illnesses (i.e. greatest benefits and fewest barriers).

Two other variables often included in the model are cues to action and health motivation. Cues to action are assumed to include a diverse range of triggers to the individual taking action which may be internal (e.g. physical symptom) or external (e.g. mass media campaign, advice from others) to the individual (Janz & Becker, 1984). An individual's perception of the presence of cues to action would be expected to prompt adoption of the health behaviour if the other key beliefs are already established in their mind. Health motivation refers to more stable differences between individuals in the value they attach to their health and their propensity to be motivated to look after their health. Individuals with a high motivation to look after their health should be more likely to adopt relevant health behaviours (i.e. more health protecting and less health risking behaviours).

The HBM has provided a useful framework for investigating health behaviours and has been widely used. It has been found to successfully predict a range of behaviours. For example, Janz and Becker (1984) found that across 18 prospective studies (that is, those in which behaviour was measured later, following an earlier measurement of beliefs) the four core beliefs were nearly always found to be significant predictors of health behaviour (82%, 65%, 81% and 100% of studies report significant effects for susceptibility, severity, benefits and barriers, respectively). Some

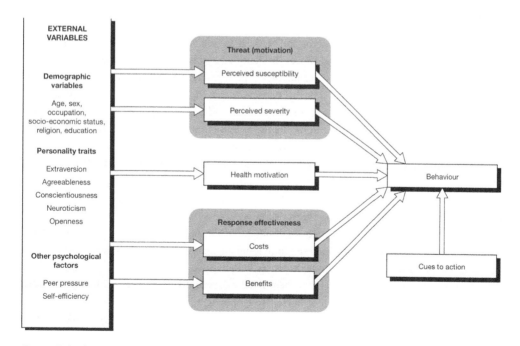

Figure 7.1 The health belief model.

studies have found that these health beliefs mediate (or explain) the effects of demographic correlates of health behaviour. For example, Orbell, Crombie and Johnston (1995) found that perceived susceptibility and barriers entirely mediated the effects of social class upon uptake of cervical screening. However, the overall evidence for such mediation is somewhat mixed. Recent research has seen the HBM applied to understanding influenza and COVID-19 vaccination (Mercadante & Law, 2021).

In addition, the HBM has inspired a range of successful behaviour change interventions. For example, Jones et al. (1987) tested an intervention designed to encourage patients visiting an "accident and emergency" service to make a follow-up appointment with their own doctor. Patients were randomly assigned to a control (i.e. routine care) group or to the intervention group. The intervention involved meeting a nurse who assessed and challenged patients' health beliefs. For example, a patient who did not feel susceptible to reoccurrence of the emergency event (e.g. an asthmatic attack) might be told of the likelihood of reoccurrence without further treatment in order to increase perceived susceptibility. Results of this randomized controlled trial showed that while only 24% of the control group subsequently attended a follow-up, a significantly greater 59% of the intervention group did so.

The main strength of the HBM is the common-sense operationalization it uses including key beliefs related to decisions about health behaviours. However, further research has identified other cognitions that are stronger predictors of health behaviour than those identified by the HBM, suggesting that the model is incomplete. This prompted a proposal to add "self-efficacy" (see Chapter 8 and below) to the model to produce an 'extended health belief model' (Rosenstock et al., 1988) which has generally improved the predictive power of the model (e.g. Hay et al., 2003).

Protection motivation theory

Protection motivation theory (PMT; Norman et al., 2015) is a revision and extension of the HBM which incorporates various appraisal processes identified by research into coping with stress (see Chapter 3). In PMT, the primary determinant of performing a health behaviour is protection motivation or intention to perform a health behaviour (see Figure 7.2). Protection motivation is determined by two appraisal processes: threat appraisal and coping appraisal. Threat appraisal is based upon a consideration of perceptions of susceptibility to the illness and severity of the health threat in a very similar way to the HBM. Coping appraisal involves the process of assessing the behavioural alternatives which might diminish the threat. This coping process is itself assumed to be based upon two main components: the individual's expectancy that carrying out a behaviour can remove the threat (response efficacy); and a belief in one's capability to successfully execute the recommended courses of action (self-efficacy).

Together these two appraisal processes result in either adaptive or maladaptive responses. Adaptive responses are those in which the individual engages in behaviours likely to reduce the risk (e.g. adopting a health behaviour) whereas maladaptive responses are those that do not directly tackle the threat (e.g. denial of the health threat). Adaptive responses are held to be more likely if the individual perceives him or herself to be facing a health threat to which he or she is susceptible and which is perceived to be severe and where the individual perceives such responses to be effective in reducing the threat and believes that he or she can successfully perform the adaptive response. So, for example, smokers will try to quit smoking when they believe

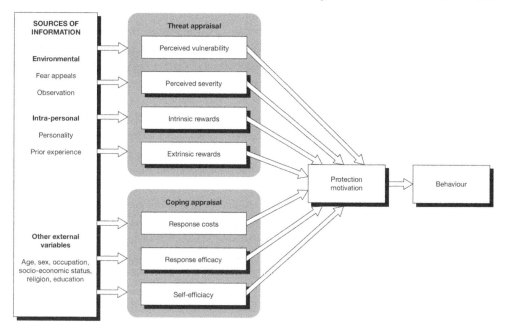

Figure 7.2 Protection motivation theory.

themselves to be susceptible to smoking-related illnesses which they think to be serious and where quitting smoking is perceived to be effective in reducing the threat and perceived to be something they have confidence they can achieve. The PMT has been successfully applied to the prediction of a number of health behaviours (for a recent review see Norman et al., 2015). Recent research has used the PMT to help understand protective behaviours taken in response to the threat of COVID-19 (Kowalski & Black, 2021).

Theory of planned behaviour

The theory of planned behaviour (TPB) was developed by social psychologists and has been widely applied to understanding health behaviours (Conner & Sparks, 2015). It specifies the factors that determine an individual's decision to perform a particular behaviour (see Figure 7.3). Importantly this theory added "perceived behavioural control" to the earlier theory of reasoned action (Ajzen & Fishbein, 1980) which continues to be applied (Ajzen, 2001; Fishbein & Ajzen, 2010). The TPB proposes that the key determinants of behaviour are intention to engage in that behaviour and perceived behavioural control over that behaviour. As in the PMT, intentions in the TPB represent a person's motivation or conscious plan or decision to exert effort to perform the behaviour. Perceived behavioural control (PBC) is a person's expectancy that performance of the behaviour is within their control and confidence that they can perform the behaviour. PBC is similar to Bandura's (1982) concept of self-efficacy used in the PMT and the extended HBM.

In the TPB, intention is itself assumed to be determined by three factors: attitudes, subjective norms and PBC. Attitudes are the overall evaluations of the behaviour by the individual as positive or negative (and so include beliefs about benefits and barriers included in the HBM). Subjective norms are a person's beliefs about whether significant others think they should engage in the behaviour. PBC is assumed to influence both intentions and behaviour because we rarely intend to do things we know we cannot and because believing that we can succeed enhances effort and persistence and so makes successful performance more likely (see Chapter 8). Thus, according to the TPB, smokers are likely to quit smoking if they form an intention to do so. Such an intention to quit is likely to be formed if smokers have a positive attitude towards quitting, if they believe that people whose views they value think they should quit smoking, and if they feel that they have control over quitting smoking.

Attitudes are based on behavioural beliefs, that is, beliefs about the perceived consequences of behaviours. In particular, they are a function of the likelihood of a consequence occurring as a result of performing the behaviour and the evaluation of that outcome (i.e. "Will it happen?" and "How good or bad will it be?"). It is assumed that an individual will have a limited number of consequences in mind when considering a behaviour. Thus, a positive attitude towards quitting smoking will result when more positive than negative consequences are thought to follow quitting. Subjective norm is based on beliefs about salient referents' approval or disapproval of whether one should engage in a behaviour (e.g. "Would my sexual partner approve?", "Would my best friend approve?"). These beliefs are weighted by the "motivation to comply" with each salient other on this issue (e.g. "Do I care what my sexual partner/best friend thinks about this?"). Again, it is assumed that an individual will only have a limited number of referents in mind when considering a behaviour. Thus, the more people (whose approval is seen to be important) who are thought to approve of the action, the more positive the subjective norm. Judgements of PBC are influenced by control beliefs concerning whether one has access to the necessary resources and opportunities to perform the behaviour successfully, weighted by the perceived power, or importance, of each factor to facilitate or inhibit the action. These factors include both internal control factors (information, personal deficiencies, skills, abilities, emotions) and

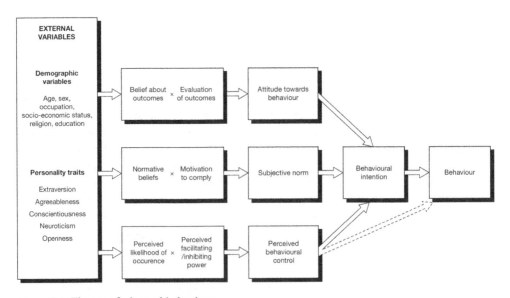

Figure 7.3 Theory of planned behaviour.

external control factors (opportunities, dependence on others, barriers). As for the other types of beliefs it is assumed that an individual will only consider a limited number of control factors when considering a behaviour. So, for example, in relation to quitting smoking, a strong PBC to quit smoking would be expected when a smoker believes there are more factors that facilitate than that inhibit quitting smoking, especially if the inhibiting factors do not have strong effects on the feasibility of quitting.

The TPB has at least two advantages over the extended HBM. First (as in PMT), health beliefs are seen to affect behaviour indirectly, in this case through attitude and intention. Thus, the model outlines a mechanism by which particular beliefs combine to influence motivation and action. Second, the model takes account of social influence on action. The TPB has been widely tested and successfully applied to the understanding of a variety of behaviours (for reviews see Ajzen, 1991; Conner & Sparks, 2015). For example, in a meta-analysis of the TPB Armitage and Conner (2001) reported that across 154 applications, attitude, subjective norms and PBC accounted for 39% of the variance in intention, while intentions and PBC accounted for 27% of the variance in behaviour across 63 applications. Intentions were the strongest predictors of behaviour, while attitudes were the strongest predictors of intentions (see McEachan et al., 2011 for a review of applications of the TPB to health behaviours).

The TPB has also informed a number of interventions designed to change behaviour. For example, Hill, Abraham and Wright (2007) employed a randomized controlled trial to test the effectiveness of a TPB-based leaflet compared to a control in promoting physical exercise in a sample of school children. The leaflet condition compared to the control condition significantly increased not only reported exercise but also intentions, attitudes, subjective norms and PBC. Additional analyses indicated that the impact on exercise was mediated (i.e. partly explained) by the increases the leaflet had produced (compared to the control group) in intentions and PBC.

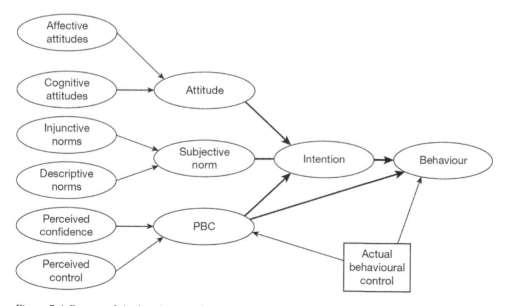

Figure 7.4 Reasoned Action Approach.

Recent work with the TPB (see Conner & Sparks, 2015) has divided attitude, subjective norm and PBC each into two components to form the Reasoned Action Approach (RAA; Fishbein & Ajzen, 2010; Figure 7.4). Attitude is divided into an affective or experiential component and a cognitive or instrumental component. The first concerns beliefs and evaluations about how it will feel to perform the behaviour while the second includes beliefs and evaluation about other consequences. So, for example, quitting smoking might be perceived as both unenjoyable (affective evaluation) but beneficial (cognitive evaluation). As well as subjective norms (defined above), the two-factor model includes descriptive norms. Descriptive norms refer to perceptions of what others are doing (e.g. "all my friends are doing it") rather than beliefs about others' approval of the target individual performing the behaviour. For example, a smoker might believe that important others approved of him or her quitting but those other individuals to have not quit smoking themselves. PBC is divided into perceived control (or autonomy) and perceived confidence (or capability). So, for example, one might perceive that quitting smoking is within one's control but not feel confident that one can easily quit smoking. The latter factor is most like self-efficacy and has been found to be the stronger predictor of intentions and behaviour in meta-analyses of the RAA (McEachan et al., 2016). Recent research has applied the RAA to understanding compliance with behaviours recommended to prevent the transmission of COVID-19 in the UK (Norman et al., 2020).

Social cognitive theory

In social cognitive theory (SCT; Bandura, 1982) behaviour is held to be determined by three factors: goals, outcome expectancies and self-efficacy (see Figure 7.5). Goals are plans to act and can be conceived of as intentions to perform the behaviour (see Austin & Vancouver, 1996; Luszczynska & Schwarzer, 2015). Outcome expectancies are similar to behavioural beliefs in the TPB but here are split into physical, social or self-evaluative depending on the nature of the consequences considered. Thus, in this model, beliefs about others' approval (subjective norms in the TPB) are grouped with beliefs about other consequences. Self-efficacy is the belief that a behaviour is or is not within an individual's control and is usually assessed as the degree of confidence the individual has that they could still perform the behaviour in the face of various obstacles. This is very similar to PBC in the TPB and particularly the perceived confidence component in the two-factor TPB. Bandura has recently added socio-structural factors to his theory. These are factors assumed to facilitate or inhibit the performance of a behaviour and affect behaviour via changing goals. Socio-structural factors refer to the impediments or opportunities associated with particular living conditions, health systems, political, economic or environmental systems. They are assumed to inform goal-setting and be influenced by self-efficacy. The latter relationship arises because self-efficacy influences the degree to which an individual pays attention to opportunities or impediments in their life circumstances. For example, self-efficacious individuals intending to exercise might be expected to focus on exercise cues in the environment such as running or cycling routes. This component of the model incorporates perceptions of the environment as an important influence on health behaviours. In overview, the SCT predicts that quitting smoking, for example, is more likely for individuals who have a goal of quitting smoking, who perceive that various positive physical (e.g. health), social (e.g. positive regard from others) and self-evaluative (e.g. feeling good about yourself) outcomes will follow from their quitting smoking, and who perceive they have the confidence to quit smoking in the face of various obstacles.

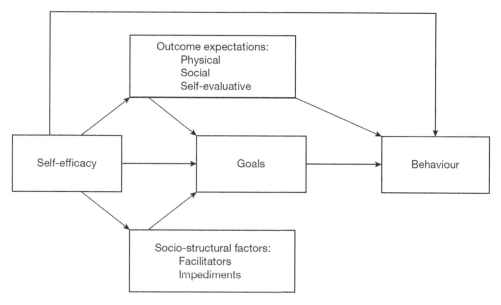

Figure 7.5 Social cognitive theory.

SCT has been successfully applied to predicting and changing health behaviours. (e.g. Luszczynska & Schwarzer, 2015). However, unlike a number of the other models we have considered, many of the applications of SCT only assess one or two components of the model rather than all components. Self-efficacy and action-outcome expectancies along with intentions have been found to be important predictors of a range of health behaviours in a diverse range of studies (for reviews see Bandura, 2000; Luszczynska & Schwarzer, 2015; see Chapter 8 on changing self-efficacy). For example, Ghazi et al. (2018) reviewed 20 interventions based on SCT to increase self-efficacy in musculoskeletal rehabilitation, reporting that they had a large effect on self-efficacy, although the review didn't examine effects on behaviour.

Stage models of health behaviour

The models considered above assume that the cognitive determinants of health behaviours act in a similar way during initiation (e.g. quitting smoking for the first time) and maintenance of action (e.g. trying to stay quit). In contrast, in stage models psychological determinants may change across such stages of behaviour change (see Sutton, 2015 for a review). An important implication of the 'stages' view is that different cognitions may be important determinants at different stages in promoting health behaviour. The most widely used stage model is Prochaska and DiClemente's (1984) transtheoretical model of change (TTM). Their model has been widely applied to analyze the process of change in alcoholism treatment and smoking cessation. DiClemente et al. (1991) identify five stages of change: pre-contemplation (not thinking about change), contemplation (aware of the need to change), preparation (intending to change in the near future and taking action in preparation for change), action (acting to change) and maintenance (of the new behaviour) (see Figure 7.6). Individuals are seen to progress through one stage to the next to eventually achieve successful maintenance. In the case of smoking cessation, it is argued that in the

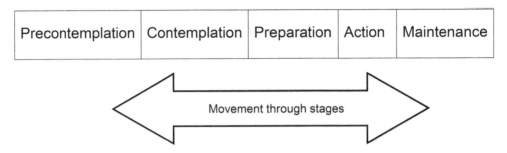

Figure 7.6 The transtheoretical model of change stage theory.

pre-contemplation stage the smoker is unaware that their behaviour constitutes a problem and has no intention to quit. In the contemplation stage, the smoker starts to think about changing their behaviour, but is not committed to try to quit. In the preparation stage, the smoker has an intention to quit and starts to make plans to quit. The action stage is characterized by active attempts to quit, and after six months of successful abstinence the individual moves into the maintenance stage. This stage is characterized by attempts to prevent relapse and to consolidate the newly acquired non-smoking status.

While the model is widely applied, the evidence in support of stage models and different stages is relatively weak (see Sutton, 2015). Sutton (2000) concludes that the distinctions between TTM stages are "logically flawed" and based on "arbitrary time periods". Moreover, even Prochaska and DiClemente's own data do not suggest that smokers typically progress through the TTM stages. For example, in one study, Prochaska et al. (1991) found that only 16% of participants progressed from one stage to the next without reversals over a two-year period and that 12% moved backwards during the same period! In addition, it has proved especially difficult to support the key prediction that there are different determinants of behaviour change in different stages. The best evidence for stage models would be where we showed that interventions matched to individuals' stage of change were more effective in producing behaviour change than interventions mismatched to an individual's stage (although see also Abraham, 2008). So, for example, in a matched intervention outcome expectancies might be targeted in individuals in the contemplation stage, while self-efficacy was targeted in individuals in the action stage, and this would be reversed in a mismatched intervention. Unfortunately, few such matched–mismatched studies have produced evidence supportive of stage models (see Littell & Girvin, 2002 for a systematic review of the effectiveness of interventions applying the TTM to health-related behaviours). Thus, at present, research findings do not support the added complexity and increased cost of stage-tailored interventions. West (2005) in reviewing stage models has suggested that work on the TTM should be abandoned.

It is difficult to usefully categorize people as "pre-contemplators" or those "in preparation" because people frequently cycle between such states as their motivation to change shifts. Nonetheless, an individual at a particular time may be more focused on deciding whether or not to act or on ensuring that they act on a prior decision to act (i.e. an intention). This is captured by the terms "motivational phase" and "volitional phase", respectively. This two-phase conception of action readiness suggests that health promoters need to think about how they can consolidate people's motivation to act and how they can help people to enact their intentions (see Chapters 8 and 9). In general, the social cognition models considered in this chapter have focused on the former. For example, the TPB does not help us distinguish between intenders who do and do not take action. Thus, there is a need to better theorize the processes which determine which intentions are translated into action. As Bagozzi (1993) argues, the variables outlined in the main social cognition models are necessary, but not sufficient, determinants of behaviour. In other words, they can provide good predictions of people's intentions (or motivation) to perform a health behaviour, but not always their actual behaviour. This area of research has been referred to as the "intention–behaviour gap".

The Health Action Process Approach (for a review see Schwarzer & Luszczynska, 2015) is one attempt to combine the ideas from traditional SCMs like the SCT with stage models. The HAPA (see Figure 7.7) makes the distinction between motivational and volitional phases of action (i.e. the process leading up to the formation of an intention and the process after that intention has been formed). The HAPA outlines three determinants of intention in the motivational phase: risk perception refers to the individual's perceived susceptibility to the health threat; outcome expectancies refer to the perceived consequences of a behaviour and are influential in the decision to change health behaviour; action (or task) self-efficacy refers to the individual's confidence in their ability to perform the behaviour, and is also proposed to have a direct effect on initial health behaviour, independent of intention. So, the HAPA would suggest that individuals with high-risk perceptions, who believe they are able to perform a behaviour with positive outcomes will have stronger intentions. Intention is the "watershed" between initial goal setting (i.e. motivational) phase and subsequent goal pursuit (i.e. volitional) phase. As noted earlier, strong intentions do not always ensure performance of a behaviour. The HAPA

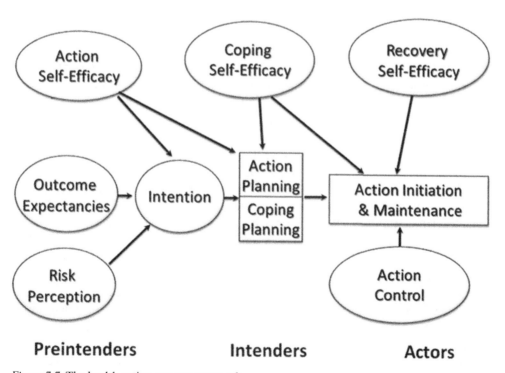

Figure 7.7 The health action process approach.

outlines a set of social cognitive variables important in the volitional phase of health behaviour: action and coping planning are important for turning intentions into behaviour. Action planning is the making of specific plans (e.g. implementation intentions) that help people enact their intentions (e.g. "If I have a gap between lectures, then I will go for a run"). Coping planning is the making of specific plans to overcome anticipated barriers that may hinder individuals from enacting their intentions (e.g. "If it is raining when I plan to go for a run, then I will go to the gym instead"). Maintenance (or coping) self-efficacy is the belief that one has the capability to cope with such barriers. Such coping is important in the volitional phase. The HAPA also outlines three components of action control important to the maintenance of behaviour: self-monitoring (i.e. monitoring ongoing levels of performance of the behaviour), awareness of standards (i.e. being aware of the desired level of performance) and self-regulatory effort (i.e. making effort to perform the behaviour as much as intended). In addition, recovery self-efficacy (i.e. perceptions that you have the capability to get back on track after a setback or lapse) is also influential in relation to maintenance of behaviour.

Zhang et al. (2019) provides a meta-analytic review of 96 HAPA studies showing strong effects for each of the components on behaviour. The HAPA has also been used as a basis for interventions to change health behaviour. For example, Rollo and Prapavessis (2020) reported a HAPA-based planning intervention to reduce sedentary behaviour in the workplace with significant effects on action planning, coping planning and action control plus behaviour.

FOCUS BOX 7.4

Deciding between social cognition models

Although a great deal of research has been devoted to testing individual social cognition models, little research has compared the relative predictive power of different SCMs. For example, Reid and Christensen (1988) found that while the HBM explained 10% of the variance in adherence among women taking tablets for urinary tract infections to a tablet regimen, the variance explained increased to 29% when cognitions specified by the theory of reasoned action were added.

Another approach to the variety of SCMs is to integrate them. This may be valuable, especially since many include similar cognitions. For example, commentators agree that the key cognitions prominently include intention, self-efficacy and outcome expectancies (or attitudes). An important attempt to integrate these models was made by Bandura (SCT), Becker (HBM), Fishbein (TRA), Kaufen (self-regulation) and Triandis (theory of interpersonal behaviour) as part of a workshop organized by the US National Institute of Mental Health in response to the need to promote HIV-preventive behaviours. The workshop sought to "identify a finite set of variables to be considered in any behavioral analysis" (Fishbein et al., 2001: 3). They identified eight variables which, they argued, should account for most of the variance in any (deliberative) behaviour. These were organized into two groups. First were those variables which were viewed as necessary and sufficient determinants of behaviour. Thus, for behaviour to occur an individual must: 1) have a strong intention; 2) have the necessary skills to perform the behaviour; and 3) experience an absence of environmental constraints that could prevent behaviour. The second group of variables were seen to primarily influence intention, although it was noted that some of the variables may also have a direct effect on behaviour. Thus, a strong intention is likely to occur when an individual: 4) perceives the advantages (or benefits) of performing the behaviour to out-weigh the perceived disadvantages (or costs); 5) perceives the social (normative) pressure to perform the behaviour to be greater than that not to perform the behaviour; 6) believes that the behaviour is consistent with his or her self-image; 7) anticipates the emotional reaction to performing the behaviour to be more positive than negative; and 8) has high levels of self-efficacy.

Figure 7.8 illustrates this integrated model.

If you were trying to identify the determinants of condom use, which cognitions would you focus on? Would this be any different if you were trying to predict smoking cessation?

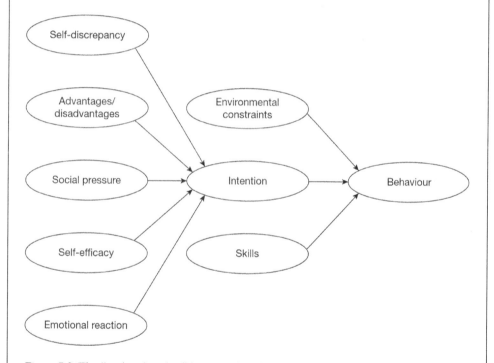

Figure 7.8 The "major theorists" integrated social cognition model.

Other models applied to health behaviours

The capability, opportunity, motivation–behaviour (or COM-B) "model" is a "summary" that integrates the insights from the various SCMs and the integrated model considered earlier, plus further insights those from other models (Michie & Wood, 2015). It's lack of specificity may be seen as a significant weakness and it is perhaps best viewed as a summary of influences rather than a model of health behaviours. Capability roughly maps on to self-efficacy seen in the PMT, SCT and TPB, while motivation maps on to behavioural intentions seen in the same three models. Opportunity is not found in these models but maps onto the absence of environmental constraints that could prevent behaviour seen in the integrated model. Each of the three "predictors" are seen as direct determinants of behaviour (see Figure 7.9). The COM-B has received some attention although it's value in relation to identifying targets for interventions to change behaviour needs to be clarified. It is interesting to note that the COM-B provides no explicit role for cognitive factors that are so prominent in other SCMs.

Other models have attempted to consider the cognitive influences on behaviour alongside other more automatic processes. The SCMs considered here can be characterised as focusing on the reflective influences on health behaviour. Dual process models suggest that alongside these reflective influences are non-reflective influences on behaviour. The Reflective-Impulsive Model (RIM; Strack & Deutsch, 2004) is one important dual process model. In the RIM, two separate but interacting systems are distinguished that together guide behaviour: a reflective and an impulsive system. The reflective system includes the reasoned, conscious and intentional Influences on behaviour and is represented by the SCMs we considered earlier. The impulsive (or automatic) system consists of associative clusters that have been created by temporal or spatial coactivation of external stimuli, affective reactions and associated behavioural tendencies. Once an association or link is established in the impulsive system then a simple perceptual input can automatically trigger an affective evaluation and associated behaviour. Sheeran et al. (2016) provide a useful review of these impulsive processes in relation to health behaviours. The relative power of reflective and implicit influences on health behaviours is an important area for research.

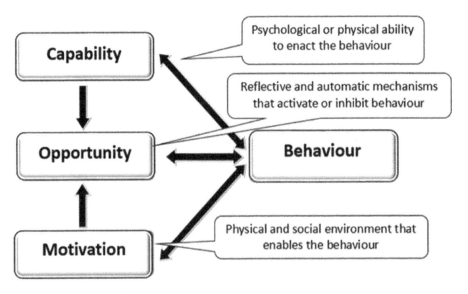

Figure 7.9 Capability opportunity motivation–behaviour model.

FOCUS BOX 7.6

COVID-19 protection behaviours: prediction and change

Over the last few years research attention has focused on trying to reduce the spread of COVID-19. One focus has been on behaviours that reduce the spread of the virus and also on bolstering COVID-19 vaccination uptake rates. Norman et al. (2020) used the RAA to predict compliance with a set of protection behaviours (limiting leaving home, keeping at least two metres away from other people when outside and when inside shops, not visiting or meeting friends or other family members, and washing hands when returning home). It was only capacity/self-efficacy that significantly predicted engaging in each of the behaviours. While Schüz et al. (2021) showed that the power of different components of the RAA to predict engaging in these COVID-19 protection behaviours varied between different demographic groups. In particular, intentions were weaker predictors and autonomy was a stronger predictor in more compared to less deprived groups. This would suggest the need for targeted interventions.

In relation to COVID-19 vaccination uptake, Norman et al. (2022) used an extended PMT to predict uptake in a UK sample. Protection motivation/intentions was the strongest predictor of uptake. While intentions were most strongly correlated with injunctive norms, maladaptive response rewards, and self-efficacy. Each of these factors might represent useful targets for interventions to change vaccination uptake through promoting intentions. In an experimental study, Capasso et al. (2021) showed that messages targeting cognitive attitudes and positive anticipated affective reactions (i.e. feeling pride) were associated with stronger intentions to get vaccinated against COVID-19 in an Italian sample.

A critical appraisal of SCMs

The use of SCMs to predict health behaviour has a number of advantages and disadvantages. Below we outline the main advantages of a social cognition approach before considering a range of specific and more general criticisms that have been made of this approach.

There are four clear advantages of using SCMs to predict and understand health behaviours. First, they provide a clear theoretical background to any research, guiding the selection of cognitions and providing a description of the ways in which these constructs combine in order to determine health behaviours. Second, because the models have been repeatedly tested, they provide reliable and valid measures of selected cognitions (for example, see Ajzen's website for guidance on developing TPB measures at www.people.umass.edu/aizen/tpb.html). Third, SCMs provide us with a description of the motivational and volitional processes underlying health behaviours. As a result, they add to our understanding of the proximal determinants of health behaviour and, because of this, they, fourth, identify key targets for interventions designed to change motivation (i.e. mechanisms of action; see Chapter 8).

The use of SCMs could also limit our understanding of health behaviour. For example, because SCMs provide clearly defined theoretical frameworks, their use may lead to the neglect of other cognitions. For example, moral norms (i.e. doing what you think is the right thing to do) are not included in the main SCMs but have been shown to be important in behaviours such as blood donation (Godin et al., 2005). Another limitation of SCMs is that while they usefully identify cognition change targets, they commonly do not specify the best means to change such cognitions. Moreover, an over-exclusive focus on SCMs may lead to the neglect of other potentially effective behaviour change interventions, such as increased taxation or legislation, which may not or may not have their effects through the cognitions specified by the SCMs (see Chapter 9).

In the health psychology area there has been one widely cited critique of SCMs written by Ogden (2003) with a response by Ajzen and Fishbein (2004) (see also Fishbein & Ajzen, 2010; Greve, 2001; Norman & Conner, 2015; Sniehotta et al., 2014 and associated commentaries). Ogden's (2003) critique is based on a review of 47 empirical studies published in four main health psychology journals over a four-year period and focuses on the HBM, PMT and TRA/TPB. Ogden raised four issues: use in developing interventions, interpretation of empirical testing, analytical versus synthetic truths and mere measurement. Ogden first concluded that SCMs were useful to researchers and ". . . to inform service development and the development of health-related interventions to promote health behaviors" (Ogden, 2003: 425). However, she also made three key criticisms. First, she argued that SCMs cannot be empirically tested, that is, confirmed or disconfirmed. She supported this point by pointing out that researchers do not conclude that they have disconfirmed SCMs when they find that one or more of the theory's constructs do not predict the outcome measure or that the findings do not explain all or most of the variance in intentions or behaviour. Ajzen and Fishbein (2004) highlight that the logic of this argument is unsound. For example, in the case of the TPB, numerous descriptions of the theory make clear that the extent to which each of the cognitions predicts intentions or behaviour is a function of the population and behaviour under study. For a specific behaviour and population one or more antecedents may indeed not be predictive, without disproving the theory. For example, social approval may be crucial to some health behaviours but not to others. Thus, finding that a particular cognition is not relevant to a particular behaviour does not disconfirm the theory. However, finding that none of the cognitions specified by the theory predicted useful proportions of the variance in intention or behaviour across behaviours would indeed disconfirm the theory. In fact, available evidence suggests that the theory is very useful, explaining on average 40–50% of the variance in intention and 21–36% of the variance in behaviour across studies (Conner & Sparks, 2005; McEachan et al., 2011).

Ogden also claimed that the theories contain only analytic truths (as opposed to synthetic or empirical truths that are based on evidence) because the correlations observed between measured cognitions are likely to be attributable to overlap in the way the constructs are measured. She claimed that this argument extends to measures of behaviour because these are often based on self-report. This interpretation of the literature has been disputed for two main reasons. First, it is not at all apparent that this explanation would account for the observed patterns of correlations among cognitions that are commonly reported in the literature. Second, high levels of prediction of behaviour are also found with objective measures of behaviour that do not rely on self-report and thus cannot be biased in the way Ogden describes. For example, Armitage and Conner (2001) in their meta-analysis of the TPB showed that intention and perceived behavioural control still accounted for an impressive 21% of variance in behaviour when behaviour was objectively measured across a number of studies (see also McEachan et al., 2011 who reviewed prospective tests of the TPB to a range of health behaviours using either self-reported or objectively measured behaviour).

This examination of the percentage of variance explained by SCMs has discouraged some health psychologists. For example, Mielewczyk and Willig (2007: 818–819) in reviewing this evidence conclude that 'the TPB is therefore unable to account for around 60% of the variance in intentions and for up to almost 80% of that in behaviour. Since the SCM approach is directed purely at providing explanations of variance in outcomes, the extent of that unexplained across such a large body of literature is highly damning'. This pessimism is unfounded for a number of reasons (see Abraham et al., 1998, for a useful discussion). First, as Sutton (1997) notes, the percentage of variance explained by any model, including physiological models of symptom appearance, is directly related to the reliability of the measures employed. The maximum variance that can be accounted for will always be the square root of the product of the two reliabilities. Thus, there are inherent measurement limitations on the percentage of variance that any model can explain. Second, when cognition and behaviour measures are not "compatible" (i.e. do not refer to the identical action, target, time and context), the R^2 will be reduced (Ajzen & Fishbein, 1980). Similarly, if the number of response options used to measure cognitions and behaviour is not equal (e.g. if attitude is measured on a seven-point scale and behaviour on a three-point scale), this will also reduce R^2. Finally, when sampling biases lead to a restricted range in either the independent (cognition) or the dependent (behaviour) variable compared to the actual range in the population (e.g. if the sample drink more alcohol than the sampled population) then the observed R^2 will underestimate the real cognition–behaviour relationship. Thus, it is methodologically unrealistic to expect predictive models to explain 100 per cent of the variance in measures of behaviour.

We would claim that explaining 21% of the variance in objectively measured behaviours is "impressive" (rather than "damning") because of the potential for behaviour change intervention that this figure represents. Rosenthal and Rubin (1982) translate percentages of explained variance into expected increases in outcome or success rates using their "binomial effect size display". This approach indicates that even when 19% of the variance in behaviour is explained we would expect an increase in that behaviour from 28% in a control group to 72% in an intervention group (who had adopted the cognitions that explained the 19%). This would indeed be an impressive finding for any evaluation of a behaviour change intervention (see Godin & Conner, 2008, for an examination of different indices of the intention–behaviour relationship for physical activity). Of course, changing the cognitions specified by the SCMs is a challenging endeavour (see Chapter 9) but the predictive success of SCMs strongly indicates that models such as the TPB can specify change targets that (if successfully changed) could make important differences to the prevalence of health behaviours in the population and, thereby, public health. Consequently, after reviewing available evidence, and providing guidance for behaviour change interventions in the UK National Health Service, the National Institute of Health and Clinical Excellence (2007: 10–11) noted that "a number of concepts drawn from the psychological literature are helpful when planning . . . behaviour change with individuals". This list included "positive attitude", "subjective norms", "descriptive norms", "personal and moral norms", "self-efficacy", "intention formation" and "concrete plans".

Finally, returning to Ogden's critique, she suggested that measuring such cognitions as the TPB suggests prompts their creation rather than simply recording pre-existing thoughts and perceptions. As Ajzen and Fishbein (2004) point out this is a common concern in questionnaire and interview studies. Recent research has in fact supported this concern. The effect has been referred to as the "Question-Behaviour Effect" meaning that measurement by itself prompts behaviour change. The strongest effects appear to be associated with the measurement of intentions. In Sherman's (1980) original demonstration of the effect, one group of participants was asked to predict how likely they would be to perform a socially desirable or socially undesirable behaviour (volunteering for the American Cancer Society or singing the Star-Spangled Banner down the phone, respectively) while a second group made no prediction about their behaviour. The results indicated that participants asked to predict their behaviour were more likely to perform the socially desirable behaviour (31% versus 4%) and were less likely to perform the undesirable behaviour (40% versus 68%) compared to control participants making no prediction. Recent research has shown that completing a TPB questionnaire about blood donation led to a 6–9% increase in attendance of blood donation 6–12 months later compared to groups who did not complete such a questionnaire (Godin et al., 2008). Other research has shown the question-behaviour effect can be used to change behaviours such as health screening attendance and influenza vaccination (Conner et al., 2011). Reviews of the question-behaviour effect indicate a significant but small effect on subsequent behaviour (Rodrigues et al., 2015; Wilding et al., 2016; Wood et al., 2015). However, rather than invalidating the use of SCMs, these findings point to the need for the use of more sophisticated designs to distinguish measurement and predictive effects, e.g. including conditions without baseline (time 1) questionnaires for comparative purposes. Moreover, the question-behaviour effect suggests that SCMs are indeed tapping psychological processes crucial to behaviour change.

The intention–behaviour gap

The intention–behaviour gap refers to the fact that intentions are far from perfect predictors of behaviour. In this section we review two areas of research exploring this gap. The first focuses on the stability of intentions across time while the second examines the volitional processes that might be important in determining whether intentions get translated into action.

Intention stability

In the vast majority of applications of SCMs the predictors of behaviour are measured by questionnaire (at time 1) and then behaviour is measured at a second time point, thereby employing a prospective survey method. One important requirement of such a design is that the measured constructs (e.g. attitudes) will remain unchanged between the measurement and the opportunity to act. So, for example, in using the TPB the assumption is that intentions to exercise will remain the same from when the (time 1) questionnaire is completed to the time points at which the respondent has the opportunity to engage in exercise. This is one of the limiting conditions of the TPB. However, cognitions including intentions may indeed change in this time period and such change provides one important explanation of the intention–behaviour gap. Several studies have now demonstrated that the intention–behaviour gap is indeed reduced for individuals with intentions that are more stable over time. For example, Conner, Norman and Bell (2002) found that intentions were stronger predictors of healthy eating over a period of six years when these intentions were stable over a six-month time period. These findings show that intention stability moderates the relationship between intention and behaviour.

A number of other factors have been found to influence the size of the intention–behaviour gap (see Conner & Norman, 2022 for a review). For example, anticipating feeling regret if one does not perform a behaviour or perceiving a strong moral norm (that is, believing that one is morally obliged to act) have both been found to significantly reduce the intention–behaviour gap (see Cooke & Sheeran, 2004 for a review). Like Conner et al. (2002), Sheeran and Abraham (2003) found that intention stability moderated the intention–behaviour relationship for exercising but, more importantly, found that intention stability mediated the effect of other moderators of the intention–behaviour relationship, including anticipated regret and intention certainty. This suggests that the mechanism by which a number of these other moderators may have their effect on intention–behaviour relationships is through changing the temporal stability of intentions. Hence, factors that might be expected to make individual intentions more stable over time would be expected to increase the impact that these intentions have on behaviour and so reduce the intention–behaviour gap.

Recent research has seen exploration of a number of other moderators of the intention–behaviour relationship. These have mainly focused on properties of intentions. For example, Conner et al. (2016) showed that when a behavioural intention was prioritized over other goals it was more predictive of behaviour. A subsequent study showed that getting participants to prioritize one or two health behaviours led to greater engagement with those behaviours without changing engagement in related health behaviours (Conner et al., 2022). Avisha et al. (2019) examined how realistic intentions were based on considerations of the expectations that the behaviour could be performed. Across a series of studies more realistic intentions were shown to be better predictors of engaging in different health behaviours. Future research could usefully explore the combined effects of these different moderators of the intention–behaviour relationship and the extent to which they all have their effects through changing the temporal stability of intentions.

FOCUS BOX 7.7

Impact of socioeconomic status on the intention–behaviour gap

A variety of studies have reported that as socioeconomic status increases engagement with health enhancing behaviours like exercise also increases while engagement with health risking behaviours like smoking decreases. This could be because of weaker intentions to engage in health enhancing and stronger intentions to engage in health risk behaviours in lower socioeconomic status groups, although there is little evidence to support this view. A more interesting possibility is that lack of available resources in lower socioeconomic status groups interferes with their ability to translate healthy Intentions into health behaviours (e.g. intending to exercise more or smoke less). This would be a moderating effect of socioeconomic status on the intention–behaviour relationship and would help explain the large intention–health behaviour gap in lower socioeconomic status groups. Conner et al. (2013) showed such a moderation effect for physical activity, breastfeeding and smoking initiation, in each case the intention–behaviour relationship was significantly weaker in the lower socioeconomic status group compared to the high socioeconomic status group. This finding would suggest that interventions targeting intentions in lower socioeconomic status groups need to be supplemented by interventions designed to tackle the problems have in enacting such intentions (e.g. by providing better access to exercise facilities). More recent research has shown similar effects for various health behaviours including COVID-19 protection behaviours (Schüz et al., 2021).

If you were trying to increase physical activity in lower socioeconomic status groups what strategies would you use to try to increase intentions to exercise and reduce the intention–behaviour gap?

Implementation intention formation

A variety of factors which affect the enactment of intentions have been investigated including personality traits, self-efficacy and planning. For example, we noted in Chapter 6 that conscientious individuals may possess skills that help them to enact their intentions (see Chapter 8 for more on self-efficacy and Chapter 9 for more on planning). However, another factor may relate to the nature of the intention formed.

Gollwitzer (1993) makes the distinction between goal intentions and implementation intentions. While the former is concerned with intentions to perform a behaviour or achieve a goal (i.e. "I intend to do x"), the latter is concerned with if-then plans which specify an environmental prompt or context that will determine when the action should be taken (i.e. "I intend to initiate the goal-directed behaviour x when situation y is encountered"). The important point about implementation intentions is that they commit the individual to a specific course of action when certain environmental conditions are met. Prestwich et al. (2015) note that to form an implementation intention, the person must first identify a response that will lead to goal attainment and, second, anticipate a suitable occasion to initiate that response. For example, the person might specify the behaviour "go jogging for 20 minutes" and specify a suitable opportunity "tomorrow morning before work". Gollwitzer (1993) argues that, by making implementation intentions, individuals pass control of intention enactment to the environment. The specified environmental cue prompts the action so that the person does not have to remember or decide when to act.

Prestwich et al. (2015) provide an in-depth review of both basic and applied research with implementation intentions. For example, Milne, Orbell and Sheeran (2002) found that an intervention using persuasive text based on protection motivation theory prompted positive pro-exercise cognition change but did not increase exercise. However, when this intervention was combined with encouragement to form implementation intentions, behaviour change was observed (see Gollwitzer & Sheeran, 2006, for a meta-analysis of such studies; Prestwich et al., 2015 for a review of the use of implementation intentions to change health behaviours). Thus, implementation intention formation moderates the intention–behaviour relationship demonstrating that two people with equally strong goal intentions may differ in their volitional readiness depending on whether they have taken the additional step of forming an implementation intention. Implementation intention formation has been shown to increase the performance of a range of behaviours with, on average, a medium effect size. Implementation intentions appear to be particularly effective in overcoming a common problem in enacting intentions, that is, forgetting. Provided effective cues are identified in the implementation intention (i.e. ones that will be commonly encountered and are sufficiently distinctive), forgetting appears to be much less likely. Implementation intentions also appear to help individuals resist negative health behaviours (e.g. smoking initiation in adolescents, Conner & Higgins, 2010; Conner et al., 2019) and recent research has suggested that pairs of individuals can form joint implementation intentions that can be particularly effective (referred to as collaborative implementation intentions, Prestwich et al., 2012).

Summary

There is considerable variation in who performs health behaviours. Demographic differences explain part of this variation, although such factors are not easily modifiable. Various modifiable cognitions have been identified which explain differences in who performs health behaviours. Key cognitions include intentions, self-efficacy and outcome expectancies (or attitudes). Cognitions have been incorporated in a number of social cognition models (SCMs) that describe the key cognitions and how they are interrelated in the determination of behaviour. The most important SCMs include the health belief model, protection motivation theory, theory of reasoned action/theory of planned behaviour/reasoned action approach and social cognitive theory. These models focus on the cognitive antecedents of motivation. Stage models attempt to describe the process of behaviour change from first consideration to maintenance of change but there is limited evidence to suggest that people remain in stable stages of action readiness over time. While SCMs have a number of advantages, criticisms of SCMs suggest the need for further sophistication in the testing of such models. SCMs are limited in their capacity to explain why some intentions are translated into behaviour while others are not. Various factors explaining this intention–behaviour gap have been explored and the important role of the temporal stability of intentions has been identified. Research has also investigated volitional processes which facilitate the enactment of intentions. Implementation intentions, that is, if-then plans situating an intended action in a specific context, have been shown to reduce the intention–behaviour gap.

Key concepts and terms

- Critique of SCMs
- Health behaviours
- Health belief models
- Implementation intentions
- Intention–behaviour gap
- Mere measurement
- Protection motivation theory
- Self-regulation
- Social cognition models (SCMs)
- Social cognitive theory
- Stage models
- Theory of planned behaviour
- Transtheoretical model of change

Sample essay titles

- Critically evaluate the use of social cognition models in understanding health behaviours.
- Compare and contrast the health belief model and the theory of planned behaviour as explanations of why people do and do not perform a range of health behaviours.
- What do we know about the antecedents of intention? Discuss with reference to available empirical evidence.

Further reading

Book chapters

Abraham, C., Norman, P., & Conner, M. (2000). Towards a psychology of health-related behaviour change. In: P. Norman, C. Abraham, & M. Conner (Eds.), *Understanding and changing health behaviour: From health beliefs to self-regulation.* (pp. 343–369). Switzerland: Harwood Academic.

Conner, M., & Norman, P. (2015). Predicting and changing health behaviour: A social cognition approach. In M. Conner & P. Norman (Eds.), *Predicting and changing health behaviour: Research and practice with social cognition models* (3rd Edn.; pp. 1–29). Maidenhead: Open University Press.

Norman, P., & Conner, M. (2015). Predicting and changing health behaviour: Future directions. In M. Conner & P. Norman (Eds.), *Predicting and changing health behaviour: Research and practice with social cognition models* (3rd Edn.; pp. 391–430). Maidenhead: Open University Press.

Journal articles

Ajzen, I. (2015). The theory of planned behaviour is alive and well, and not ready to retire: A commentary on Sniehotta, Presseau, and Araújo-Soares. *Health Psychology Review, 9*(2), 131–137. https://doi.org/10.1080/17437199.2014.883474

Ajzen, I., & Fishbein, M. (2004). Questions raised by a reasoned action approach: Reply on Ogden (2003). *Health Psychology, 23,* 431–434. https://doi.org/10.1037/0278-6133.23.4.431

Ogden, J. (2003). Some problems with social cognition models: A pragmatic and conceptual analysis. *Health Psychology, 22,* 424–428. https://doi.org/10.1037/0278-6133.22.4.424

Sheeran, P., Klein, W.M.P., & Rothman, A.J. (2017). Health behavior change: Moving from observation to intervention. *Annual Review of Psychology, 68,* 573–600. https://doi.org/10.1146/annurev-psych-010416-044007

Sniehotta, F.F., Presseau, J., & Araujo-Soares, V. (2014). Time to retire the theory of planned behaviour. *Health Psychology Review, 8,* 1–7. https://doi.org/10.1080/17437199.2013.869710

8 Changing cognitions to establish motivation

Changing cognitions to establish motivation

In Chapter 7 we discussed cognitions (such as beliefs, attitudes and intentions) that distinguish between people who do, and do not, follow health advice. Measuring cognitions can allow us to *predict* behaviour. In this chapter we focus on interventions designed to *change* the cognitions that underpin and bolster motivation and, thereby, help people change their health-related behaviour patterns.

Chapter plan

Learning about a health risk can change people's attitudes, intentions and actions. Therefore, provision of accessible and easily understood *information* is critical to health promotion. Information is evaluated by the receiver. When information is understood, but judged to be (i) mistaken, (ii) personally irrelevant or (iii) implying action that is difficult or costly, it may be ignored. Health promoters need to *persuade* individuals and groups to take action that protects health. Successful persuasion depends on anticipating how recipients will perceive and respond to persuasive attempts. Successful persuasion is likely to result in *attitude change* and, as we saw in Chapter 7, attitudes provide an important foundation for motivation to change behaviour patterns. When people feel they *cannot* make a change they are unlikely to pursue it. Consequently, communicating the possibility of behavioural control and high self-efficacy, is crucial to prompting sustainable motivation and the translation of intentions into action. Persuasion depends on presenting people with convincing and attention-getting arguments suggesting that do-able actions that will lead to attainable, valued outcomes. In this chapter, we will consider how motivation can be bolstered and changed.

This chapter is divided into in five sections.

1. Providing information.
2. Persuading others.
3. Changing attitudes.
4. Enhancing self-efficacy.
5. From motivation to behaviour change in healthcare delivery

DOI: 10.4324/9781003171096-12

Learning outcomes

When you have completed this chapter you should be able to:

1. Describe how information and advice should be presented to maximise its impact on health-related motivation and action.
2. Explain why trust in workplace management is important to healthcare professionals' motivation and optimal performance.
3. Discuss why credibility and consistency are crucial to public health messaging.
4. Explain how social influence techniques can be applied to optimise the impact of health promotion on recipients' motivation, in mass media, one-to-one and group communication.
5. Explain how the manner in which messages are processed (that is, the degree of cognitive elaboration) determines which message features have most impact on attitude change.
6. Illustrate the importance of self-efficacy to motivation, health behaviour and explain how self-efficacy can be enhanced.
7. Integrate your understanding of persuasion and motivation to provide evidence-based advice on how health promoters can maximise health-protective attitude and behaviour change.

Providing information

Credibility and trust

When people are informed of a health risk by a trusted source and believe they can easily protect themselves from the risk, they are likely to take protective action. For example, media coverage about food scares such as Bovine Spongiform Encephalopathy (BSE) lead to widespread changes in behaviour, including beef purchase (e.g. Tyler, 2001). Inaccurate information can also promote behaviour change. For example, when, in 1998, a highly regarded medical journal (The *Lancet*) published an article linking the measles, mumps and rubella vaccine (MMR) with autism and inflammatory bowel disease, MMR vaccination uptake fell and cases of measles increased. Although, the validity of the research was subsequently denounced by the journal's editor, the majority of the authors and the UK prime minister! (see *The Guardian*, Tuesday February 24, 2004) it proved difficult to rebuild public confidence in the safety of MMR. Further research found no immunological response differences in children with and without autism (Baird et al., 2008) but four years later vaccination uptake levels remained lower than the optimal 95% level. This example emphasises the power of a credible, or believable, source. When scientists and government ministers provide flawed scientific explanations, it can be difficult to restore trust in scientific findings.

Similarly when supposedly trustworthy sources provide contradictory information or when advice is thought to serve the interests of the source such as profit-making companies or ambitious politicians, information may not be believed. People may interpret phrases such as, "there is no cause for concern", as, "there must be a problem". Or "this is dangerous" to mean "just more state interference". There is an ethical imperative for health professionals, scientists and governments to check that information available to the public is accurate and not, in any way, misleading. In addition, there is a need to ensure that information is accurate and evidence-based to maintain ongoing credibility. By ensuring that messaging is consistent and evidence-based we can minimise trust breakdowns. This would have been helpful during the COVID-19 pandemic but, unfortunately, important evidence-based advice was often swamped by conflicting advice by leaders and experts (Nagler et al., 2020).

Source credibility may also be enhanced by presenting two-sided arguments. Presenting the disadvantages as well as the advantages of a product or recommended action has been found to be more persuasive because two-sided presentations increase the perceived credibility of the source (e.g. Crowley & Hoyer, 1994; Eisend, 2006). This may be especially true for skeptical audiences. Two-sided arguments may also increase the perceived novelty of the message which, in turn, enhances attention and interest and so may promote positive attitude change (Eisend, 2007). Thus, being open about the costs or side effects of a recommended action may be more effective in changing attitudes and intentions because the audience is more likely to believe that the highlighted benefits are real.

Communication credibility and trust is also critical to the effective management of health services. Okello and Gilson (2015) conducted a systematic review of how trusting workplace relationships influenced motivation among healthcare professionals. These researchers concluded that trusting workplace relationships encourage social interactions and cooperation among professionals and enhance their intrinsic motivation to perform well in everyday work. Importantly, the provision of good quality care for patients seems to be improved by workplace relationships that are supportive and respectful. By contrast, poor interpersonal workplace relationships and distrust in workplace management have the opposite effects, reducing health professionals' performance and their quality of care for clients or patients. These findings have critical implications for managerial style. To promote excellent healthcare services, we need to ensure that healthcare managers are credible and trustworthy sources of information and guidance.

Similarly, in health promotion, we need to persuade members of the public that health experts and political leaders are credible and trustworthy. When this fails, as when political leaders downplayed the health threats of COVID-19, this undermines evidence-based health promotion. Interestingly, endorsement of misinformation about COVID-19 was greatest among those who relied on the internet for information and had high trust in information found on social media (Filkuková, Ayton, Rand & Langguth, 2021). This emphasises the need to create consistent, credible, trustworthy, evidence-based sources of health information that can be contrasted with the misinformation people may find on social media. You may remember Diogenes's wall (see Chapter 1). What is the equivalent in our media-rich societies? How can we provide trustworthy evidence-based information to help people maintain and protect their health?

Making information accessible and easy to understand

Information can only change motivation and behaviour if people can access it and understand it. So, providing accurate information in the right place for the target audience is crucial. Information providers need to know where and when the target audience will seek information before designing an information campaign. Will the target audience seek information online or from an information leaflet? When will the information be relevant, for example, before taking a new medication? Preliminary research with the target audience can answer such questions and so guide effective information provision. Such research is sometimes called *elicitation research* (see Chapter 9).

Information providers must also ensure that what they say is easily understood. For example, if patient information leaflets provided with medications are written in tiny writing and include technical terms patients do not understand then they are not likely to be read or to enhance adherence. Ease of comprehension is partly determined by what the recipient already knows. If you want to give someone good directions (e.g. in a city) you need to understand what landmarks they already know. Yet evidence suggests that health professionals often overestimate patients' knowledge and, therefore, their ability to understand health-related information. For example, Hadlow and Pitts (1991) found that while the vast majority of doctors were able to select correct clinical definitions of conditions such as stroke, eating disorder and depression only 18%, 30% and 32% of patients were able to do so, respectively. We need simple explanations of medical (and unfamiliar terms) in information designed for the general population.

Text can be more or less difficult to read depending on the words used. The level of reading difficulty can be assessed using a variety of measures. For example, the Flesch Reading Ease (FRE; Flesch, 1948) measures the average number of syllables in words used and the average sentence length. A score between zero and 100 is generated with higher scores denoting easier texts. Text with higher scores is also easier for readers to scan before they read in detail and this may be especially important for online texts. A score of 67–70 is acceptable for literate adults but even higher scores can be achieved. Media professionals regularly edit text to achieve good readability. For example, the most popular newspaper in the UK is said to have a reading age of nine.

Considerable effort is required to ensure that health information is readable by the vast majority of the population. For example, a survey of more than 1,000 leaflets provided by palliative care units in the United Kingdom and Ireland (Payne, Large, Jarrett & Turner, 2000) found that 47% were printed in less than font 12 and that two thirds had poor readability scores as assessed by the FRE, implying that they would only be understood by 40% of the UK population. More recently, the National Health Service in the UK concluded that content on their websites required a reading age of 16 and that 80% of UK adults were not reading at this level (Robinson & Savic, 2019). The NHS now recommends that its websites should be readable by the average 9–11-year-old and both the NHS and National Institutes for Health in the USA have provided guidance on presenting readable online information. By implementing such guidance, we can help people find easy-to-understand and persuasive information. For example, the NHS provide examples on how to rewrite advice so that is more accessible to most people (Robinson & Savic, 2019). No matter how information is presented, whether on websites, in leaflets or in text messages, it is critical that the message is easy to understand by the audience it is intended for.

Providing wanted information

Health professionals tend to underestimate patients' desire for information. Even when facing bad news and potential terminal diagnoses, evidence indicates that patients want to know as much as possible (e.g., Jenkins, Fallowfield & Saul, 2001) – but what do they want to know? Coulter, Entwistle, and Gilbert (1999) reviewed 54 sources of information, including information leaflets and listened to patients in focus groups to discover what kind information patients wanted. Results showed the sources of health information reviewed often did not provide the information wanted by patients. These researchers generated a list of 22 questions that patients commonly want answered (reproduced in Activity Box 8.1) and recommended that that patient information resources be written and revised to ensure that they answer these questions.

ACTIVITY BOX 8.1

What do patients want to know?

Coulter, Entwistle, & Gilbert (1999) suggest that patients typically want answers to the following questions:

What is causing the problem?
Am I alone? How does my experience compare with that of other patients?
Is there anything I can do myself to ameliorate the problem?
What is the purpose of the tests and investigations?
What are the different treatment options?
What are the benefits of the treatment(s)?
What are the risks of the treatment(s)?
Is it essential to have treatment for this problem?
Will the treatment(s) relieve the symptoms?
How long will it take to recover?
What are the possible side effects?
What effect will the treatment(s) have on my feelings and emotions?
What effect will the treatment(s) have on my sex life?
How will it affect my risk of disease in the future?
How can I prepare myself for the treatment?
What procedures will be followed if I go to hospital?
When can I go home?
What do my carers need to know?
What can I do to speed recovery?
What are the options for rehabilitation?
How can I prevent recurrence or future illness?
Where can I get more information about the problem or treatments?

Examine the UK NHS website (https://www.nhs.uk/). Do you think this website provides the answers to patient questions identified by Coulter et al. (1999). For example, have a look at the section on diabetes. How readable is the website? Do you have ideas for improving this website? You can send your feedback to the NHS!

Organising information

We have noted that to be persuasive information needs to be (i) easy-to-understand, (ii) wanted by the target audience and (iii) presented in the right context, by (iv) trustworthy sources.

In addition information providers can make information easier to understand and use by *organising it in a manner that is easy to process*. Providing information in a logical order facilitates processing. For example, clarifying the cause of an illness before explaining how a treatment works can help a patient understand why the treatment is necessary or why it should be administered as recommended. Telling the audience what you are about to tell them can also enhance recall. This foreshadowing technique is often referred to as "explicit categorisation". For example, a nurse might say "First, I am going to tell you what I think is wrong. . . . now I'm going to tell you about the treatment. . . . etc." Highlighting and repeating important points also helps people pay particular attention to them ("this is important so I'm going to say it again . . ."). Finally, when giving advice, it is important to be specific, e.g. "you need to lose 5 kilograms" is much easier to interpret than, "you need to lose weight". In foundational research, Ley et al. (1976) wrote a manual for GPs explaining these simple techniques and assessed patient recall for information provided in consultations with four GPs before and after they read the manual. Results showed that recall increased from 52–59% across the four doctors at baseline to 6–80% after the GPs had read the manual. These five simple presentation techniques (logical order, explicit categorisation, specific advice, emphasising and repeating important points) make information easier to process and recall.

Visual aids can make written materials easier to understand. For example, an experiment conducted by Kools, van de Wiel, Ruiter, Crüts and Kok (2006) showed that participants who read text describing asthma care extracted from a health promotion leaflet had poorer comprehension of the text than participants who read the same text modified by the addition of *graphic organisers* (including the one in Figure 8.1). Pre-testing of such materials is important to ensure that they are appropriate for the target audience.

The way in which risk information is presented determines how it affects motivation and action. For example, as we shall see in Chapter 10, risk information can be more or

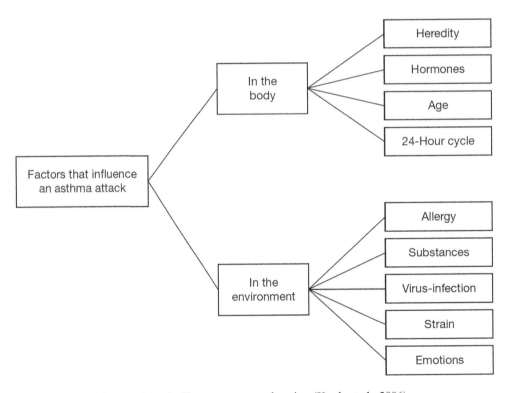

Figure 8.1 Graphic organisers facilitate text comprehension (Kools et al., 2006)

persuasive depending on whether it is framed in terms of gains or losses (even when the same information is included).

Information knowledge and motivation

Unfortunately, information is often not enough to change behaviour because even those who understand and have a good knowledge of the consequences of their actions fail to follow advice. Why? Can you think of a health-related behaviour that you know you should change? Why have you not changed it?

Using meta-analysis (see Research Methods Box 8.2), Sheeran, Abraham and Orbell (1999) examined psychosocial factors (see Chapter 7) associated with heterosexual condom use in 121 empirical studies. Effect sizes for 44 separate correlates of condom use could be calculated. These analyses revealed an average weighted correlation of 0.06 (a small effect size) for the relationship between knowledge and reported condom use. Thus, increasing knowledge by itself is unlikely to be enough to promote condom use. By contrast, the average weighted correlations for attitude towards condom use (0.32), others' approval of use (0.37) and intention to use (0.43) were of medium effect size. These findings indicate that changing perceived social approval and attitudes towards condoms is much more likely to impact on heterosexual condom use, than changing knowledge. Sheeran et al. concluded that these results "provide empirical support for conceptualising condom use in terms of . . . an extended theory of reasoned action" (p. 126), and argued that these correlates specify important targets for safer sex promotion. A similar meta-analysis of studies applying the theories of reasoned action and planned behaviour (see Chapter 7) to condom use confirmed the utility of these theories as models of cognitive antecedents of condom use (Albarracín, Johnson, Fishbein & Muellerleile, 2001). Thus, for many behaviours, changing key cognitive antecedents of motivation is a critical first step towards behaviour change. This is unlikely to be achieved by providing information alone. Nonetheless accurate information is critical to consideration of change. Information is prerequisite but not enough to ensure persuasion.

RESEARCH METHODS BOX 8.1

Meta analysis

Meta analysis allows researchers to examine the average size of associations (or differences) between two measures or conditions across a series of studies. When combining effect sizes (e.g. the size of an association between two measures) across studies it is important to weight studies for the number of participants because a finding based on 100 participants is likely to be more reliable than one based on 10. For example, if a correlation study found that knowledge and behaviour were correlated at $r = .05$ amongst a sample of 100 people and another study found the correlation to be $r = .07$ amongst a similar sample of 100 people then the average weighted correlation ($r+$) would be 0.06, across these two studies. However, if the second study had only recruited a sample of 50 then $r+$ would be 0.0425. In this way, meta-analyses allow researchers to combine results across studies to calculate average "effect sizes". Cohen (1992) has provided guidelines for interpreting the size of sample-weighted average correlations ($r+$) suggesting that $r+ = .10$ is "small", $r+ = .30$ is "medium", while $r+ = .50$ is "large".

Meta analyses can be also used to estimate the average impact that behaviour change interventions (see Chapter 9) have on a particular outcome (such as physical activity levels). In this case, the most usual measure is d (rather than r). d is calculated by subtracting the behavioural outcome score of one condition from another and dividing this by the standard pooled deviation, that is, the standard deviation for both conditions combined (Hedges & Olkin, 1985). For example, if, at follow up, those who had received an intervention were found to exercise three times a week on average while those in a no-intervention control group exercised only 1.5 times a week on average, and there was an overall standard deviation of 1.5 this would generate a d value of 1.0. Cohen (1992) suggests that ds of 0.2 are "small" while ds of 0.5 are of "medium" size and ds of 0.8 are "large" effect sizes. Thus, this would be a large and impressive effect size. This is not surprising because in this example, the intervention doubled the rate of the target behaviour compared to the control group – indicating an unusually successful intervention.

Persuading others

How can we overcome resistance to change? How can health professionals move from providing information to persuading people to look after their health. Persuasion is social influence (a person or group influencing another) and there is a considerable body of research on how social influence works. For example, Cialdini and Sagarin (2005) discuss key characteristics of influence, including reciprocity (offering something of value), social validation (showing that the messages are supported by others who matter to the audience), consistency (not contradicting oneself), liking (ensuring that the audience likes the source) and authority (showing that the source is well informed). Pratkanis (2007) extended this list to include 107 potentially effective social influence tactics, including, being a credible source, being empathetic, using flattery, agenda setting, using metaphor, story-telling, fear appeals and making people feel guilty. Here we will consider some key principles that need to be followed when trying to motivate someone to change their behaviour.

Message framing

Prospect theory (Tversky & Kahneman, 1981) predicts that people process information differently depending on whether it relates to losses (or costs) or gains (or benefits). Specifically, people tend to be "risk averse", that is, they want to avoid risk, when thinking about gains but, when thinking about potential losses, people tend to be open to taking risks, or risk seeking. Consequently, a behaviour which is not associated with risk may seem more attractive when thinking about gains (because we want to avoid risk when thinking about gains) while a behaviour which is perceived to be risky may be more attractive when people are thinking about losses or costs (when people favour risk). Preventive behaviours including condom or sunscreen serve to reduce the risk of ill health and so tend to be perceived as low risk. By contrast, detection behaviours such as breast or testicular self-examination are thought to be high risk because, despite the potential long-term benefits, there is an immediate risk of discovering a worrying problem. It has been predicted, therefore, that health promotion information about preventive behaviours will be most effective when it focuses upon potential gains while health promotion information about detection behaviours will be most effective when it focuses upon potential losses or costs (see Rothman & Salovey, 1997). There is some evidence to support this. For example, Detweiler, Bedell, Salovey, Pronin and Rothman (1999) presented messages to beachgoers that either emphasised gains associated with sunscreen use (e.g. "If you use sunscreen with SPF 15 or higher, you increase your chances of keeping your skin healthy and your life long") or losses associated with not using sunscreen (e.g., "If you don't use sunscreen with SPF 15 or higher, you decrease your chances of keeping your skin healthy and your life long). They found that those who read the gain-focused messages were more likely to redeem a coupon to collect sunscreen. Moreover, this (gain-focused) group were more likely to intend to use sunscreen with a sun protection factor of 15 and to apply it repeatedly.

However, framing effects do not always produce the desired effects on motivation and behaviour. One of the main reasons is that not all preventive behaviours are perceived as low risk and not all detection behaviours are perceived as high risk. For example, consider parents' decisions to have their children vaccinated against measles, mumps and rubella using the combined MMR injection. It is likely that following the publication of the (refuted) report linking MMR vaccination with autism and inflammatory bowel disease parents' perceived this preventive behaviour as high risk and therefore, might be more likely to respond to loss-focused messages rather than gain-focused messages. Abhyankar, O'Connor and Lawton (2008) tested this hypothesis and found, as predicted, a loss framed message (e.g. "By not vaccinating your child against mumps, measles and rubella, you will fail to protect your child against contracting these diseases") was more effective in increasing women's MMR vaccination intentions than a gain-focused message (e.g., "By vaccinating your child against mumps, measles and rubella, you will be able to protect your child against contracting these diseases"). Similarly, when a detection behaviour is perceived and leading to a safe or certain outcome, then a gain-focused message is likely to be most effective. A study by Apanovitch, McCarthy and Salovey (2003) found that women who felt safe about the outcome of a HIV test, because they considered themselves to be at no risk were more likely to report having the test six months after watching a gain-focused video message compared to those who watched a loss-focused message.

Other factors influence the extent to which messages are processed. For example, the degree to which an individual is involved with, or interested in, an issue influences the effectiveness of gain and loss-focused messages. Rothman, Salovey, Antone, Keough and Martin (1993) found that framed messages only worked as expected for people who were concerned with the target health behaviour (e.g. skin cancer detection). The extent to which a person holds a positive or negative attitude towards to the target health behaviour (see Chapter 7) is also important. In a study of intentions to use hormonal male contraception, O'Connor, Ferguson and O'Connor (2005), found that the hypothesised framing effects were only observed in men with a positive attitude towards the behaviour. Thus personal involvement and positive attitudes facilitate framing effects and thereby moderate the relationship between framing and motivation.

Framing information and advice in terms of benefits or gains is important to persuasion and how any recommended action is perceived. For example, low risk behaviours may be more likely to be prompted by emphasising gains. There are, however, no universal rules. Framing effects should be pre-tested on the target audiences before materials are produced. This should show the way health threats are described, including metaphors used. For example, should a health threat be conceptualised as an enemy with whom we are at war, a monster to be defeated or a natural disaster (Wicke & Bolognesi, 2020)? Again this emphasises the importance of elicitation research (see Chapter 9).

Social influence: personal motives and principles

People want accurate information about reality. When we see other people looking behind us, we sensibly turn around to see what's there. This type of influence has been referred to as *informational influence* (Deutsch & Gerard, 1955) and is one source of expert power (French & Raven, 1960). If we believe someone else is better informed and better able to predict what will happen then they have the potential to exert informational influence over us. For example, we might be influenced by a nurse's advice.

We also want to have good relationships with others (sometimes referred to as the *affiliation motive*). This is an important foundation of our feelings of self-worth, or self-esteem, so these motivations combine to facilitate *normative influence*. For example, we are reluctant to lose friends' approval so may be are willing to do what they want rather than following our own preferences. In doing so we are subject to normative influence.

Research supports a series of principles concerning social influence processes. First, as we have seen, ensuring that the message source is perceived to be *credible and expert* enhances persuasive impact. Our perception of a message source also depends on *how we categorise ourselves* in relation to the source (whether this is an individual or group). People seen as similar to ourselves or belonging to the same group are more likely to be liked, viewed positively and able to validate our experiences (Turner, 1991). Therefore, these people have a greater potential to exert normative influence. Consequently, it has been proposed that peers (people belonging to the target audience) are the most persuasive communicators. However, evidence indicates that this is only true if these communicators are also seen to be experts. Those perceived to be expert and whose beliefs, gender and ethnicity match ours may be most persuasive (Durantini, Albarracín, Earl & Gillette, 2006).

Cognitive dissonance theory (Festinger, 1957) proposes that we are motivated to maintain a consistent view of the world because cognitive inconsistency creates dissonance which is inherently unpleasant. Consequently, when the opinions of others or persuasive messages appear consistent with what we already believe, they are more likely to be persuasive. So, *consistency*, that is, ensuring that a health message does not contradict existing beliefs, commitments or obligations (and thereby generate cognitive dissonance) is an important feature of persuasive communication. Therefore, starting with what we know others will agree with is a good approach.

A third related principle is the perception of *consensus*. If a proposed change is supported by or adopted by others, we are more likely to want to join in. So believing that others are performing an action that we are considering (that is holding a positive descriptive norm – Rivis & Sheeran, 2003 – see Chapter 7) is likely to facilitate persuasion and bolster motivation. This may be even more persuasive if we categorise ourselves as belonging to the same group as those adopting the change (e.g. "other people like you have already adopted this behaviour") because such identification is likely to enhance the self-worth impact of the message. Thus, informational influence (and to some extent normative influence) can be strengthened by three key features of persuasive messages: (1) source credibility and expertise; (2) perceived consistency with current world view; and (3) perceived consensus/ identification.

People we like and identify with can exert greater normative influence over us. Thus, persuasion is more likely when the source is seen as enjoying a *good relationship or good image* with the target audience. This emphasises the importance of good social and communication skills among professionals involved in face-to-face health-promotion activities and of enhancing the brand value of organisations offering health advice such as the National Health Service in the UK. We tend to like those who offer us things of value so people are more open to social influence from those who have provided something for them. Therefore, *reciprocation*, through offering services or products that are seen as valuable may be a useful way of encouraging a target group to listen to health-related advice. In addition, we value approval so believing that those who are important to us approve of a particular course of action (i.e. holding a positive subjective norm, see Chapter 7) is likely to facilitate persuasion and affect motivation. Thus, normative influence can be strengthened by three key features of persuasive messages: positive relationships, reciprocation and the approval of valued others.

Persuasion in groups

Both informational and normative influence are important in group dynamics. Persuasion within groups differs depending on whether it is persuasion by the majority (more than half the group), called conformity (Asch, 1952) or conversion to a minority view or action. Majority influence or *conformity* is strengthened by consensus. A large and consistent majority exerts considerable informational and normative influence. By contrast, a minority challenges our usual assumptions and leads us to evaluate the contrast between majority and minority views (Moscovici, 1976; Moscovici & Lage, 1976). *Conversion* to a minority view does not work through consensus influence and is determined instead by what minority members do. If members of a minority group are seen to be consistent, committed, confident and fair they can prompt others to think carefully about their alternative position. This systematic consideration and evaluation of the minority view means that, when minorities are persuasive, the belief and attitude changes resulting from conversion is likely to be longer-lasting and less subject to counter persuasion than conformity influence (Martin, Hewstone & Martin, 2007).

Persuasion and influence in groups has important applied implications because group discussions are regularly used by researchers and health services. Discussions in focus groups and so-called "citizen's juries" are regularly used to discover what people want and the results used to draw conclusions about public opinion and popular policy development. One problem associated with this methodology is that the way in which groups are managed and facilitated may affect what people say. For example, the questions posed and choices offered shape responses. Moreover, powerful majorities or confident and committed minorities may limit the number of viewpoints considered through conformity and conversion. This raises the questions of whether focus groups are a good way to sample beliefs (e.g. in elicitation research) and how they should be run to ensure that what group members say expresses what they believe.

Groups can be very supportive and influential for those managing long-term illnesses, such as diabetes. The group experience can offer social validation ("yes that's exactly how I feel") and expert advice from others who have similar experiences (Borek et al., 2019a). Sharing experiences and problems with others who are seen to have high credibility because they are dealing with the same challenges builds trust. In trusting relationships, advice and feedback is more likely to be considered carefully, and processed using the central route (see below). Consequently, communication in peer groups can change beliefs and attitudes, influence and behaviour patterns, including optimising self-care (see Borek et al., 2019a for a review and framework of factors that determine how effective such groups are). We return to the role of groups in changing behaviour in Chapters 9 and 10.

Obedience and informed decision making

We have seen how important the source of a message is to persuasion. Holding legitimate authority is an especially powerful attribute in relation to social influence. When people occupy a role in which they accept that another person has the right to make decisions about what they do, they are more easily persuaded. This was powerfully demonstrated in Milgram's (1974) experiments in which he showed that people would deliver (what they thought were) electric shocks to others to a much greater extent than was predicted, so long as they accepted the experimenter (ordering the shocks) as a legitimate authority figure. Following this work, Rank and Jacobson (1977) investigated nurses' obedience to an apparent order from a medical doctor to administer a drug in a too large a dose, so apparently giving the patient a drug overdose. The research demonstrated that nurses were less likely to obey the mistaken order if they were familiar with the drug and had time to confer with other nurses. This emphasises a more general point relevant to all those involved in healthcare decisions, namely, being well informed and having time to confer prior to decisions is likely to minimise mistakes. This also emphasises the importance of trusting relationships at work.

Overcoming resistance to change

Persuasion is important because people may not want to change even when change will bring benefits. Persuasion can be challenging when people do not want to change, in part because we do not like being told what to do! We can view persuasive communications as threatening or unbelievable and we feel that it is too difficult to change everyday routines in the face of competing demands. *Reactance* (Brehm, 1966) is an emotional response to attempts at coercion, prohibition and regulation. Reactance leads people to take the opposite view to that imposed and motivates people to do the opposite of what is recommended. So, if persuasive communication is to avoid reactance, it needs to be carefully prepared for the target audience and begin with points of agreement.

We have noted the importance of perceptions of the message source and how this relates to the way in which persuasive communication is delivered. Explicit, and especially unwelcome, persuasive attempts may be resisted. Even tone of voice and other non-verbal indicators of power within a relationship can undermine social influence in one-to-one settings. For example, Ambady et al. (2002) taped surgeons' consultations with patients and, on the basis of ten-second clips, rated dominance and concern in their voices (regardless of content). Higher dominance and lower concern were significantly associated with whether or not surgeons had previously been involved in malpractice claims initiated by their patients! This has important implications for doctor-patient communication which we consider in Chapter 10. In an analogous manner, governments need to persuade populations that public health legislation is in the public interest before enacting such legislation (e.g. necessitating seatbelt wearing in cars or banning smoking in public places). Otherwise, enforcement may be costly and there is a risk that unpopular legislation may be overturned. Reassuring a target audience that what is offered is caring and practical advice which is in their own interest is a crucial foundation for persuasion. Reactance and resistance can be minimised by presenting persuasion attempts as choices, and by highlighting the ease with which change can be managed. Highlighting what people can do is likely to be more effective than telling them what they should not (e.g. "you can choose to be smoke free", "you can choose to eat a healthy diet and feel and look better") (Knowles & Rinner, 2007).

ACTIVITY BOX 8.2

Design a brief set of arguments that could be used to persuade young people to donate blood, drawing on evidence-based principles of persuasion.

An alternative could be designing a set of arguments that would persuade young men to always use condoms.

In either case, think about the preparatory actions that the person needs to take to ensure that they succeed with the planed action.

Attitude change

Evaluating action positively, that is, holding a positive attitude towards the action is critical to change. Consequently, *attitude change* is a key target for those wishing to persuade others to adopt healthier lifestyles.

Message processing and attitude change

Attitude change is dependent on how a recipient responds to a persuasive message. For example, some evaluative responses are based on superficial impressions while others are the result of systematic consideration. This has important implications for persuasion. Petty and Cacioppo (1986) argued that, although we are all motivated to hold valid attitudes which help us make reliable predictions about our reality (hence the power of informational influence), we can have more or less motivation and capacity to devote to the systematic processing of messages we receive. They refer to the amount of systematic processing devoted to a message as "cognitive elaboration" and, consequently, their model is known as the "elaboration likelihood model" (ELM).

The ELM refers to systematic processing of messages as *central route processing* and processing of messages in a superficial manner as *peripheral route processing*. Central route processing involves greater cognitive elaboration and the meaning of the message is critical to persuasion. By contrast, peripheral route processing involves little systematic processing (low cognitive elaboration) so characteristics other than meaning are more likely to determine whether or not a message is persuasive.

When people are under time pressure, do not understand a message, think that the issue is not relevant to them or are distracted by something else they may evaluate a message on the basis of simple cues rather than considering its meaning in detail. For example, people use rules or decision-making heuristics to evaluate messages. These include, "expertise = accuracy", that is, she's an expert so what she says must be right, or "consensus = correctness", that is, if so many people agree they must be right and "length = strength", that is there are lots of arguments so it must be true. Sometimes situational constraints force people into peripheral route processing. For example, the message may be presented quickly with many distractions, as is the case in many screen advertisements.

In addition, individual differences mean that some people are more or less likely than others to engage in systematic processing. For example, Chaiken (1980) identified people who agreed or disagreed with the length = strength heuristic (using agreement with questionnaire items such as, "the more reasons a person has for some point of view the more likely he/she is correct"). These people were then presented with a message containing six arguments in favour of cross-course, end-of-year examinations for students. However, the message was described to participants as either containing ten or two arguments (although it always contained the same six arguments). The results showed that those who endorsed the length = strength heuristic were more likely to be persuaded when the message was described as having ten arguments than were those who did not endorse the heuristic.

Central route (systematic) processing is unlikely when recipients who do not understand a message. Figure 8.2 shows results from a study by Wood, Kallgren and Mueller Preisler (1985). Amongst message recipients with poor knowledge, attitude change was almost as likely whether a message contained weak or strong arguments because the ability to engage in systematic, central route processing was compromised by lack of knowledge. These recipients relied on peripheral processing and so failed to differentiate between strong and weak arguments. By contrast, those with good knowledge differentiated clearly between strong and weak arguments and were only persuaded by the former. These results emphasise the importance of knowledge (and quality information) in allowing people to evaluate messages about their health. Similarly, those who are confident that their responses to a message are correct are more likely to be persuaded (Petty, Briñol & Tormala, 2002). Of course, if recipients are more confident that their rejections or negative appraisals of the message are correct, then they are even less likely to be persuaded! Enhancing recipients' knowledge, encouraging them to be confident in their own judgements and providing quality information are all critical to persuasive public health messaging.

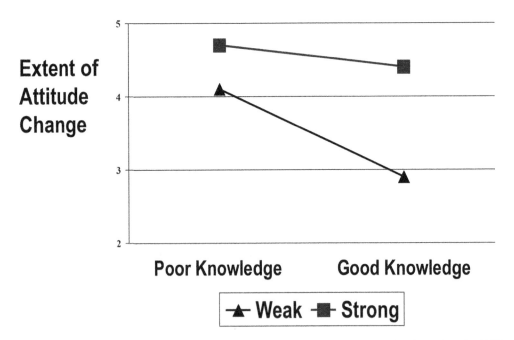

Figure 8.2 Prior Knowledge and the effect of argument strength on persuasion (Wood et al., 1985)

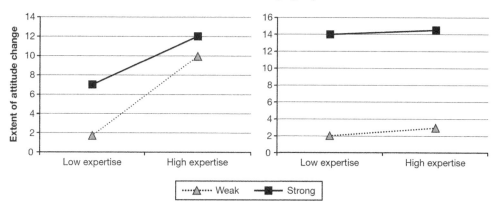

Figure 8.3 The impact of expertise on persuasion by strong and weak arguments under conditions of low (left) and high (right) personal relevance (Petty & Cacioppo, 1986)

When people have time to process messages, or make time because they regard the message as personally relevant, they are more likely to engage in systematic processing so that the meaning of the message is more important than other characteristics. Figure 8.3 shows how perceiving the message source to be an expert has different effects depending on whether recipients regard a message as high or low in personal relevance. The low-relevance participants are strongly affected by perceived expertise and are more persuaded by an expert (rather than inexpert) source whether strong or weak arguments are used. However, for those who see the message as personally relevant (and so engage in systematic processing) only the quality of argument determines persuasion. Strong arguments are persuasive for this group, regardless of source expertise. Even an expert cannot persuade this group using weak arguments. This does not mean that source expertise in unimportant but rather that for those with the ability and motivation to engage in systematic processing, poor quality arguments cannot be compensated for by the impression of expertise. This again emphasises the importance of equipping the population with high quality information and education about health. This, in turn, has implications for early teaching of biology, psychology and health in schools.

The ELM proposes that persuasion occurs through both central and peripheral routes simultaneously but that one or the other route will be dominant depending on factors such as message-relevance. Individual characteristics also affect whether people are likely engage mainly in systematic processing. For example, some people have a high "need for cognition" and so, in general, are motivated to devote more cognitive resources to central route processing (Briñol & Petty, 2005).

Overall then, research suggests that if you do not have strong arguments then you are better discouraging systematic processing and relying instead on numerous arguments, consensus and perceived expertise. Perhaps fortunately, attitude changes resulting from peripheral route processing are less likely to be stable (that is, long lived) and more likely to further change due to counter persuasion. Whereas attitude change resulting from systematic (central route) processing is more likely to be stable and to influence behaviour. Consequently, health promoters should encourage systematic processing by ensuring appropriate prior knowledge, emphasising personal relevance, providing distraction-free presentations, using repetition, and encouraging confidence in people's own judgement. Strong attitudes can be defined are those the person feels are more important to them *and* those they feel most certain about. These attitudes are more likely to predict future actions (Conner et al., 2022). So, ideally health promotion should aim not just to change attitudes but to promote strong, pro-health attitudes and, thereby influence health behaviour patterns. All of the advice above is critical to furthering this aim.

If we want to change people's behaviour we need to marshal all the tools discussed above in our persuasive communication strategies

Having facilitated systematic processing we must ensure that our persuasive messages are easily understood and composed of strong arguments, if we are to change beliefs, attitudes and behaviours.

ACTIVITY BOX 8.3

Identify three screen-based advertisements which illustrate application of evidence-based principles of persuasion, including those that use distraction to undermine central route processing.

Enhancing self-efficacy

Perhaps you have *not* changed the health-related behaviour you thought of earlier? Perhaps you thought it would be too difficult to change. *Self-efficacy* (SE) is the belief that we have the ability and resources to succeed in achieving a goal, despite environmental barriers. It is feeling confident that you can make the change even when you understand that it may be challenging. Perceived behavioural control and SE are important prerequisites of intention (see Chapter 7). SE promotes intention *and* performance so consideration of SE enhancement bridges our discussion of changing motivation (this chapter) and behaviour (Chapter 9). SE is important to many areas of health psychology. For example, in Chapter 3 we discussed how secondary appraisals determine our experience of stress. When we believe we can competently manage a demand, it becomes a challenge, otherwise it is a stressor. SE can sometimes depend on perceived social support (see Chapter 5). We believe we can manage a demand because we know others will help us.

Self-efficacy and performance

SE is correlated with performance across a range of behaviour patterns including academic performance and health-related behaviours (Bandura, 1997). For example, in a meta-analysis (see Research Methods Box 8.1) of 114 studies of SE and work-related performance, Stajkovic and Luthans (1998) found an effect size of $d = .82$ which corresponds to an increase of 28% in performance due to higher SE. This is an impressive effect size. Such findings recommend SE-enhancing interventions to improve work performance. Unfortunately, high SE can also lead people to be overly optimistic about their capacity to change and so does not always predict behaviour change. This is especially true when people are trying to break unwanted habits. It is very important to bolster SE amongst those intending to change but it is not always enough (see Chapter 9)

While there is little evidence for distinct stages of behaviour change (see Chapter 7), people face different challenges as they progress from adoption (e.g. jogging for the first time) through to establishment of habits (e.g. jogging regularly three times a week). So, SE-enhancing interventions should target challenges relevant to particular target audiences. To facilitate this, different types of SE measures have been defined. For example, Schwarzer and Luszczynska (2015) distinguish *action SE* (believing one can succeed in completing a planned behaviour), from *maintenance SE* (believing one can maintain the action over time) and *recovery SE* (believing one can adopt the behaviour again after a relapse) (see Zhang, Zhang, Schwarzer & Hagger, 2019 for a meta-analysis).

People who believe they can succeed set themselves more challenging goals. They exert more effort, use more flexible problem-solving strategies and are more persistent *because* they believe they will eventually succeed. By contrast, low SE undermines striving. High SE also minimises stress (because of favourable secondary appraisals, for example, "I can do this, it's a challenge" (see Chapter 3). This enhances skilled performance. Moreover, high SE facilitates concentration on the task at hand rather than concerns about personal deficiencies or exaggeration of task demands (Wood & Bandura, 1989), thereby, minimising anxiety during performance. SE determines how people conceptualise a task, how confident they feel during performance, how persistent they are in the face of setbacks, how much effort they invest, and how they feel about themselves during performance. Consequently, targeting SE in behaviour change interventions can strengthen motivation and result in behaviour change. This is critical to public health policy implementation (see e.g. a study of handwashing during the COVID-19 pandemic, Luszczynska et al., 2022).

Self-efficacy and health

As well as affecting performance, SE levels affect health directly by moderating the impact of potential stressors on physiological systems. Low SE in the face of demands generates stress which elicits a variety of damaging physiological responses (see Chapter 2). These include the release of catecholamines into the bloodstream, such as adrenalin and cortisol, from the adrenal gland. This, in turn, increases heart rate, blood pressure, sugar levels and blood flow to large muscle groups. SE changes have been found to be associated with catecholamine activation (Bandura, 1997) providing a plausible mechanism by which SE levels alter the physiological impact of demands on the body. It is unsurprising, therefore, that that high SE is associated with *less* down-regulation of the immune system in response to stressors (Wiedenfeld et al., 1990). So, believing you can succeed in the face of challenging demands has positive effects on biological functioning and health because high SE reduces unnecessary activation of the sympathetic nervous system.

It has also been argued that intermittent (as opposed to chronic) stress responses may "toughen" physiological systems by dampening down stress responses over time (Dienstbier, 1989). In other words, periodic increases in sympathetic nervous system arousal train the body to respond less extremely to subsequent stressors. However, this effect depends on these intermittent stressors being perceived as challenges (rather than threats) which, in turn, depends on high SE in relation to actions necessitated by such stressors. High SE is critical to ensuring that motivation, or intention, is translated into action in the face of demands. Consequently, promoting SE in health promotion communication is critical to behaviour change effectiveness.

Enhancing self-efficacy

Bandura (1997) argued that there are four main approaches to enhancing self-efficacy:

1. Mastery experiences.
2. Vicarious experience.

3.   Verbal persuasion.
4.   Perception of physiological and affective states.

First, and most powerful, *mastery experiences* (i.e. experience of successfully performing the behaviour) give people confidence that they can tackle new tasks because they know they have previously succeeded with similar challenges. This recommends that teachers and trainers guide learners towards success by identifying manageable tasks and only increasing difficulty as confidence and skill grow, that is by use of graded tasks (see Figure 8.4). Moreover, helping someone practice a manageable task and providing constructive feedback can consolidate skills and enhance SE. Failure undermines SE and focusing on past failure can be self-handicapping.

Second, SE can also be enhanced through observation of others' success, especially if we categorise the models as being like ourselves. For example, Bandura notes that observing failure in a model judged to have less skill than ourselves has little or no impact on SE but observing the same failure in a model judged to have similar skills undermines SE. Health promoters should conduct preliminary research into when positive and negative models are helpful to people who are establishing new goals, building SE and acquiring new skills. Positive models (that is, observation of successful others) are likely to be most SE-enhancing (e.g. in the case of physical fitness), although in *some cases*, for example when undesirable body image is salient, negative models (that is, use of models failing to establish physical fitness) may be motivating (Lockwood, Wong, McShane & Dolderman, 2005). Moreover, contrasts between current self and desired or ideal self can be motivating. Seeing oneself and distinct from what you want to be can have positive effects on changing motivation when combined with realistic goal-setting and action plans.

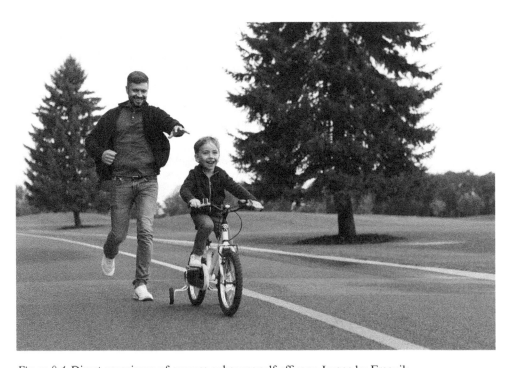

Figure 8.4 Direct experience of success enhances self efficacy. Image by Freepik.

Third, when direct experience and modelling are not available, SE can be enhanced by verbal persuasion. People can be persuaded by arguments stating that others (like them) are successful in meeting challenges similar to their own (thereby, changing descriptive norms) as well as persuasion highlighting an individual's own skills, and past success. Tailoring communication to enhance persuasiveness (as discussed in this chapter), including, optimising source trustworthiness and expertise is likely to enhance the effectiveness of such SE-promoting interventions.

Finally, our own physiological reactions and our interpretations of these reactions affects SE. Mood, stress and anxiety during performance can undermine SE. For example, although physiological arousal is normal during demanding performances, it can be interpreted as a sign of panic or incompetence. Such interpretations are likely to disrupt and undermine performance. By contrast, acknowledging arousal as a natural response to performance demands may add to excitement and commitment. So, interventions designed to reduce negative moods and anxiety and to re-interpret destructive interpretations of physiological arousal are likely to enhance SE and facilitate skilled performance.

Translating motivation into behaviour change

We have considered the use of evidence-based approaches to enhance motivation to perform health-related behaviours. In Chapter 7 we noted that motivation alone is not be enough to prompt action. Research on the intention–behaviour gap and implementation intention formation indicates that interventions focusing on post-intentional or volitional processes may be critical to prompting already-motivated people to adopt health-promoting behaviours. Consequently, the challenge for health promoters is twofold. First, generate strong and stable motivation and to facilitate goal setting through persuasive communication that can change attitudes, normative beliefs and self-efficacy. Second the help motivated people to develop volitional capacities by bolstering self-efficacy, goal-setting, prompting implementation intention formation (if-then planning) and skill development. The aim is to generate strong and stable motivation that is more likely to shape people's behaviour over time. As we shall see in Chapter 9, this is likely to involve helping people prioritise health goals in the face of many other demands.

Growing healthcare demands from ageing populations, poor adherence to healthcare advice in terms of e.g. diet, physical activity and sleep and the, consequential increasing prevalence of long-term illnesses (see Chapter 11) has meant that health services have found it increasingly difficult to offer one-to-one professional-patient models of healthcare delivery (Whelan, 2002). Group meetings can be effective behaviour change interventions when people meet together to discuss similar problems because others' lived experiences make them credible and trustworthy sources (Borek & Abraham, 2018). Group interventions can develop personal self-management skills including illness-specific competencies and decision-making skills. Evaluations of these interventions have found that they can be effective in changing health behaviour patterns and be cost effective. For example, Lorig, Mazonson and Holman (1993) found that a self-management course for patients with chronic arthritis resulted in increased self-efficacy, reduced pain and a 43% reduction in consultations with doctors. The course was delivered to groups by trained volunteers who were themselves arthritis sufferers. For patients suffering from rheumatoid arthritis, the reduction in health service usage constituted a saving of $162 per patient. Translating this 1993 figure to 2023 rates would mean the course could save about $334 per patient. Since there are more than 400,000 people with rheumatoid arthritis in the UK, this intervention has the potential to save the UK National Health Services more than £110 million, if provided for all sufferers. Other evaluations have identified a variety of healthcare gains from participation in such group-based self-management training. Barlow et al. (2002) reviewed 145 evaluations and concluded that self-management training led to increases in patients' knowledge and SE, better symptom management, adoption of appropriate coping techniques, and enhancements in health status. Other studies have found reduced hospitalisation (e.g. Lorig et al., 1999) and enhanced physical and psychological wellbeing following attendance at such courses (Wright, Barlow, Turner & Bancroft, 2003). An important general principle emerges from these studies. As Wanless (2002, see Chapter 1) pointed out, if people are not actively striving to manage their own health and illnesses then it becomes very expensive to run health services. Preventive interventions that reduce the demands on health services can improve public health and ensure that health service delivery remains affordable. Prevention is less expensive than curative treatment.

Evaluation of health interventions of this kind illustrates one area in which quantitative and qualitative research complement each other (see too Chapter 9). Quantitative research is required to assess effectiveness in terms of pre-defined criteria from healthcare usage figures, including attitudes quality of life and behavioural measures. Qualitative research typically uses interviews can examine the perspective of the user in detail (see e.g. Borek et al., 2019b). In such research, health promotion researchers need to focus on detailed similarities and differences between people's accounts of their challenges and their experiences of interventions. Qualitative process evaluations (see Chapter 9) of an intervention might, for example, reveal which intervention approaches were especially valued or disliked by participants and also highlight the range of individual responses in terms of cognition, emotional and behavioural responses. The results of such research can help intervention designers understand why some users respond positively while others do not. This can provide valuable guidance on intervention refinement and implementation. Qualitative analysis of interview data can also reveal positive or negative experiences not previously considered by researchers and, thereby, imply new theoretical advances and/or new outcome. For example, an intervention targeting motivation change might be found work, in part, by generating new identities with matching goals. Such insights into mechanisms of change can help refine the delivery of health-care interventions.

Influenced by the results of quantitative and qualitative evaluation research, the UK Department of Health developed the Expert Patient Programme (EPP) in 2001 and this still operates as an NHS Foundation Trust (https://www.nelft.nhs.uk/epp/) This is a generic self-management training intervention designed to empower patients to effectively manage long term health conditions and associated symptoms. The aim of EPP was to facilitate patients becoming key decision-makers in the treatment process and gaining greater control over their lives through improved resourcefulness and self-efficacy, as well as reducing health service demand. EPP was based closely on the previously-evaluated Chronic Disease Self-Management Course (Lorig et al., 1999; see too Bandura, 1997) which developed from the successful interventions with arthritis patients.

An EPP course comprises six weekly structured self-management training sessions delivered to groups of 6–15 patients with heterogeneous health conditions, led by trained, lay tutors with chronic health conditions. Patients also receive a self-help manual containing further information. The programme includes information provision and cognitive and behavioural modification techniques as well as action planning, problem solving, dealing with depression, nutrition, and exercise. Course sessions are held in community settings and tutors are volunteers, thus keeping administration costs low. Early evaluations were encouraging. Barlow, Wright, Sheasby, Turner, and Hainsworth (2002) observed a number of benefits including increased SE in managing symptoms, reduced fatigue and depressed moods, and better communication with doctors. Moreover, benefits were sustained 12 months after attending an EPP course. Similarly, a randomized-controlled trial found improvements in SE and psychological wellbeing, together with reduced anxiety and greater levels of physical activity, at six months follow-up (Kennedy et al., 2007).

Abraham and Gardner (2009) used interviews and qualitative research to explore how EEP groups worked and found that quality information provision, especially face-to-face information exchange as well as in-group instruction and modelling of physical skills. For example, showing how to conduct and exercise or use a piece of equipment. Help with personal goal setting, using graded tasks (one step at a time), self-monitoring (recording and tracking how well one is doing with goal achievement) and goal review (for example, resetting a goal that is too difficult at present) were seen to be some of the most helpful components of EPP groups. Teaching and adoption of these self-management strategies also depended on establishment of an empathic and self-validating interpersonal content, that is a friendly group in which all members felt they were listened to. The importance of social context in groups designed to promotive cognitive and behaviour change was further emphasised by Borek et al. (2019b). We will return to the role of group interventions in changing health-related behaviour patterns in Chapter 9.

Key terms introduced in Chapter 8 (in order of appearance)

- Information accessibility
- source credibility
- elicitation research
- Flesch Reading Ease measure
- explicit categorisation
- graphic organiser
- average weighted correlation
- effect size
- social influence
- informational influence
- normative influence
- self-categorisation
- cognitive dissonance
- consensus
- conformity
- conversion
- obedience
- reactance
- choice

- attitude change
- cognitive elaboration
- central and peripheral route processing
- decision-making heuristic
- need for cognition
- self-efficacy
- mastery experience
- graded tasks
- vicarious experience
- verbal persuasion
- perception of physiological states
- Expert Patient Programme
- quantitative and qualitative research
- focus groups

Summary of main points addressed in Chapter 8

Health-related information is likely to be persuasive when provided by credible and trustworthy sources.

Health-related information needs to be accessible, minimise use of jargon, be easily readable and answer questions relevant to the target audience. Simple techniques, including logical order, explicit categorisation and repetition enhance recall.

Persuasion is a form of social influence which can be understood in terms of underlying motives. We are motivated to access valid sources of information; this facilitates informational influence. We are also motivated to feel positively about ourselves and to have good relationships with others. This facilitates normative influence. Informational influence is strengthened by source credibility, expertise, consistency and consensus. Normative influence is strengthened by positive relationships, reciprocation and approval. Persuasion in groups can be understood in terms of conformity and conversion (in the case of minority influence). Avoiding prohibition and presenting advice as easy-to-implement choices can minimise reactance.

Attitude change based on systematic (or central route) processing is more stable and less susceptible to counter persuasion than attitude change following from peripheral route processing. Central route processing is more likely when people are informed, motivated (e.g. they think the message is relevant to them) and have the capacity to process messages (e.g. distraction-free time to consider arguments). During central route processing the meaning or quality of arguments is critical to persuasion.

Self-efficacy is correlated with performance across a range of behaviour patterns but tends to be behaviour-specific. SE leads to greater effort, persistence and flexible responding. SE promotion needs to correspond directly to the challenges faced by individual actors and target audiences. SE can be enhanced by mastery experiences, vicarious experience (i.e. modelling), verbal persuasion and perception of physiological and affective states.

Recommendations for further reading

Journal articles

Bandura A. (2004). Health promotion by social cognitive means. *Health Education and Behavior*, *31*(2), 143–164. doi: 10.1177/1090198104263660

Filkuková, P., Ayton, P., Rand, K. & Langguth, J. (2021). What should I trust? Individual differences in attitudes to conflicting information and misinformation on COVID-19. *Frontiers in Psychology*, *12*, 588478. doi: 10.3389/fpsyg.2021.588478

Petty R. E., Cacioppo, J. T. (1986) The elaboration likelihood model of persuasion. In L. Berkowitz (Ed.) *Advances in Experimental Social Psychology, 19*, (pp. 123–205). New York: Academic Press. doi.org/10.1016/S0065–2601(08)60214–2

Wood, W. (2000). Attitude change: Persuasion and social influence. *Annual Review of Psychology*, *51*, 539–570. doi.org/10.1146/annurev.psych.51.1.539

Illustrative essay titles

1. Information isn't enough: health psychology research recommends a new approach to health promotion.

2. Why do people *not* believe evidence-based, public health advice? What can be done to deliver persuasive public health messaging?

3. Attempts to persuade people to avoid unhealthy behaviours often fail. How can health promoters persuade people to look after their health more effectively?

4. What lessons can health promoters learn from the psychology of attitude change?

5. Why is self-efficacy important to health and health-related behaviour and how can health promoters enhance self-efficacy?

9 Changing behaviour
Intervention design and evaluation

Changing behaviour: intervention design and evaluation

From Hippocrates' advice on diet, to Diogenes' wall (see Chapter 1) to modern public health policy, we strive to help people look after their health, including adherence to proven treatments (see Chapter 10) and avoidance of foreseeable health risks. Yet, despite many centuries of health promotion, global public health is not improving.

This chapter is divided into six sections:

1. Evidence-based health promotion.
2. Specifying behaviours, target groups and informational, cognitive and skill deficits.
3. Targeting feelings and fear to change behaviour.
4. Identifying change components in intervention design.
5. Developing and evaluating behaviour change interventions.
6. Beyond individual behaviour-change interventions.

Learning outcomes

When you have completed this chapter you should be able to:

1. Discuss how constructs highlighted by social cognition models can be used to make health promotion materials more effective.
2. Identify key questions to be answered by elicitation research prior to intervention design, referring to the "Information, Motivation and Behavioural Skills" model.
3. Explain how particular intervention components can target key change mechanisms and so address cognitive, behavioural or deficits in a target population.
4. Discuss when fear appeals may or may not be effective with reference to Protection Motivation Theory and illustrate the importance of carefully-designed theory-based materials.
5. Critically discuss progress made towards identifying theory-based change techniques linked to change mechanisms.
6. Describe key phases in the design and evaluation of behaviour-change interventions.

DOI: 10.4324/9781003171096-13

7. Discuss the limits of behaviour change interventions that focus on individual change and discuss alternative community and population approaches.
8. Explain the importance of the "Social Ecological" model to understanding and implementing behaviour-change interventions.

Evidence-based health promotion

In Chapter 7, we reviewed models describing cognitions that strengthen motivation. For example, the Health Belief Model and Protection Motivation Theory. When such explanatory models are found to predict behaviour, they can be used to guide the design of behaviour-change interventions. For example, we might design health promotion messages to emphasise individuals' susceptibility to infection and subsequent health problems (drawing on the Health Belief Model and Protection Motivation Theory). If we design interventions that can change cognitions found to predict behaviour then we may be able to promote motivational and behavioural change. In a meta-analysis of 204 studies that used experimental methods to change participants' normative beliefs, attitudes and self-efficacy, Sheeran et al. (2016) found that these cognition changes gave rise to medium-sized changes in intention (ds = .48–.51) and small to medium-sized changes in behaviour (ds = 38–.47) (see Research Methods Box 8.1 explaining d values). This strongly suggests that precise targeting of the cognitive underpinnings of motivation (see Chapter 8) can contribute to the effectiveness of behaviour change interventions. This is evidence-based, behaviour-change intervention design.

Psychologists have attempted to integrate social cognition models (e.g. Abraham, Sheeran & Johnston, 1998) and in Chapter 7, we described the Fishbein et al. (2001) proposal for an integrated explanatory framework. This is a helpful step forward, especially if applied psychologists can adopt a consensual terminology so that change mechanisms (e.g. believing one is susceptible to an anticipated event) and experimental methods used to change them can be understood in same way across studies. Hagger & Hamilton (2020) emphasise the need for progress on, "the definitions of constructs and . . . the relations among them . . . if they are to have value in . . . informing behaviour-change interventions" (p. 219). Without theoretical consensus and specificity of theoretical definitions the science of behaviour change is unlikely to provide a reliable evidence base for health promotion practice.

A health psychologist designing health promotion messages might ask, "is the target audience (e.g. adults in the population) motivated to undertake the target behaviour (e.g. wearing a face mask in public to reduce the risk of COVID-19 infection)"? If the answer to this question is "no" or "not strongly", further questions follow. Do they accept that they are susceptible to infection? Do they believe that the consequences of infection could be severe for them? Do they believe that masks are effective in reducing infection risk? Do they believe others will approve or disapprove of them wearing a mask? Do they believe that wearing a mask will have consequences for their social identity or relationships with others. For example, if mask wearing is perceived to have implications for self-presentation and as well as self-protection then both these motivations will be important to the design of persuasive interventions (Cha, Ku & Choi, 2023). These questions can then direct research (e.g. using interviews and questionnaires) to identify why motivation is weak and what messages are most likely to bolster that motivation. Such research, undertaken prior to the design on interventions, is referred to as elicitation research.

Once elicitation research has been completed further work is needed to develop health promotion materials that are salient to the target audience. In particular, messages that will attract and keep their attention and be persuasive. This will also involve a selection of credible sources of persuasion. We discussed some of these challenges in Chapter 8 in relation to providing information, persuading others, changing attitudes and enhancing self-efficacy. Precise targeting of evidence-based messaging is critical to effective health promotion.

If we do not undertake elicitation research then well-intentioned interventions may not promote health behaviour change or health. Abraham, Krahé, Dominic and Fritsche (2002) surveyed widely-available leaflets promoting condom use. The content of each leaflet, that is, the arguments and messages used, were categorised. In general, leaflets devoted most content to providing information on the transmission of sexually-transmitted infections (STIs), people's susceptibility to acquiring STIs, the effectiveness of condom use and on encouraging professional contact. This is a reasonable approach but is it evidence-based? We know that knowledge alone and perceived susceptibility are weak correlates of condom use. Sheeran et al. (1999) reported average weighted correlations with condom use of 0.06 for measures of knowledge and measures of perceived susceptibility. Even perceived condom effectiveness was found to have an average correlation of only 0.10 with condom use. So, the cognitions targeted most frequently by the majority of leaflets were not those found to be those most strongly correlated with condom use. By contrast, cognitions found to be stronger correlates of condom use, such normative beliefs about others' approval, attitudes and self-efficacy were targeted less frequently by leaflets. The researchers identified 20 core messages that corresponded to the cognitions significantly associated with condom use in previous studies. Seventy-five percent of leaflets included less than half of these cognition-matched messages. However, a small number of illustrative leaflets were identified which included between 15 and 18 of the 20 core messages, demonstrating that safer sex promotion leaflets can include a range of messages matched to the cognitions found to predict condom use. Overall, however, the design of these leaflets was not based on elicitation research and did not target the strongest correlates of condom use. Unfortunately, the design of health promotion materials is not always evidence-based. Abraham, Southby, Quandte, Krahé and van der Sluijs (2007) found that leaflets designed to reduce alcohol consumption (across three European countries) failed, in general, to incorporate the range of messages suggested by prior research into the determinants of risky drinking. If health promotion messages are not evidence-based or are not matched to the needs of the target group then, even if the messages are persuasive, they may not lead to the desired behaviour change.

A key health problem, globally, is the growing prevalence of being overweight or obese. For example, in the UK, 10% of children are obese by the age of five and this rises to 23% by the age of eleven. Moreover, children are more likely to be obese if they live in deprived areas and this gap between rich and poor obesity levels is widening. Among adults in England, 64% are either overweight or obese (Baker, 2023). Being obese makes it more likely that one will die earlier, contract type 2 diabetes, suffer from high blood pressure and experience heart attacks and strokes (World Health Organization, 2021). Diabetes alone costs the UK National Health

Service over £1.5 million (1.89 million USA dollars) *an hour*. This constitutes 10% of the UK NHS budget (https://www.diabetes.co.uk/cost-of-diabetes.html). So, obesity represents a critical and expensive public problem. How could evidence-based health promotion mitigate this problem?

We noted in Chapter 8 that different types of messages may be more or less salient to target audiences and may have more or less effect on beliefs and motivation. Can food labelling change consumers' selection of food products and, thereby, assist with healthy eating? Many types of food labelling have been considered. These include traffic light systems which indicate unhealthy products using red symbols and healthy products using green symbols. In Australia health stars are used with up to five stars indicating greater healthiness. Calorie counts indicating the calorie content to the product have also been used, as have Physical Activity Calorie Equivalent (or PACE) labels which tell the person how far they would have to walk to "burn off" the calorie content of the product. Whatever labelling system is used it needs to be eye-catching and simple to interpret. So, can health psychology research make recommendations about what kind of food labelling would be most effective in shaping consumers healthy food choices? Kunz, Haasova, Rieß and Florack (2020) tested traffic light labelling among Austrian consumers choosing dessert products. They found that these labels promoted stronger intentions to purchase lower-sugar products. While this is encouraging, a narrative review considering 65 studies of different food labels reported mixed findings and called for further better-quality studies (Braesco & Drewnowski, 2023). PACE labelling is easy to understand, especially to the individuals with low socioeconomic position or/and with low health literacy levels and limited knowledge about nutrition (Cramer, 2016). A meta-analysis (Daley et al., 2020) of 15 studies comparing PACE labelling to other types of food labelling found that PACE labelling resulted in significantly fewer calories being selected by consumers, relative to comparator labelling. Moreover, PACE activity-based labelling has been found to increase physical activity levels and decrease time spent in sedentary activities (Deery et al., 2019). Future, large-scale randomised controlled trials could provide definitive advice to governments on the effectiveness of food labels on food purchases. This would be an example of experimental health psychology research having direct implications for public health policy.

Specifying behaviours, target groups and informational, cognitive and skill deficits

Defining behaviours and target groups

When designing behaviour change interventions, it is important to be specific about the definition of *the target behaviour*, e.g. in the case of exercise, how many times a week, for what duration and at what intensity do we want people to exercise? Similarly, for complex behavioural sequences, interventions may be need to target a set of preparatory behaviours. For example, if we want young men to use condoms we may first need to ensure that they have access to condoms and that they view carrying condoms as an action likely be approved of by their peers. So most behaviour-change interventions need to target a series of actions. Having condoms available is prerequisite to using them. Therefore, if elicitation research suggests that young men are not carrying condoms then accessibility and carrying interventions need to developed.

It is also important be clear about *who* exactly an intervention will target. For example, an intervention designed to reduce unwanted teenage pregnancies may not target the average teenager but young men and women who are most likely to have unprotected intercourse at a young age. This is important because sub-groups differ in their knowledge, cognitions, motivation and skills. As we note in Chapter 10, when we provide information it is critical that it is the information wanted by the target group. Similarly, emphasising susceptibility to a health threat in communication with groups that already accept their susceptibility is unlikely to generate change. Imprecision in defining the target group or understanding what they already believe may lead to mismatched interventions, that may be ineffective.

Targeting informational, cognitive and skills deficits

The Information, Motivation and Behavioral skills model (IMB; Fisher & Fisher, 1992; see Figure 9.1) provides a useful planning tool. This model acknowledges the potential importance of quality information provision (see Chapters 8 and 10) and encompasses cognitive components of motivation shared with the Theory of Planned Behaviour and Social Cognitive Theory (see Chapter 7). In addition, this model highlights the importance of skills required to translate motivation into action which we focus on in this section.

A number of successful behaviour change interventions have been based on the IMB and some of these have been evaluated using long term follow up (e.g. at 12 months in the case of Fisher, Fisher, Bryan & Misovich, 2002). For example, the model was used in the design of an effective group-based intervention (see Chapters 8 and 10) to help patients with long-term pain reduce reliance on opioid drugs (Sandhu et al., 2023). Chang, Choi, Kim and Song (2014) report a systematic review of 12 IMB intervention evaluation studies. See Focus Box 9.1 for an illustration of targets and methods. The IMB emphasises that skills are required to translate motivation into behaviour and highlights the need to assess informational, cognitive and skills deficits amongst the target group prior to intervention design. The model proposes that health psychologists need to discover, through elicitation research, whether the (precisely-defined) target group lack any behaviour-relevant information, whether the key determinants of motivation (e.g. normative beliefs attitudes and self-efficacy) are strongly held among the target group (as discussed above) and whether the target group lack skills required to translate motivation into behaviour.

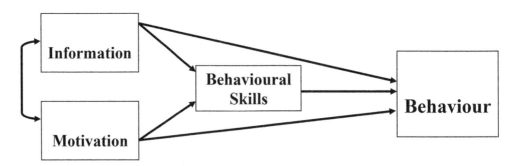

Figure 9.1 The Information-Motivation-Behavioral Skills model (Fisher & Fisher, 1992)

Three types of core skills can be considered. First, *self-management skills*. These cognitive skills empower people to consider long-term consequences of current action, evaluate their behaviour patterns, set new goals, including setting graded tasks, prioritise goals in the face of other demands, plan action before and during goal-relevant experiences and prompt appropriate effort when opportunities present themselves. Implementation intention formation (see Chapter 7) and self-efficacy enhancement (see Chapter 8) involve self-management skills. This type of skill training may involve conscious rehearsal of the skill followed by practice over time with a view to longer-term habitual initiation. For example, Schinke and Gordon (1992) describe a culturally-specific intervention including a self-completion book using comic strip characters and rap music verse to encourage effective safer sex management amongst black teenagers. The aim was to develop self-monitoring and planning skills as well as verbal resources which can be used to control and disrupt scripted interaction that could lead to unprotected sex. The acronym SODAS, standing for Stop, Options, Decide, Act and Self-praise, was used in this training. The first step, "stop" explicitly elicits anticipated regret ("stop and think what these choices could really mean for you today, tomorrow . . . and for years to follow") – while the fourth step, "act" involves the reader in generating implementation intentions concerning five types of verbal responses which can be used when they are subjected to social pressure. If self-management skills are lacking, then informational and persuasive campaigns may be ineffective because they do not empower the target group to translate motivation into action.

Second, *motor skills* may also be lacking among the target group. For example, correct condom use depends upon a basic understanding of infection control as well as the manual skills involved in opening and using a condom without damaging it. Similarly, before using a gym, people need to be taught to use exercise machines. Certain medication regimes require patients to learn to use devices such as inhalers or needles and patients and medical staff may need instruction in simple skills such as hand washing as part of infection control in hospitals (Boyce & Pittet, 2002). Thus, analysis of any health behaviour targeted in an intervention should involve an assessment of the skills required and the extent to which the targeted recipients are proficient, or lacking, in these skills. Of course, technological advances can make the skills involved in health behaviours easier to learn. Extra-fine needles make it easier for diabetics to inject themselves, alcohol wipes make hand washing easier and the development of a once-a-day single pill for HIV control makes adherence much easier than if patients have to take many pills each day! So, skill deficits can highlight a need for organisational or technological change to support behaviour change.

Third, we require *social skills* to mange behaviour and seek others' support for change. For example, the skills to negotiate condom use with a reluctant partner or the skills to explain why we will not share alcoholic drinking sessions or eat traditional but unhealthy foods. The social skills required depend on the target behaviour and the social resources available to individuals planning change. During skill-training, instruction, demonstration, opportunities for practice and feedback are all important to facilitate new skills being used habitually.

Assertiveness training (that is, being able to express one's own wants and needs in an honest and non-aggressive manner) and negotiation skills are often prerequisite to managing interactions arising out of behaviour change. Assertiveness training may help people develop the skills they need to negotiate change with others (González-Yubero, Lázaro-Visa & Palomera, 2021). By explaining one's needs and goals carefully to others and being consistent over time, one may help others accept a change or make changes themselves. For example, *Negative Feelings*

Assertion can be used to communicate how other's actions are upsetting us without using aggressive challenges. This kind of assertive statement is made up of four parts;

1. A description of the other person's behaviour: *"When you . . .".*
2. Clarification of how it affects your plans: *"that . . .".*
3. A description of your feelings: *"and I feel . . .".*
4. The assertive description of what you want: *"I would like you . . .".*

For example, "When you watch television in our bedroom late at night, that affects my sleep and I feel frustrated and undermined. I would like you to read a book instead, or watch television in the living room" or "When you bring home fast-food for dinner, that derails my diet goals and I feel undervalued and upset. I would like you to stop bringing unhealthy foods home". This is just one of a number of assertiveness techniques that people can be taught when negotiating change with others (Speed, Goldstein & Goldfried, 2018).

In summary, it is important to assess core skills among the target group and deliver matching skills training (where skills are poor or absent) to improve the effectiveness of behaviour-change interventions.

FOCUS BOX 9.1

IBM-based intervention targeting identified deficits

In an intervention designed to reduce the risk of HIV infection amongst college students, Fisher et al. (1996) included intervention components to address deficits in information, motivation and skills identified in elicitation research amongst US college students. Some of the targets they identified and the methods they used to achieve them are considered below.

Information Component: A slide show and large group discussion presented and consolidated information on HIV transmission and prevention, the risk from different sexual behaviours, the effectiveness of condoms, where to buy condoms near campus, safer sex decision-making rules, HIV testing, and facts and myths about HIV/AIDS.

Motivation Component: Small-group discussions led by a peer educator, followed by large group discussions led by a professional health educator and incorporating a video narrated by HIV positive individuals were designed to provide persuasive arguments targeting key cognitions. In particular, perceptions of personal susceptibility to HIV and attitudes and subjective norms relating to condom use were targeted.

Skills Component: Negotiation self-efficacy was enhanced using peer-led role plays demonstrating safer sex communication. Students were encouraged by educators to practice safer sexual behaviours (e.g. condom handling skills and negotiation role playing) at home. Perceived effectiveness of condom use and self-efficacy in relation to condom use were bolstered by using a video in which peers modelled correct handling and use. In addition, group discussions were used to identify potential problems and reinforce newly-learned negotiation skills.

After you finish reading this chapter return to this focus box and think about other intervention components that could have been included in this intervention.

Targeting feelings and fear to change behaviour

Many health promotion interventions target what we believe, that is, our cognitions. Others target how we feel. For example, by prompting people to anticipate the regret they may feel if they do not act we may be able to facilitate the translation of motivation into action (Abraham & Sheeran, 2003). Similarly, by teaching people how to use if-then plans to respond to their feelings we may be able to empower them to protect themselves from undermining feelings. Sheeran, Aubrey and Kellett (2007) instructed people to make if-then plans to control anxiety about attendance at initial psychotherapy appointments. Participants were promoted to resolve that, "As soon as I feel concerned about attending my appointment, I will ignore that feeling and tell myself this is perfectly understandable". This instruction constitutes a cognitive skill intervention that limits the impact of anxiety on future plans. This simple and easy to administer intervention, resulted in 75% attendance in the intervention condition compared to 63% in the no-intervention control group. This is an important and potentially cost-saving outcome for such a simple planning intervention. People can also be taught to use such plans to bolster self-efficacy and effort during goal striving. For example, 'If I feel I cannot manage my goal, I will remember that I have been successful before and redouble my efforts to succeed".

In a meta-analysis of 306 experimental studies of interventions designed to change emotional responses, Webb, Miles & Sheeran (2012) highlighted the potential effectiveness of distraction techniques ($d = .27$) and suppression of expression of emotion (as in Sheeran et al., 2007) ($d = .32$) but not suppression of experience of emotion. Using perspective taking to reappraise emotional experiences was found to be effective ($d = .45$). These findings suggest that further elicitation and experimental research is needed to optimise intervention strategies that focus on feelings (Conner, Williams & Rhodes, 2020).

Inducing fear to change behaviour

Public health campaigns frequently deploy messages which highlight health risk and health threat and then recommend protective action. Such campaigns can be based on the Health Belief Model and Protection Motivation Theory. Some of these interventions are designed to frighten the target audience. These are fear appeals.

In their meta-analysis of 127 papers, Tannenbaum et al. (2015) concluded that fear appeals promote change in attitudes, intentions and behaviours, showing average small to medium effect sizes ($d = .29$). They also conclude that fear appeals are more effective when messages also target perceived efficacy (that is the belief that the recommended action will protect from the threat), emphasise susceptibility and severity and when one-time-only (not repeated) action is required. So, fear appeals work optimally in very specific circumstances.

Another meta-analytic review, of six studies that assessed both susceptibility and efficacy beliefs, (Peters, Ruiter & Kok, 2013) concluded that interventions emphasising threat alone (that is, perceived severity of consequences) were only effective when perceived efficacy (that is, the belief that the recommended action would protect effectively) was strong. This study also concluded that interventions that promote efficacy are more effective when the gravity of the threat is acknowledged. These findings strongly imply that elicitation research is needed before deploying fear appeals. For example, how does a health threat emphasising the severity of lung cancer work among current smokers who have low self-efficacy in relation to quitting? Peters et al. (2013)

suggest that such interventions could backfire because, if the smoker sees no possibility of quitting, then the campaign may raise anxiety which may encourage further smoking. This is, of course, very different to promoting a vaccine which has been shown to be effective and is readily available to a targeted population, especially since this only requires occasional responses.

Protection Motivation Theory specifies that fear appeals should incorporate threat and efficacy messages emphasising perceived susceptibility and severity as well as the effectiveness of the recommended protection and self-efficacy enhancement. Collectively, these messages should prompt protective intentions. Such threat-inducing messages can enhance systematic processing of subsequent messages (as might be expected because of enhanced personal relevance – see ELM in Chapter 8). For example, Das et al. (2003) found that fear appeals generated favourable cognitive responses and consequent attitude change if participants felt susceptible to the threat (see too Witte & Allen, 2000). One limitation of this approach is that fear appeals may miss cognitions that are strongly correlated with the target behaviour. For example, if normative beliefs about others' approval are important to young vapers and these are not targeted by an anti-vaping campaign, a core component of vaping motivation may be missed. So, as well as fully deploying Protection Motivation Theory, fear appeals may need to be based on wider more integrative theories to effectively target the underpinnings of motivation in particular target groups.

Fear appeals may also fail to persuade. Two types of failure have been identified. First, if people are not persuaded that the threat is relevant to them this may undermine attitudes towards the recommended preventive action. For example, target recipients think, "this is relevant to other people but not to me". Second, if people do not believe they can protect themselves (i.e., they have low self-efficacy) they tend to protect themselves psychologically through defensive cognitive responses (see Chapter 8 on reactance and Chapter 5 on coping). When defensive processing (sometimes called fear control) occurs, then recipients may dismiss the message as untrustworthy – rejecting it altogether – or rejecting its relevance to them (Ruiter, Abraham & Kok, 2001). When perceived efficacy and self-efficacy are more salient than perceived threat (e.g. "I know I can protect myself against the threat") then positive motivational and behavioural change are likely. However, when self-efficacy is weak ("it's a threat I cannot manage") then coping is likely to be defensive. So, fear appeals need to incorporate a strong and persuasive threat, that is, perceived severity information (to affect subsequent processing) as well as strong efficacy and self-efficacy messages if they are to be effective (Witte, 1992; Witte & Allen, 2000; Peters et al., 2013). Note too that the framing of risk awareness messages can be important (see Chapter 8).

Self-affirmation and fear appeals

The emotional impact of threat messages may be reduced by affirming the person before the message. "Self-affirmation" reduces the need to defend the self against threat and so may promote message acceptance. For example, one might prompt message recipients to think about positive aspects of themselves. Affirmed participants have been found to be more convinced by threat information and more willing to accept risk or severity of threat (Steele, 1988). For example, in a study conducted by Harris and Napper (2005) male participants in a self-affirmation condition wrote about their most important value, why it was important and how it affected their everyday lives. Participants engaging in health-risk alcohol consumption who had been affirmed in this way reported greater ease of imagining developing breast cancer and higher perceptions of personal risk, suggesting that self-affirmation facilitated acceptance of personal risk (by reducing defensive processing). These high-risk, self-affirmed participants were found to have greater intentions to reduce their alcohol consumption at four-week follow up, compared to controls. In a very similar way, it appears that, by enhancing self-efficacy before presenting threat information, can facilitate acceptance of threatening messages (Floyd et al., 2000). Functional magnetic resonance imaging (fMRI) tracking neural processes associated with affirmation during exposure to potentially threatening health messages indicates that self-affirmation may change how our brains respond to threatening messages (Falk et al., 2015) suggesting that affirmation of core values may have positive effects by empowering at-risk individuals to acknowledge the self-relevance and value of threatening messages.

Here too elicitation research is required to provide clear insights into the responsiveness of different target groups. Examining the effects of self-affirmation on older teenagers before they were presented with messages highlighting heart-disease consequences of not exercising for 60 minutes a day, Good, Harris, Jessop and Abraham (2015) found that self-affirmation had different effects on sub-groups. For relatively inactive participants, self-affirmation was associated with increased persuasion. However, for those who were moderately active (but still not meeting recommendations), self-affirmation led to less persuasion. So, while self-affirmation can increase the acceptance of health threat messages, for some people, the open-mindedness it induces may decrease persuasion. Making assumptions without elicitation research can lead to ineffective or even counter-productive interventions.

FOCUS BOX 9.2

Promoting smoking cessation

The illustrations below are typical of those used in many anti-smoking campaigns (including those used on cigarette packets). How do these materials correspond to PMT specifications?

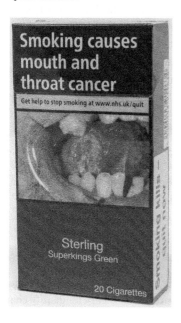
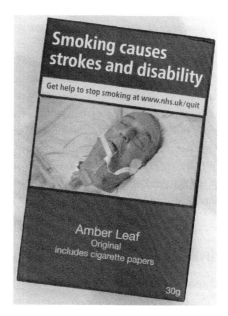

Most smokers want to give up and have tried to quit so motivation is not usually the main barrier to behaviour change. Instead, most smokers feel low self-efficacy in relation to quitting. The materials shown above do not help bolster smokers' self-efficacy so smokers may dismiss them (e.g. "that won't happen to me") resulting in no health benefit. Compare these to the "Get Unhooked" campaign below. This appeal offered smokers help by first acknowledging how unpleasant being "hooked" on cigarettes was and by promising help in quitting.

Given what you know about fear appeals and smoking which approach would is most worth pursuing and how would you design appropriate elicitation research?

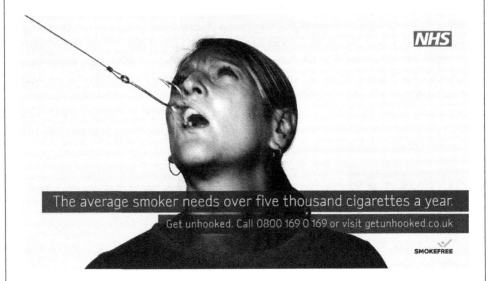

Smoking cessation also illustrates the biopsychosocial nature of health-related behaviour. Evidence suggests that participation in smoking cessation groups which employ verbal persuasion as well as teaching self-management skills increases the chances of successful quitting and abstinence over six months. Moreover, because of the nicotine-based dependency helping maintain smoking, use of nicotine replacement therapy Zyban (Bupropion hydrochloride which dampens appetite) is also effective. However, the most effective treatment is the combination of behaviour cessation groups and either nicotine replacement therapy or Zyban. This combination has been found to increase successful six-month abstinence rates fourfold over those among smokers who receive no help (West, McNeill & Raw, 2000). By taking account of a variety of key cognitive determinants, important self-management and social skills and critical biochemical processes, a package of intervention components can be combined to tackled complex and difficult-to-change behaviours.

Identifying change components in intervention design

Specification of change mechanisms is crucial to the advance of any science. When we develop a theory that can predict cognition, emotion or behaviour, we can use that theory to identify change mechanisms and test whether we can induce changes that corresponds to theoretically-specified mechanisms by conducting experiments. See, for example, the application of cognitive dissonance theory in Box 9.3. When such experiments show that our theory-based manipulation creates predicted changes then we have identified a potentially effective approach to behaviour change.

FOCUS BOX 9.3

Using cognitive dissonance to promote condom use

Cognitive dissonance theory proposes that we are strongly motivated to avoid and eradicate contradictions in our world views. Consequently, it should be possible to motivate change by generating salient contradictions between beliefs and actions. In an experiment conducted by Stone, Aronson, Crain, Winslow and Fried (1994) participants were randomly allocated to one of four conditions: (1) receiving information about condom use (information only); (2) receiving information and giving a talk promoting condom use that might be used in school health education (commitment); (3) being made aware of past failures to use condoms by recalling these failures (failure awareness) and (4) a combination of the commitment and failure awareness conditions. All participants were then given an opportunity to buy condoms cheaply. As Figure 9.3 shows, significantly more people in the combined commitment and failure awareness condition bought condoms (82%) than in the failure awareness condition (50%) or the commitment condition (34%). The study also emphasised that information alone is often not enough to prompt behaviour change because significantly fewer people in the information only condition bought condoms (44%). This study illustrates how, applying cognitive dissonance theory, a cognitive contrast was created between people's representation of health protective action (which they were committed to by becoming an advocate of condom use for school students) and their own riskier health behaviour.

Can you think of applications of this approach to behaviour change? How would you use such cognitive contrasts in a behaviour change intervention?

Cognitive Dissonance Promotes Condom use.

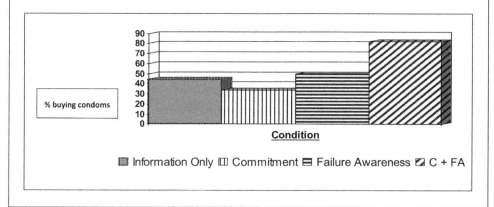

Imagine we want to increase people's self-efficacy (see Chapter 8) in relation to cooking tasty meals using fresh vegetables. Following Bandura's advice, we might show participants a video of someone like themselves preparing such a meal (providing vicarious experience) and use persuasive statements, providing instruction and telling them that this is easy, and that they, and people like them, can learn how to do this quickly. We would then want to test: (1) whether the intervention changed self-efficacy (so confirming our proposed change mechanism), (2) that, e.g. over the next month, intervention participants cooked more vegetarian meals than a randomly assigned no-intervention control group (i.e., the intervention changed behaviour) and (3) that, within the intervention group, changes in self-efficacy were predictive of vegetarian cooking, that is, self-efficacy mediated the intervention effect (see Research Methods Box 3.1 on mediation and moderation effects). If all three hypotheses were supported by experimental results, we would have developed a theoretically-based, potentially-effective intervention with a clearly explained change mechanism. This is the basis of an experimental approach developing a science of behaviour change Rothman and Sheeran (2021) advocate such an experimental approach and also consider moderator effects. These might include the type of behaviour and the degree of behaviour change attempted, the type of intervention delivery and the context (e.g. how and where the intervention is delivered) as well as target population characteristics (e.g. socioeconomic, gender or personality characteristics). Such an integrated theoretical framework underpinning by experimental research can generate the evidence needed to optimise the effectiveness of behaviour-change interventions

Abraham & Michie (2008) developed a list of 26 categories of "change techniques." These were generated by categorising the content of 195 interventions to promote physical activity, as described in published evaluation studies. In general, these categories could be identified reliability by independent coders by reading the intervention descriptions. The aim of this work was to lay the foundations for a consensual set of definitions of approaches to behaviour change that would guide behaviour-change practitioners in the design and description of behaviour-change interventions. As the authors note, "a common terminology in terms of which intervention content can be understood and compared across interventions, behavioural domains, and research teams. . . . would clarify links between inclusion of techniques and theory-specified change processes" (p.385). This remains an important aim for scientists working towards a science of behaviour change.

Many similar listings have been created. There are three general problems with all current lists. First, while the listed categories are often referred to as "techniques", they are very rarely descriptions of "change techniques" that could be implemented and replicated. One of the 26 categories of "change techniques" identified by Abraham and Michie was named, "provide information on consequences". This was defined as providing information on the benefits and costs of action or inaction, that is, using messages describing what consequences are likely if a person does or does not act in a particular way. Abraham and Michie note that this type of change technique can be derived from a number of theories that specify attitude change as a precursor of motivation, including the Theory of Planned Behaviour, Social Cognitive Theory and the IMB. This approach has also been using predictive and experimental studies (e.g. Conner & Sparks, 2015; Hill et al., 2007; Norman et al., 2020 – see Chapter 7). Of course, this theory-based approach needs to be translated into clearly-defined, replicable techniques. How exactly will any particular health promotion campaign emphasise consequences (see our discussion of fear appeals above). Nonetheless, this is a useful category because it maps onto mechanisms of change specified by empirically-tested theory. We know that when target audiences are unaware of consequences then information high-lighting such consequences can change attitudes and, thereby, motivation and behaviour (see Sheeran et al., 2016, above, and Chapter 7). Elicitation research can be used to clarify what particular techniques and types of delivery (e.g. texts versus leaflets and what message sources) are likely to be most effective for particular audiences.

A second problem with these listings is that their authors often refer to them as "taxonomies". Yet unlike, taxonomies developed in other sciences, such as biology, there is usually no nesting of categories, beginning with broad categories and then specifying ever more specific descriptions of techniques. In general they are just lists of categories with little conceptual structure.

A third problem is that the mix of categories often contains quite different types of categories. Consider one of the most recent and comprehensive listings. Knittle et al. (2020) include 123 categories of change techniques. There is a lot of helpful advice in this paper such as suggestions to talk problems over with friends and family and there are some interesting ideas in this list. Nonetheless, the categories themselves are of quite different types and not linked to theory-based change mechanisms. The first technique category is "agenda mapping" and the last is "prayer". Does "agenda mapping" refer to the research on goal prioritisation in behaviour change (Conner, Wilding, Prestwich et al., 2022)? This is unclear. If we advise prayer then what psychological changes (and, therefore, benefits for the person) are we expecting. Do we expect increased self-efficacy, higher self-esteem or mood change? There is no link between these categories and psychological change mechanisms.

Other categories include, "adding objects to the environment" and "restructuring the physical environment". Is adding objects to the environment a sub-category of restructuring the physical environment and what kind of techniques, relying on what kind of mechanisms of change, do these categories refer to? If someone wears a step-counting watch to monitor their physical activity does that count as "an object"? As Presseau, Ivers, Newham, Knittle, Danko and Grimshaw (2015) reported when trying to apply such categories that, "there may be a need to characterise what specifically is 'restructured' and/or 'added' to be helpful in replication efforts" (p.8). In other words, we need much more "technique" specific categories if we want to develop potentially testable behaviour-change techniques.

Finally, Knittle et al. (2020) also list "credible source" as a category of change techniques. We know that credibility of message sources is important to the impact they have on target audiences (see Chapter 8). So, highlighting this point is useful but this is not a category of types of techniques. Any technique involving persuasive communication can be delivered by a more or less credible source. Therefore, this is a different kind of category. It refers to one aspect of optimising the effectiveness of persuasive messages. It does not refer to a set of techniques.

Developing integrated theoretical framework supported by experimental evidence that specifies change mechanisms that can be precisely targeted by specified change techniques is the basis of any science and is much needed in health psychology. This remains a critical challenge for future health psychology research (Hagger, Cameron, Hamilton, Hankonen & Lintunen, 2020). Unfortunately, there is much work to be done to translate available listings of categories of techniques into such an integrated, theoretically-coherent framework linked to change mechanisms.

In summary, health psychology needs a detailed categorisation of psychological change mechanisms based on an integrated theoretical framework. This could provide a foundation for a precisely-defined, theoretical and evidence-based categorisation of change technique types that can be used to prompt psychological and behaviour changes. Other scientific disciplines, including biology, illustrate how such taxonomies can be developed.

Accurate and detailed reporting of intervention designs

An experimental science of behaviour change will require examination of intervention content in detail to identify unique techniques applied and identification of change mechanisms. This means that, as in other sciences, health psychologists need to keep detailed manuals describing all evaluated interventions. This is essential to replication and to accumulation theoretical understanding across experiments. Unfortunately, there are problems with the reporting of behaviour-change evaluations in the social science literature. Detailed descriptions of the interventions and their implementation are often unavailable. Indeed, many published intervention descriptions focus primarily on modes of delivery or the type of person delivering the intervention (Davidson et al., 2003), rather than the techniques employed. Descriptions such as "counselling sessions", "classes", "discussion groups", "peer-led laboratories", give no indication of the change techniques included. Comparisons of intervention descriptions published in peer reviewed journals and detailed manuals suggest that perhaps a third of technique types are omitted from published descriptions, suggesting that we cannot understand the content and design of behaviour change interventions from the current scientific literature (Abraham & Michie, 2008). In addition, process evaluations revealing the mechanisms by which interventions generate their effects, and for whom, are often not conducted. This undermines the possibility of replication and limits our understanding of the mechanisms involved. Abraham Johnson, de Bruin and Luszczynska (2014) discuss these problems and provide advice to the editors of scientific journals on how such reporting problems can be resolved. They draw on recommendations made by an international group of behaviour change scholars constituting the Workgroup for Intervention Development and Evaluation Research (WIDER); work that built on recommendations by Davidson et al. (2003). Albrecht et al. (2013) have developed a checklist to assess the quality of reporting of interventions using these recommendations.

Developing and evaluating behaviour-change interventions

In this section we briefly consider key methodological aspects of designing, refining, implementing and evaluating behaviour-change interventions. We focus on ten tasks defined and discussed by Abraham and Denford (2020) based on the Intervention Mapping Framework (Bartholomew Eldredge et al., 2016). These are presented in Table 9.1.

Working through these tasks necessitates careful planning, consultation and pre-testing, followed by design refinement and gradual scale-up towards widespread use. Different types of research can generate the evidence needed at each stage. Exploratory or elicitation research, is required at the beginning when needs are being assessed and the key challenges defined. As we have discussed, it is important to know what the target audience believes and what they want to know. Epidemiological and medical research may also be important when prioritising change targets (see tasks 1 and 3). Again, as we have discussed, experimental psychological research is essential to tasks 4 and 5. Detailed qualitative and observational research is likely to facilitate intervention pre-testing and refinement. Then, of course, we need to evaluate interventions to discover if they have the potential

Table 9.1   Ten tasks involved in the design, development, implementation and evaluation of behaviour-change interventions

1. Understand and define the problem (including assessing the needs of target groups).
2. Clarify how behaviour change can ameliorate or resolve the problem.
3. Identify which group/s of people need to change which behaviours, or behaviour patterns, and at what level.
4. Understand behavioural antecedents (that is, change mechanisms), including the contexts and cues that prompt targeted behaviour patterns for each targeted group.
5. Design interventions/intervention components that can alter some, or all, of these behavioural antecedents and regulatory mechanisms.
6. Pilot, or pre-test, intervention prototypes to discover whether they are acceptable, feasible and affordable.
7. Refine and develop the intervention with those who will implement and experience it to optimise fidelity of implementation and effectiveness.
8. Implement the intervention and identify and minimise embedding problems.
9. Evaluate efficacy by investigating whether the intervention shows evidence of changing targeted antecedents and behaviours.
10. Evaluate effectiveness by testing the intervention in new contexts and scaling up to target new groups or populations.

to change behaviour (efficacy evaluation) and if they can change behaviour at-scale, that is, have public health implications (effectiveness evaluation) (tasks 6–10). Finally, research into how interventions have their effects is critical to implementation and transfer of interventions form one context to another (tasks 7–9).

Intervention planning

The process of planning interventions and managing them from design, through implementation to evaluation is complex. The first step is a *needs assessment* which involves ascertaining if and how a target group need to change and precisely specifying the target behaviour. This is not always easy. We have noted the high costs of increasing obesity at a global level. Those who are overweight have increased morbidity and mortality risks which greatly increases demand for, and cost of, health services. Tasks 1 and 2 are relatively easy to define, but task 3 presents challenges. Who should be targeted and at what level (see Figure 9.2)? It might be important to prioritise those most in need (e.g. those who are most obese), or those with high blood glucose levels who, through sustained behaviour change can avoid diabetes. Or, perhaps we should target children and their parents. Should we focus on national legislation, community-based interventions to make healthy food affordable or on health promotion targeting individual responsibility? Should governments be "lobbied" to change the content of food and drink products or ensure improved labelling? Should communities be empowered to change how take-away outlets prepare food products (Hillier-Brown et al., 2017), or should restaurants and bars be helped to make some foods and drinks more prominent or available? Should schools be helped to promote new dietary and physical activity habits among children (Lloyd et al., 2018)? Or, perhaps, greater participation in physical activity should be promoted through work place changes (Abraham & Graham-Rowe, 2009). See Activity Box 1. In each case different challenges arise but to tackle this problem we need to consider multiple interventions that are carefully planned and evaluated across levels.

ACTIVITY BOX 9.1

How can we help people change their diet?

In 2017, it is estimated that 11 million years of life were lost to due to premature mortality caused by poor diet across 195 countries (GBD 2017 Diet Collaborators, 2019). How would you design behaviour change interventions to improve the diet of the UK population? Consider the models discussed in Chapter 7, the psychology of persuasion discussed in Chapter 8 as well as the social–ecological model and the ten-step model discussed in this chapter.

Tasks 4 and 5 ideally result in a "logic model" (Moore et al., 2015) that clarifies the aims of the intervention, the theory-defined mechanisms it targets (perhaps at different levels, see Figure 9.2), as well as the intervention techniques that are intended to directly impact those mechanisms. In addition, we need to specify interim changes (the anticipated mediators e.g. self-efficacy) as well as the targeted outcomes (e.g. a change in cooking and eating behaviour patterns). A logic model is not a theory but a bespoke map of what an intervention is designed to change and how it will work. There are many components to a logic model (McLaughlin & Jordan, 1999; Kellogg Foundation, 2004). At the simplest level, a logic model would define change mechanisms (e.g. a fear-based communication) that would lead to anticipated interim changes such as enhanced susceptibility, increased perceived severity of risks and increased self-efficacy in relation to avoidance of risk which would be, tested by mediation analyses and, for example, lead to increased likelihood of attending for vaccination.

Once the intervention is designed, it will need refinement in collaboration with those who will deliver it and those who will receive it. If such piloting and refinement research is not undertaken the intervention may never be used. So, tasks 6, 7 and 8 are critical to the development of interventions that can make a difference to health. For example, how do young adults with type 2 diabetes respond to information about the potential blindness and the importance of retinopathy screening (Lake et al., 2018)? Such stakeholder involvement in the refinement of interventions before implementation is critical to ensuring potential effectiveness (Hudson et al., 2020; Luszczynska et al., 2020).

Intervention evaluation

Initial evaluation may be conducted using qualitative interviews to establish whether individuals benefited form an intervention and how this worked. Then small trials may assess efficacy, that is the potential to induce behaviour change. Finally, at-scale randomised controlled trials are needed to establish whether an intervention has the capacity to enhance public health and to establish the cost effectiveness of the intervention (Cockcroft, 2019). See Sandhu et al. (2023) in further reading for an illustration. Randomisation can control for confounding variables but sometimes it is necessary to randomise at group level (e.g. randomising schools, classes, doctors' surgeries etc.). In these cases, a statistical technique known as multi-level modeling can control for systematic biases that might pre-exist between groups (e.g. some classes happen to be more active than others).

Where randomisation is impossible, matched groups need to be carefully scrutinised to ensure that differences other than exposure to the intervention are not responsible for observed group differences. Note too that inclusion of groups which do not complete pre-intervention measures can control for the mere measurement effect (see Chapter 7). Many excellent guidelines for the design, ethics, and conduct of RCTs are available (e.g. Deaton & Cartwright, 2018).

For successful interventions, an effect size can be calculated (e.g. a *d* value) to indicate how effective the intervention was. Anticipating the likely effect size is important to conducting a pre-evaluation power analysis. This is necessary to ensure enough participants are included to detect any change that the intervention generates. In calculating power and in interpreting observed post-intervention differences attrition rates (i.e., number of participants who drop out of the study) need to be considered. For example, if an intervention requires persistence and 50% of those in the intervention group drop out then, even if the intervention is very successful amongst the 50% who persist (compared to no-intervention controls) the overall impact of this intervention will be limited. Intention-to-treat analysis is recommended in such instances. This approach includes all randomised participants in the analyses and counts drop outs as showing no change. Note what a difference this makes when attrition in the intervention group is high.

Validated measures of behaviour are required to evaluate behaviour-change interventions (e.g. condom use or exercise levels). In addition, psychological measures are needed to track and understand change mechanisms. These include psychological determinants theorised to be involved in the change process upon which the design is based (e.g. measures of attitudes, normative beliefs). If expected changes in such determinants occur in a successful intervention then the inclusion of these measures allows *mediation analyses* to be conducted, thereby testing whether the theoretical account of change mechanisms is supported by evidence.

Interventions may be differentially successful for different groups (e.g. men versus women or those high in conscientiousness verses those low in this trait). Such *moderation* analyses can tell us for whom the intervention was effective but again require appropriate pre-intervention power analysis. Finally, health outcome measures (such as weight loss or STI rates) are valuable to check the hypothesised link between behaviour change and health enhancement. For example, behaviour-change interventions focusing on increasing physical activity or promoting a healthy diet may weight participants in intervention and control groups before and after interventions (e.g. Luszczynska *et al.*, 2007).

When an intervention is *not* effective, it is important to know whether it failed because it was not capable of generating the predicted effects (and mediation analyses can help clarify this) or because it was not delivered as designed (e.g. classes were not taught as described in the manual or participants did not read or attend the intervention). To answer this question a *process evaluation* is required (Moore et al., 2015). This involves examining whether the intervention is being delivered as intended *during* the delivery. This is referred to as fidelity analysis (see e.g. Lambert et al., 2017). For example, those delivering and receiving the intervention may be interviewed and surveyed regarding their experience of the intervention. Classes or intervention groups may be observed and examined for fidelity to design, that is, whether those delivering the intervention (e.g. teachers or nurses) are doing what the intervention designers planned. If, for example, an intervention is found to have worked for some groups but not others and it is also observed that the difference between groups was fidelity of delivery then it would be clear that the intervention works – but only when delivered strictly according to prepared manuals. Process evaluations establish the context in which an intervention can be effective, the change mechanisms that it impacts and how it is implemented in practice and how well the implementation matches the intervention plan. Without process evaluations, we cannot, for example, distinguish between failure of impact and failure of delivery.

Evaluating utility and sustainability of interventions

Even well-designed, effective, competently-evaluated interventions may have little impact on health if they are not adopted by their target audience or incorporated into routine care by health-care professionals. To be adopted, interventions need to be useful to adopters, easy to implement, sustainable and affordable in the setting in which they have been tested. Glasgow, Bull, Gillette, Klesges and Dzewaltowski (2002) and Green and Glasgow (2006) discuss how we can evaluate these intervention features using the RE-AIM (reach, effectiveness, adoption, implementation and maintenance) framework (discussed by Luszczynska et al., 2020).

Reach refers to how many of the target population were involved in an evaluation and how representative they were. For example, if an intervention was evaluated using economically advantaged participants then questions would arise as to whether it would also be effective for economically less advantaged people – or, for example, with those with more severe health problems. *Effectiveness* relates to the range of effects an intervention might have. For example, even if it changed behaviour – did it enhance overall quality of life or have any unintended consequences (e.g. did participants find it onerous or upsetting)? *Adoption* refers to whether the users (e.g. nurses, teachers, managers, members of the public) are persuaded of the utility of the intervention. This is likely to depend on how easy it is to implement, whether they or their clients like it and whether it is compatible with their other main goals (Paulussen, Kok & Schaalma, 1994). For example, interventions are unlikely to be used if adopters cannot afford them. Understanding this adoption and diffusion process is critical to the overall impact of any intervention (Rogers, 2003). *Implementation* refers to the ease and feasibility of faithful delivery. If an intervention is complex, expensive or requires specialist training or teams of people to deliver it then it is less likely to be sustainable in real-world settings. *Maintenance* refers to the longer term sustainability of the intervention in real-world settings. For example, if an organisation or community does not have the resources to deliver an intervention then, no matter how effective, it will be dropped over time. Similarly, if implementation problems are encountered then even if the intervention is retained it may be changed and adapted to the setting which may mean altering change techniques critical to its initial effectiveness, so rendering it ineffective. These practical, real-world considerations are as important as observed *d* values, if health behaviour change is to impact population health.

Beyond individual behaviour-change interventions

Social influences on health behaviours operate at different levels.

Psychologists tend to focus on the individual processes involved in behaviour change but behaviour change is embedded in, and must be understood in terms of social context. Bartholomew, Parcel, Kok and Gottlieb (2006) advocated a "social ecological" model (p.9) of change which includes individual and social determinants of behaviour and recognises different levels of intervention (see Figure 9.2). These levels include individual behaviour change (the focus of this chapter), interpersonal behaviour change (including how relationships change can be managed, see e.g. assertiveness training), organisational change and community change. Ruiter, Crutzen, de Leeuw & Kok

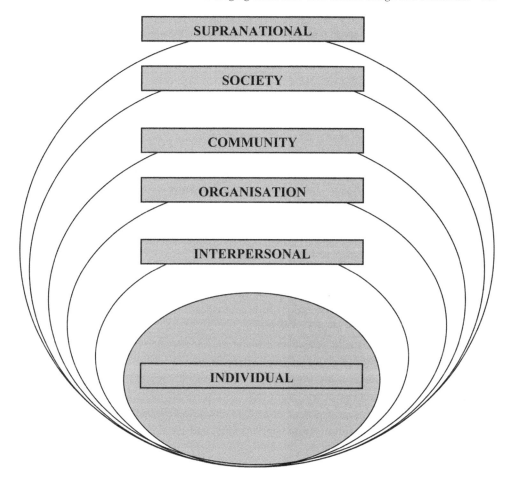

Figure 9.2   The Social Ecological model: Levels of behaviour-change intervention (Bartholomew et al., 2006)

(2020) use this model to argue convincingly that interventions operating at these different levels may need to draw upon theories explaining change mechanisms operating at different levels. So change technique types need to be categorised, not only at the individual level but also at intrapersonal (for example, changing how relationships are managed), organisational and community levels.

Organisational interventions include changing policies and practices to increase productivity or improve the safety, health, or quality of life of employees (Nielsen, Randall, Holten & González, 2010) as well as attempts to change individual behaviour through organisational change, including worksite interventions (Abraham & Graham-Rowe, 2009) and school-based interventions (Denford, Abraham, Campbell & Busse 2017). An understanding of intergroup processes and organisational change is needed to design and implement such interventions (see e.g. Pearson et al., 2015 for a discussion of school-based, health promotion interventions). Organisational rules, norms and resources may create stress (see Chapter 4) and impede health-related behaviour change. Consequently, worksite interventions may, for example, aim to integrate physical activity into employees' days including exercise breaks and promotion of walking and stair use or change the availability of healthy food and/or how food is labelled (e.g. Engbers et al., 2005). Worksite interventions focusing on exercise have been found to be effective in increasing physical activity and fitness as well as promoting weight loss among participants (King, Carl, Birkel & Haskell, 1988; Proper et al., 2003).

We saw in Chapter 4 how relative poverty arising from the distribution of wealth within a country can affect health. The management of taxation and benefit systems have large effects on health and longevity within countries (Wilkinson, 1996). Such change requires action by legislators. Consequently, in certain cases, effective health promotion necessitates lobbying politicians and legislators and presenting the results of research to decision makers in government. For example, in the UK in 2007, smoking in public places was banned and it became illegal to sell tobacco to people below the age of 18 years. Evaluating a similar legislative change, Sargent, Shepard and Glantz (2004) found that myocardial infarction admissions to a hospital in Montana, USA fell significantly over six months during a smoking ban in public places, while at the same time, surrounding areas (without a smoking ban) experienced non-significant increases. Of course, we may also need international legalisation because taxation in one country is unlikely to effective if unhealthy products can easily be imported from other countries.

Lack of resources, lack of skills and social norms at community level can also sustain health risk behaviours. Consequently, interventions to promote health behaviours need to be based in, and engage, communities. This involves meetings and discussion with local people and organisations. It may also entail persuading local government to change policies, enforce existing legislation or provide new resources. In addition, such interventions may utilise local media campaigns and educational programmes. This work merges health psychology practice with community development work. Community development seeks to involve people in identifying local assets and needs and facilitating action to create or acquire new resources and/or skills. It is based on choice and participation and aims to extend opportunities and social justice for people in particular communities.

Community interventions to promote health behaviours may target specific behaviours or a range of related behaviours. For example, such interventions might target buying more fruit and vegetables and could involve campaigns to establish a local fresh produce market and/or the provision of vouchers to make healthier products more affordable to poorer people. In Chapter 8, we considered the UK Expert Patient Programme (EPP), which, while implemented nationally, targets those with chronic illness in particular communities. More comprehensive interventions may target a range of health-related behaviours. For example, the North Karelia Project which began in Finland in 1972 included education on smoking, diet and hypertension using widely distributed leaflets, radio and television slots and education in local organisations. Voluntary sector organisations, schools and health and social services were involved and training was provided for personnel in various contexts. The intervention included education of school students about the health risks of smoking and the social influences which lead young people to begin smoking as well as training for students in how to resist such social influences. This comprehensive intervention was found to be effective on a range of indices including reduction in smoking and serum cholesterol levels. For example, 15 years later, smoking prevalence was 11% lower amongst intervention participants compared to controls (Vartiainen, Paavola, McAlister & Puska, 1998).

In a review of evaluations of comprehensive community interventions (including the North Karelia Project), Hingson and Howland (2002) found that greater effectiveness was observed when interventions: (1) targeted behaviours with immediate health consequences such as alcohol misuse or sexual risk taking; (2) targeted young people to prevent uptake of health-risk behaviours; (3) combined environmental and institutional policy change with theory-based behaviour-change interventions and (4) involved communities themselves in intervention design.

We have seen the important role that social support can play in moderating stress (in Chapter 5). Interpersonal processes are often critical to prompting and sustaining individual behaviour change. Behaviour change motivation can be undermined when it is disapproved of or resisted by valued others, including family members or opinion leaders. Consequently, additional social support can enhance the effectiveness of interventions both in initiating and maintaining behaviour change. For example, planning how barriers to change may be overcome or the signing of behavioural contracts are change techniques which are facilitated by interpersonal interaction. Moreover, community and worksite interventions (e.g. EPP) may provide social support by establishing buddy systems or support groups in which two or more people work together to support initiation and/or maintenance of behaviour change. Thus, establishing how interpersonal processes influence a target behaviour and assessing skills in managing relevant social interactions and available social support is important when designing interventions (e.g. consider the focus on resisting social influence included in the North Karelia Project).

The social ecological model of behaviour change emphasises that a critical step in planning individual-level behaviour-change interventions, is an assessment of the levels at which social and societal change mechanisms shape individual behaviour patterns (Ruiter et al., 2020). Without such assessment, interventions may not target the most relevant or influential antecedents of the target behaviour. These may differ across groups defined, for example, in terms of socioeconomic status, age, gender, ethnicity or culture. Such assessments may highlight the need to intervene at individual, interpersonal, organisational, community, national, or even international levels to change mechanisms that sustain health-compromising behaviours.

Key terms introduced in Chapter 9 (in order of appearance)

- Change mechanisms.
- Traffic-light labelling.
- PACE labelling.
- Information Motivation and Behavioural skills model.
- Elicitation research.
- Self-management skills.
- Motor skills.
- Social skills.
- Fear appeals.
- Social-ecological model of change.
- Needs assessment.
- Multi-level modelling.
- Intention-to-treat analysis.
- RE-AIM framework.
- Intervention development.
- Process and outcome evaluation.

Summary of main points addressed in Chapter 9

A health psychology perspective on changing behaviour involves needs assessment including analyses of the social process affecting a behaviour as well as the motivational and skills and information, motivational and skills deficits among the target population. Theories, supported by predictive evidence that specify relevant change mechanisms are crucial to selection of appropriate change technique types, combined in multi-technique interventions. These need to be delivered using audience-appropriate materials, developed though collaboration with those who will deliver ad receive interventions. Interventions need to be evaluated for efficacy and effectiveness and, using process evaluations, to assess the validity of theoretical understandings of change mechanisms that can lead to behaviour change.

Illustrative group exercises (e.g., over two class sessions)

Choose a health behaviour (e.g., dietary change) and design an evidence-based intervention to promote this behaviour amongst a specific target group. See Activity Box 9.1.

Draft a plan on how to intervene to enhance fitness amongst employees in a desk-based organisation. Identify the defining features of your intervention and draw upon the ten-task framework.

Select a set of (e.g. ten) published intervention evaluations and assess them in terms of the quality of evaluation and RE-AIM criteria (reach, effectiveness, adoption, implementation, maintenance). On the basis of your analysis, how useful do you think these interventions are likely to be in improving health or healthcare practice?

Recommendations for further reading

Journal articles

Luszczynska, A., Szczuka, Z., Abraham, C., Baban, A., Brooks, S., Cipolletta, S., Danso, E., Dombrowski, S. U., Gan, Y., Gaspar, T., de Matos, M. G., Griva, K., Jongenelis, M. I., Keller, J., Knoll, N., Ma, J., Miah, M. A. A., Morgan, K., Peraud, W., Quintard, B. . . . Wolf, H. (2022). The interplay between strictness of policies and individuals' self-regulatory efforts: Associations with handwashing during the COVID-19 pandemic. *Annals of Behavioral Medicine, 56*(4), 368–380. https://doi.org/10.1093/abm/kaab102

O'Connor, D. B. (2020). The future of health behaviour change interventions: Opportunities for open science and personality research. *Health Psychology Review, 14*(1), 176–181. doi: 10.1080/17437199.2019. 1707107.

Sandhu, H. K., Booth, K., Furlan, A. D., Shaw, J., Carnes, D., Taylor, S. J. C., Abraham, C., Alleyne, S., Balasubramanian, S., Betteley, L., Haywood, K. L., Iglesias-Urrutia, C. P., Krishnan, S., Lall, R., Manca, A., Mistry, D., Newton, S., Noyes, J., Nichols, V., Padfield, E. . . . Underwood, M. (2023). Reducing opioid use for chronic pain with a group-based intervention: A randomized clinical trial. *JAMA, 329*(20), 1745–1756. https://doi.org/10.1001/jama.2023.6454

Books

Hagger, M., S., Cameron, L., D., Hamilton, K., Hankonen, N. & Lintunen, T. (2020, Eds.). *The handbook of behaviour change*. Cambridge: Cambridge University Press.

Chapters

Abraham C. & Denford S. (2020) Design, implementation and evaluation of behavior change interventions: A ten-task guide. In *The Cambridge handbook of behaviour change.* M Hagger & K Hamilton (Eds.) Cambridge University Press.

Ruiter, R., A., C., R., Crutzen, de Leeuv E. & Kok, G. (2020). Changing behaviour at the interpersonal, organizational community and societal levels. In *The Cambridge handbook of behaviour change.* M Hagger & K Hamilton (Eds.) Cambridge University Press.

Illustrative essay titles

1. How can health psychology inform the design of health promotion campaigns?
2. What works in health behaviour change interventions? Discuss with reference to empirical research.
3. What evidence-based, change techniques can health-behaviour change designers use in developing effective interventions?
4. How can health psychologists develop reliable and valid taxonomies of change mechanisms and change techniques?
5. How can organisational and policy interventions affect population health?

PART 5

Applied health psychology

10 Working with clients and patients

Working with clients and patients

Chapter plan

The chapter is divided into four sections.

1. Deciding to consult.
2. Adherence and concordance.
3. Managing consultations.
4. Health psychology in practice.

Learning outcomes

When you have completed this chapter you should be able to:

1. Discuss who is most likely to consult healthcare services and explain why.
2. Identify key predictors patient adherence and discuss how adherence can be maximised.
3. Describe key tasks that need to be completed during healthcare consultations with patients.
4. Identify key components of patient-centred consultations and discuss the findings of research into their effects on patients' wellbeing and health.
5. Identify the competencies that practising health psychologists need to demonstrate in order to provide safe and evidence-based services.

Deciding to consult

People frequently experience symptoms but do not consult health services. Estimates vary, but 50–75% of the population experience one or more symptoms of ill health in any two-week period (Demers, Altamore, Mustin, Kleinman & Leonardi, 1980; Porter, 2004). Yet, as Porter (2004) notes, about one third of these people do nothing about their symptoms, about one third self-medicate using over-the-counter medications or alternative therapies. Only about one-third

DOI: 10.4324/9781003171096-15

consult their medical practitioner. Even when healthcare is free at the point of delivery there is no one-to-one correspondence between symptom recognition and consultation. This is problematic because people who need healthcare may not seek help and so worsen their prognosis. Moreover, a substantial proportion of those who do consult have only minor symptoms which do not require medical intervention.

Why do people consult?

Consultation prompts have been identified (Porter, 2004; Zola, 1973). Unsurprisingly, these include symptoms that persist, especially if these are perceived to be serious and are believed to be amenable to treatment. Symptoms which interfere with important goals or are seen to reduce attractiveness, are also more likely prompt consultation. Advice from others is also an important trigger. Finally, ease of access to services and having time (e.g. away from work or child care) also makes consultation more likely. In a study of 1,210 people, Berkanovic Telesky, and Reeder (1981) found that 64% reported symptoms over one year. These researchers used multiple regression to discover which of a range of prompts were most strongly associated with consultations following symptom identification. Results showed that respondents who had greater numbers of long-term health problems, were older, had a regular doctor or had greater social support were more likely to consult ($rs = .02–.19$). However, consulting was most strongly predicted by advice to consult from a member of their social network ($r = .35$), the degree to which the symptom generated disability ($r = .31$), the perceived seriousness of the symptom ($r = .56$) and, especially, the perceived efficacy of care (that is, believing that medical intervention could alleviate or eradicate the symptoms ($r = .69$). This study was based on the health-belief model (see Chapter 7) but the results also support the theory of planned behaviour emphasising the role of social norms and the perceived benefits (or efficacy) of acting (that is, positive attitudes to towards consulting). The results also emphasise the role of social support in consulting behaviour and the importance of anticipation of consultation effectiveness, that is, will it make a difference to me?

Anticipated effectiveness of consultation is an important trigger for consultation as shown in a population study of people with serious breathing difficulties which compared people who had and had not consulted. Controlling for smoking status and perceived relative severity of symptoms, attribution of wheezing to smoking and lower self-efficacy in relation to explaining breathing difficulties to a doctor differentiated between those who did and did not consult (Abraham, Costa-Pereira, du V Florey & Ogston, 1999). The importance of perceived causation was also highlighted by King (1982) who found that understanding the causes of elevated blood pressure predicted whether or not people attended for screening. Beliefs about what causes symptoms and anticipation of helpful interactions with healthcare professionals are key determinants of health service use.

Symptoms are not always clear so patients may stuggle to understand what they mean. For example, Kendrick, Higgs, Whitfield and Laszlo (1993) found that, for 60% of asthmatic patients, there was no significant correlation between ratings of severity and simultaneous peak flow measurements (of lung capacity). This 60% were not characterised by less severe symptoms (as measured objectively by peak flow) or by age or gender. The researchers concluded that a large proportion of asthmatic patients cannot reliably detect changes in their lung function. Similarly, Cantillon et al. (1997) found that, among patients who believed they could predict changes in their blood pressure, there was no significant association between patients' assessments and clinical assessments. Confidence in the ability to predict was associated with higher anxiety. When symptoms are unclear our emotional responses to symptom detection are likely to be important to health-related action, including service usage.

It is important to understand patients' reasons for consulting a healthcare practitioner so a consultation can focus on what the patient hopes for and, therefore, be judged to be worthwhile by the patient. Asking a patient, "What can I do for you today?", is more than a polite greeting. It is an initial attempt to clarify what the patient expects from the consultation. If the purpose of the visit is simple and a treatment or advice is clear then this clarification can happen quickly and advice and prescription can follow quickly. Unfortunately, asking the patient what they expect may not always reveal their hoped-for outcomes. For example, if reassurance is what is wanted the patient may be reluctant to express this for fear of being seen to waste valuable professional time. So, a key element of healthcare consultations is to identify the *real purpose* of the visit; to discover what the patient was thinking when the made the appointment (Thorsen, Witt, Hollnagel & Malterud, 2001).

It is also useful to ask why people do *not* consult? Of course, sometimes we do not consult because we expect our problem to resolve itself without treatment. Encouraging people to make informed decisions *not* to consult is an important part of healthcare provision because this can reduce expensive but unnecessary consultations. Rondet, Parizot, Cadwallader, Lebas & Chauvin (2015) found that key barriers to consulting about depressive symptoms were concerns about the negative stigma associated with depression and fears about the negative consequences of relevant treatments. Accurate and credible health information, for example, on websites or phone lines can facilitate consultation and ensure that people identify symptoms that require treatment. Of course, people fear unpleasant or unwanted effects of consultation and have concerns about the cost of care and may struggle to make time within busy schedules (Taber, Leyvan & Persoskie, 2015). So, it is equally important to minimise such barriers so that those who need to consult can do so.

Interpretation of symptoms

Leventhal and colleagues (e.g. Leventhal et al., 1997; Leventhal, Nerenz & Steele, 1984) identified five broad dimensions within which beliefs about symptoms and illnesses can be categorised. First, *identity,* the way a symptom label is related to our perception of cause and has profound implications for how we respond. "Fatigue" or "stress" have very different connotations to "cancer". Second, *cause*, refers to our understanding of the processes generating symptoms. For example, "indigestion" has very different implications to "heart attack" and believing that symptoms are due to one's own behaviour may lead to reduced motivation to seek professional help. Third, beliefs about *consequences*, including the perceived severity of symptoms. Fourth, *timeline*, people's expectations regarding the duration of symptoms and their perceptions of whether symptoms (e.g. of diabetes or asthma) are chronic or acute can have important implications for health seeking and adherence. Finally, beliefs about *control and treatment effectiveness*, including, for example, perceptions of whether the illness can be cured strongly affect help seeking. For example, Leventhal et al. (1997) found that help seeking is more likely if ambiguous symptoms are detected when someone is also stressed but only if the stress has lasted for three weeks or more. Stress may be seen as the cause of a symptom and so it may be expected to be short-lived or to have only minor consequences but if stress is perceived to be ongoing then symptoms may be regarded as more serious and long term. This model has since been extended to incorporate a wider range of beliefs including beliefs about treatment effectiveness, side effects and treatment overuse as well as beliefs specified by the Theory of Planned Behaviour (Hagger & Orbell, 2022).

Note how the findings of Berkanovic et al. (1981, see above) highlight two of the categories of beliefs proposed by Leventhal et al. (1997). The model highlighted seriousness (consequences) and perceived efficacy of care (control-treatment) and so also maps onto beliefs specified by the social cognition models we studied in Chapter 7. For example, the health belief model and the theory of planned behaviour identify beliefs about consequences as important to intention and action and the theory of planned behaviour and social cognitive theory emphasise the importance of perceived control to action. Finally, look back at Activity Box 8.1 and compare patients' questions about medication to the beliefs associated with consultation.

Personality and emotional responses affect symptom interpretation

Rietveld and Prins (1998) found that negative emotions did not affect objective measures of children's asthma but made it more likely that children would interpret normal exercise-related sensations (e.g. heart pounding and fatigue) as indicating asthma. Those experiencing more negative emotions reported greater breathlessness, regardless of objective symptoms. Patterns of emotional responding can be predicted by personality assessments (see Chapter 6) so that, for example, those high in neuroticism report more symptoms (Watson & Pennebaker, 1989). In a study of cold infections, Feldman et al. (1999) found that while neuroticism was not related to objective measures of infection, it was associated with symptom reporting amongst healthy people. Those scoring in the top third of the neuroticism distribution reported more than twice as many symptoms as those in the bottom third. The researchers suggested that greater attention to bodily sensations among those high in neuroticism could explain these results; a conclusion supported by other research (Kolk et al., 2003).

Other personality factors influence symptom detection and perception. For example, while pessimism may be bad for one's health (see Chapter 6), pessimists seem to be more accurate in assessing their health. Leventhal et al. (1997) report that self-reported ratings of health were better predictors of mortality five years later among pessimists than optimists. Controlling for age and medical history and comparing those who reported their health to be fair or poor with those who reported their health to be excellent or very good, mortality was eight times higher amongst pessimists but only 1.5 times higher amongst optimists. Here optimism moderates the relationship between self-reported health status and mortality (see Research Methods Box 5.2). Yet, while there is evidence that neuroticism leads to overreporting of symptoms, the evidence linking particular traits to over or under-reporting is suggestive rather than conclusive (van Helvoort, Merckelbach, van Nieuwenhuizen & Otgaar, 2022). Moreover, it is not clear that neuroticism itself is a useful predictor of help seeking through consultations (Holtman et al., 2021). So, it would be unwise to assume that any particular person's symptom reporting or consultation is personality driven.

Personality traits can influence decisions about service usage and adherence through specific symptom-related beliefs, that is, beliefs mediate the effect of personality on help seeking and adherence. For example, Skinner, Hampson and Fife-Schaw (2002) found that greater perceived consequences of diabetes symptoms and greater perceived effectiveness of available treatment were both associated with greater self-reported selfcare amongst young people with diabetes. Such beliefs are important both to consulting and adherence (see Berkanovic et al., 1981 and above). Skinner et al. also found that neuroticism was associated with beliefs about the consequences of diabetes but not with beliefs about the effectiveness of treatment. By contrast, conscientiousness was associated with stronger beliefs in the effectiveness of treatment. The researchers suggested that because conscientious people are more likely to engage in active problem-focused coping (see Chapter 5) they may access more information about their diabetes and its management, which in turn may result in more positive beliefs about treatment effectiveness. Conscientiousness is also associated with adherence to public health lifestyle guidance, including fruit and vegetable consumption, alcohol use, smoking and physical activity. Those high in conscientiousness may be nearly twice as likely to follow such advice (Gartland, Wilson, Lawton & O'Connor, 2021). This suggests that people low in conscientiousness may need greater support in adhering to healthcare advice.

Seeking help from health professionals and following their advice is strongly related to people's beliefs about their health. Monitoring and seeking to change such beliefs could lead to more cost-effective use of health services. Public health interventions in schools and communities that promote such understanding could change people's perspectives on health and healthcare usage (Wolferz, Arjani, Bolze & Frates, 2019). In particular, targeting beliefs concerning the consequences of lifestyle choices, the meaning of symptoms and the effectiveness of treatments could be helpful in shaping healthcare service usage.

Adherence and concordance

Adherence refers to following advice given by healthcare professionals. This can involve a variety of behaviour changes including taking preventive action (e.g. reducing alcohol consumption or changing one's diet), keeping medical appointments (e.g. screening, physiotherapy or check-up appointments), following self-care advice (e.g. caring for a wound after surgery) and taking medication as directed (in relation to dose and timing). Non-adherence is usually defined as a failure to follow advice to an extent that causes a harmful effect on health or a decrease in the effectiveness of treatment.

Most medical and healthcare interventions rely on patient adherence. For example, if a patient is prescribed antibiotics but does not take them, the consultation and advice will have no effect. Yet about 50% of patients do not take prescribed medications as recommended (Myers & Midence, 1998). Across behaviour patterns, between 15% and 93% of patients do not follow the advice of healthcare professionals and non-adherence patterns have remained high over decades (Ley, 1988; Kleinsinger, 2018). Non-adherence is observed even when its consequences are fatal. In a prospective study of heart, liver and kidney transplant patients, Rovelli et al. (1989) found that 15% were non-adherent, with non-adherence leading to organ rejection or death in 30% of non-adherent cases, compared to only 1% amongst adherent patients.

Non-adherence is problematic because it means that when healthcare professionals make accurate diagnoses and prescribe effective treatment their intervention may, nonetheless, be ineffective. Non-adherence has substantial implications for preventable deaths, preventable use of hospital services and healthcare costs. Consequences have been estimated at more than 100,000 deaths, billions of dollars a year and up to 69% of hospital admissions (Benjamin, 2012). Such estimates vary depending on what type of non-adherence is considered for what type of patient. In a systematic review of hospital admissions, Mongkhon et al. (2018) found that, across studies, the median rate of preventable hospital admissions associated with non-adherence was 4.3% of all admissions. While this is a small percentage it represents a very large healthcare cost that could be saved through persuasion in public health interventions and consultations to promote adherence.

More than 40 years ago Sackett and Snow (1979) reported that only half of patients on long-term medical regimens were adherent. Similarly, in a study of people with long-term illnesses, Fernandez-Lazaro et al. (2019) found that 44% were not adherent to treatment. These authors found that those who had received complete treatment information, had adequate knowledge about a medication regime and saw themselves as enjoying a good quality of life were more likely to be adherent. These findings indicate that consultations, especially with patients managing long-term illnesses, should ensure good understanding of recommended treatments and, if possible, optimism about treatment outcomes. Communication in the consultation is an important predictor of adherence and, therefore, of treatment effectiveness (Noble, 1988; Osterberg & Blaschke, 2005; Zolnierek & Dimatteo, 2009). Many other barriers need to be investigated including the complexity of advice and prescribed medication regimes (Andhi et al., 2023; Osterberg & Blaschke, 2005).

How can we measure adherence?

Simple self-report measures can provide good estimates of adherence (Morisky, Green & Levine, 1986) but when self-report measures are compared to objective measures, results indicate that patients tend to overestimate their adherence (Myers & Midence, 1998). Direct indicators such as analyses of urine or blood content as well as indirect objective measures such as pill counts, refill records and service usage records are also used to track adherence. In addition, indirect measures such as health improvement (e.g. weight loss, blood pressure or hospitalisation) may be employed as indicators of adherence (Roter et al., 1998, and see Lam & Fresco, 2015 for an overview).

Antecedents of adherence

Why do patients not follow advice? Patients are non-adherent for different reasons (Donovan & Blake, 1992). Some patients intend to take recommended actions but forget or find adherence too difficult. Others suspend medication or test their health or to avoid side effects that might impinge on important social events (Conrad, 1985). Some patients fear medication dependency while others disagree with the doctor's diagnosis or the prescribed treatment and deliberately take more or less than was advised. Knowing why patients do not adhere is important to designing interventions that may promote better adherence. Some key questions that influence patients' decisions to adhere are: Do I really need this treatment? Am I at risk of symptoms without doing what was advised? How effective/beneficial is the recommended action? What side effects will it have? To what extent will adherence conflict with other things I want to do? When consultations do not adequately answer these questions, patients may reach their own conclusions and decide against adherence (see Activity box 8.1).

If a patient feels her doctor is not interested in her problem or has not understood it, this will undermine confidence in the doctor's advice. Consequently, patient satisfaction is significantly correlated with adherence (Ley, 1988). For example, in a foundational study of paediatric consultations, Korsch et al. (1968) found that mothers who were very satisfied with their doctor's warmth, concern and communication were three times more likely to adhere than dissatisfied mothers. Satisfaction depends upon the patient's perception of the doctor's sensitivity, concern, respect and competence. Reducing waiting time, taking time to greet the patient in a courteous manner and engaging in friendly introductory exchanges are all likely to increase satisfaction.

Asking open-ended questions which cannot be answered "yes" or "no" and allowing the patient time to express his or her worries is also likely to make the patient feel satisfied with the consultation. Communication with practitioner is an important precursor of adherence (Osterberg & Blaschke, 2005).

Given the importance of patient satisfaction, it is important to note that doctors' own satisfaction with work is a predictor of patients' adherence. In a two-year prospective study, DiMatteo et al. (1993) found that, controlling for adherence at baseline, doctors' satisfaction with their work was a significant predictor of patient's future adherence ($r = .25$). This study also showed that doctors' self-reported willingness to answer all their patients' questions, regardless of the time involved was positively associated with adherence. Doctors who are happier in their work may be more willing to answer questions and may engender greater satisfaction in their patients. Thus, patient satisfaction may mediate the relationship between doctors' job satisfaction and their patients' adherence. Skilled healthcare professionals can optimise their patients trust, satisfaction and adherence and, thereby, their own job satisfaction.

The social context in which people live including the social support they receive also affects adherence. Indeed, adherence may partially mediate the effect of social support on health. In a meta-analysis summarising 122 studies reporting associations between social support and adherence, DiMatteo (1993) found that adherence (compared to non-adherence) was 3.6 times more likely amongst those receiving practical support than amongst those who did not have such support. Similarly, the risk of non-adherence was 1.35 times higher among patients without emotional support, compared to those receiving such support. Practical support increases self-efficacy and actual control over adherence behaviours (see the theory of planned behaviour and social cognitive theory in Chapter 7) thereby rendering recommended changes feasible. A lack of social support may also increase stress levels which may, in turn, allow less priority for adherence goals (DiMatteo, 1993). Finally, unsurprisingly, having a mental health problem, as well as the target illness, and being less well-off increases the likelihood of non-adherence. Again this emphasises the importance of communication in healthcare consultations. If patients do not fully understand recommendations or are unpersuaded of the benefits of treatments then adherence is likely to be compromised. This is likely to especially relevant for more vulnerable patients. While the evidence is not decisive, it seems that patients who have fewer resources or are more disadvantaged are more likely to be non-adherent, perhaps because they face more daily challenges (Gast & Mathes, 2019).

Can we improve adherence?

Available evidence suggests that we can improve adherence but that this may require interventions including multiple behaviour-change techniques. For example, in a meta-analysis of 153 studies evaluating the effectiveness of interventions designed to improve patient adherence, Roter et al. (1998) found that interventions significantly improved adherence compared to control conditions with small to moderate effect sizes. The researchers reached four conclusions. First, while effect sizes were small, interventions were generally effective. For example, even the smallest effect size on measures of health outcomes translated into 10% increase compared to no-intervention controls. As the researchers note, a 10% difference between an intervention and control group could "save considerable cost and suffering" (p.1150). Second, no particular intervention approach worked better than any one other but combinations were more effective than single techniques, especially if they simultaneously targeted education, behaviour-change and emotional responses.

Techniques targeting adherence behaviour included changing drug packaging, simplifying dose instructions, mailed reminders and skills development approaches. Third, adherence interventions were more effective for some conditions, especially diabetes, asthma, cancer and hypertension, suggesting that it may be easier to increase adherence for some patients than others. Finally, the researchers noted that a broader approach to identifying outcome measures could be beneficial. For example, as well as boosting adherence, interventions may affect patient satisfaction, patient understanding and quality of life. These may be important targets in themselves. This suggestion links to a more general question about the evaluation of healthcare interventions, that is, who decides what are the most appropriate outcome measures? While physical health is very important, is it always the most important outcome? Consider the definition of health we began with in Chapter 1. Overall then, healthcare professionals are more effective in encouraging patients to follow medical advice when we understand and address patients' personal reasons for consultation and their personal barriers to adherence (Thorsen et al., 2001).

In a meta-analysis, Haynes et al. (2005) examined the outcomes of randomised controlled trials which measured adherence to medication and included a clinical or health outcome (that is, whether people in the intervention condition also showed greater health benefit). For short-term prescriptions they found that four of nine interventions (44%) had an effect on both adherence and at least one clinical outcome while, for longer term treatment, 26 of 58 (45%) led to improvements in adherence but only 18 interventions (31%) led to improvement in at least one clinical outcome. The researchers concluded that for short-term drug treatments counseling, written information and a personal phone call could boost adherence, but for long-term treatments, no particular intervention type and only complex interventions led to improvements in health outcomes. Those that were successful in improving health included combinations of more convenient care, providing information, counseling, reminders, self-monitoring, reinforcement, family therapy, psychological therapy, crisis intervention, telephone follow-up and additional supervision.

Similarly, in a review of interventions to increase medication adherence, Kini and Ho (2018) considered six categories of interventions, including patient education (e.g. telephone counseling sessions), changing medication regimens (e.g. using combination pills to reduce the number of pills patients take daily), clinical pharmacist consultation for long-term illness co-management (including education and follow-up telephone calls), cognitive behavioural therapies (such as motivational interviewing by trained counselors), medication reminders (such as refill reminder calls or use of electronic drug monitors for real-time monitoring and reminding) and incentives to promote adherence (such as paying patients and clinicians for achieving disease management goals). The authors noted that effective interventions that are practical in clinical contexts include using combination pills to reduce daily pill burden (see too Andhi et al., 2023), clinical pharmacist consultation for illness co-management, and medication-taking reminders. They suggest that these interventions could increase adherence by up to 20%, potentially making a considerable difference to the effectiveness of recommended treatments and substantially reducing healthcare costs. Thus, changes in healthcare delivery can improve adherence, particularly to long-term medication.

Healthcare professionals can optimise adherence by improving patients' understanding, recall and satisfaction. Patients must understand advice before they can follow it and they must remember it beyond the consultation if it is to shape behaviour. Both understanding and recall are associated with patient satisfaction. Consequently, in foundational research, Ley proposed the model of adherence shown in Figure 10.1. Understanding is correlated with adherence ($r = 0.36$; Ley, 1988) and, in Chapter 8, we discussed how healthcare professionals can enhance patient

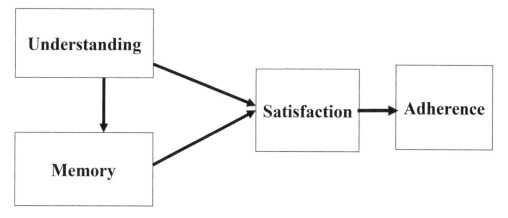

Figure 10.1. Antecedents of adherence. (From Ley, 1988)

understanding. Even when information is understood it may be forgotten. For example, in an early study, patients were found to have forgotten around half of the verbal instructions given to them, after only five minutes (Ley, 1988). We noted in Chapter 8 how recall could be improved (e.g. see our consideration of logical order, explicit categorisation, specific advice and emphasising and repeating important points).

Strategies that bolster memory for intentions and their subsequent enactment may also be used to increase adherence. For example, event-based recall is better than time-based recall (Ellis, 1998). So, trying to remember "take antibiotics twice a day" is likely to be less successful than trying to remember "take antibiotics before breakfast and before dinner". If one or more intentions have to be recalled, events can be more tightly specified, e.g. "take the blue pill before cereal and red pill with toast at breakfast". Consider the use of implementation intention formation, or if-then plans, as discussed in Chapter 7. Memory may also be enhanced by individualised feedback. For patients on long term treatment medication, adherence can be monitored (e.g. by using electronic pill containers) and combined with individualised recommendations for remembering in relation to specific events (e.g. brushing teeth) that occur when the patient tends to forget their medication. Such interventions have shown success with blood glucose control in diabetes, nebuliser use in people with obstructive lung disease, psychiatric medication, antiretroviral medication for HIV and oral anti-diabetic tablets (Rosen, Rigsby, Salahi et al., 2004). Healthcare professionals can also influence motivation and self-efficacy (see Chapter 8). For example, patients could be asked if they intend to follow advice and if they see any barriers to doing so (e.g. "Do you think you will take these tablets four times a day over the next two weeks? Can you think of anything that might prevent you taking the medication?"). Such questions provide a check on the degree to which an agreed plan has been established and its feasibility, or attainability, in the context of the patient's life. Goal setting and if-then plans may help patients implement their intentions to take medication.

From compliance to concordance

At one time adherence was referred to as "compliance" but this term was discarded because it suggested that that patients should do what they were told by doctors and that failing to do so was their responsibility. Of course, patients decide whether the advice they receive is helpful and whether or not they will follow it. So, healthcare professionals need to collaborate with, and persuade, patients if they are to shape health-behaviour patterns. It has been proposed that healthcare professionals should seek to reach "concordance", with their patients, that is, a mutual understanding and agreement about treatment and its implementation (Mullen, 1997; Pollock, 2002; Bissell, May & Noyce, 2004). For example, Bissell et al. (2004) used qualitative analyses of interviews with type 2 diabetic patients of Pakistani origin and found that some patients felt they could not discuss emotional, familial and financial factors which undermined their attempts to follow a diet appropriate to their condition. Thus, these patients were unable to discuss key barriers to achieving adherence, thereby limiting the advice their healthcare professional could offer on how to best follow a recommended diet. If healthcare professionals are to ensure that their advice is clearly understood and is relevant to their patients' lives, they will also need to discuss barriers patients may have in following an agreed plan. Consultations need to allow time for discussion and negotiation if they are to achieve good levels of concordance and so help patients to set SMART goals and If-then plans. Murdoch, Salter, Ford, Lenaghan, Shiner and Steel (2020) observed that promote goal setting among patients with multiple long-term illnesses, general practitioners need to check patients' understanding of goal-setting in the consultation, while actively aligning their discussion to patients own framing of their goal. As these authors put it "doctors and patients need to negotiate each other's perspectives."

Managing consultations

Interactions between healthcare professionals (e.g. health psychologists, medical doctors and nurses) and their patients have the capacity to affect patient understanding, patient satisfaction, patient adherence and, therefore, health outcomes. Consequently, the success and cost effectiveness of healthcare services depends critically on consultation management. Use of good communication skills in consultations has been found to affect a range of health outcomes from emotional wellbeing to blood pressure and blood sugar concentration (Stewart, 1995). Yet it is all too easy for consultations to go wrong. The Toronto Consensus Statement on Doctor-Patient Communication (Simpson et al., 1991) noted that 54% of patient complaints and 45% of patient concerns were not elicited by doctors and that in up to 50% of consultations the patient and the doctor did not agree on the nature of the main presenting problem. This may be because patients are sometimes interrupted too quickly by their doctors (e.g. within 18 seconds of speaking). Consultations serve different purposes and involve different groups of patients but key principles underlying effectiveness have been identified. This underlines the importance of clarifying the patient's own reasons for consulting (Thorsen et al., 2001).

Many models of successful doctor-patient consultations have been developed. For example, after analysing 2,500 taped consultations, Byrne and Long (1976) identified six phases which form the structure of successful consultations. They suggested that doctor: (1) establishes a relationship with the patient; (2) attempts to discover the reason for the patient's visit; (3) conducts a verbal and/or physical examination; (4) considers the diagnosis with the patient; (5) describes further treatment or investigation; and, finally, (6) ends the consultation. Byrne and Long noted that consultations can go wrong in phase two if the doctor fails to identify the true reason for consulting. Similarly, if the patient fails to understand the diagnosis in phase 4 this may affect adherence.

The more widely used Calgary–Cambridge consultation model provides a similar guide to structuring consultations (Silverman, Kurtz, & Draper, 2005). Six stages are identified: (1) *initiating the consultation* including establishing rapport (e.g. greetings and introductions) and identifying the reason(s) for the consultation (e.g. asking the patient what they would like to discuss); (2) *gathering information*, including understanding the patient's perspective (e.g. listening attentively without

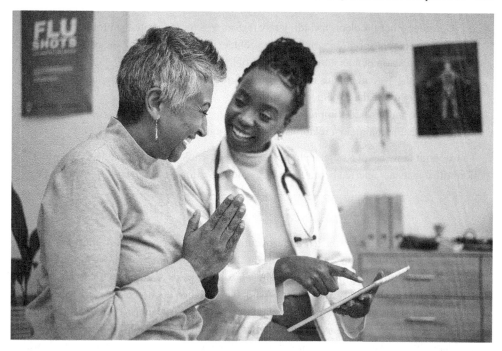

Figure 10.2. Doctor-patient interaction has is crucial to patient satisfaction, patient adherence and health outcomes.
Copyright of PeopleImages.com – Yuri A/Shutterstock.

interrupting and using open questions to clarify what has been said); (3) *building the relationship*, including showing interest using non-verbal cues and communicating appreciation of the patient's concerns; (4) *providing structure* including summarising what has been said; (5) explanation and planning, including providing the correct amount and type of information in a manner which aids recall and understanding and achieves a shared understanding and shared plan; and (6) ending the consultation. Rather than focusing on sequence, Pendleton, Schofield, Tate, and Havelock (1984) identified seven tasks that need to be successfully completed in a medical consultation. These tasks, listed in Focus Box 10.1, overlap substantially with the Byrne and Long and Calgary–Cambridge models and while developed as a learning aid for doctors could be applied to many consultations between healthcare professionals and patients.

FOCUS BOX 10.1

Seven key tasks in consultations with patients

Pendleton, Schofield, Tate and Havelock (1984) identified seven tasks that need to be successfully completed in a medical consultation.

1. Define the reason for the consultation including the nature and history of the problem, its effects and the patient's concerns and expectations.

2. Consider other problems including risk factors which exacerbate the problem.
3. Choose an appropriate action for each problem in negotiation with the patient.
4. Achieve a shared understanding of the problem(s).
5. Involve the patient in the management of problems and encourage acceptance of responsibility by the patient.
6. Use time and resources appropriately.
7. Establish and maintain a relationship with the patient.

Think about how these tasks relate to how a health psychologist would conduct a consultation with a manager referred because she was suffering serious stress at work (see Chapter 4)

Byrne and Long (1976) contrasted doctor-centred and patient-centred consultations. Doctor-centred (or illness-centred) consultations focus on eliciting information necessary for precise diagnosis and prescription of appropriate treatment. The doctor tends to dominate such consultations asking direct, closed questions which demand short factual answers which can clarify details (e.g. "Where do you feel the pain?"). In such consultations, little time is spent eliciting or understanding the patient's ideas or providing information other than instructions on medical management of the problem. By contrast, in patient-centred consultations, doctors ask more open questions which allow the patient to explain their perspective (e.g. "So what do you think is wrong?"). The doctor also allows time to reflect back what the patient has said to demonstrate understanding and/or show empathy (e.g. "you're worried about side effects") and to check that any treatment plans are acceptable to the patient. The Calgary–Cambridge model and Pendleton et al.'s seven-task model both emphasise the importance of patient-centredness in consultations because evidence suggests that patients are less likely to be satisfied and so less adherent following doctor-centred consultations. For example, after observing 865 consultations with general practitioners (or family doctors), Little et al. (2001) identified five aspects of patient-centeredness: (1) building a partnership, that is, being sympathetic, taking an interest in patients' worries and sharing planning; (2) taking an interest in the patient's life; (3) establishing a personal relationship, that is knowing the patient and their emotional needs; (4) providing health promotion, for example, addressing risk factors in the patient's lifestyle; and (5) taking a positive and definite approach including providing concrete guidance on what was wrong and when it would be resolved. They found that patient satisfaction was related to building a partnership and taking a positive approach. They also found that patients felt more enabled to deal with their problem when doctors had taken an interest in their lives, provided health promotion and adopted a positive approach. Patients also reported fewer symptoms one month after the consultation when doctors adopted a positive approach. Similarly, Howick et al. (2018) found that doctors expressing empathy and communicating positive or optimistic messages enhanced patients' health across a range of clinical conditions, and especially pain. Note how such results relate to the finding that doctor's communication style was associated with malpractice claims (see Chapter 8). It seems that patients expect partnership building and do not appreciate or benefit from doctors airing their uncertainties or concerns.

Does the presenting problem (or illness) moderate the effectiveness of consultation styles? A study by Savage and Armstrong (1990) suggests that it does. In this experimental study 200 patients were randomly allocated to two different consulting styles and followed up one week later. The styles were referred to as "sharing" ("Why do you think this has happened?", "What do you think is wrong?", "Would you like a prescription?", "What do these symptoms or problems mean to you?") and "directing" (e.g. "This is a serious problem", "You are suffering from X", "It is essential that you take this medicine", and "You should be better in X days"). In all cases patients were allowed to complete their explanation of the problem and more than 80% of those receiving each style reported that they had been able to discuss their problem well. So, phase 2 in the Byrne and Long model was completed. The researchers found that a "directing" style was associated with greater patient confidence that their doctor has understood their problem, perception of higher quality explanation by the doctor and greater reported health improvement one week later – but *only amongst patients consulting about a physical problem or receiving a prescription*. Amongst patients with a long-term or psychological illness and amongst those not receiving a prescription there was no difference between the two consulting styles. These findings mirror those of Little and colleagues emphasising that, while patients need to be listened to, they expect positive, unambiguous expert advice from doctors reflecting their medical understanding of illness and treatments. However, where the problem has no clear physical diagnosis or cannot be treated using biomedical prescriptions a sharing style is likely to be important to patient satisfaction. So, care of patients with long term illnesses needs to be different to those with acute, resolvable problems (e.g. take this antibiotic or do nothing). This is important because about half of all general practitioner appointments and two thirds of hospital outpatient appointments are with people who have long term illnesses (Department of Health, 2012).

Further insight into which aspects of patient centredness matter to patients with long term illness was provided by Michie, Miles and Weinman (2003). These researchers distinguished between measures of the extent to which healthcare professionals: (1) understand the patients' perspective and acknowledge their beliefs and emotional needs; and (2) empower patients to actively shape the consultation and its conclusions. Thirty studies of consultations with patients who had long term illnesses were divided into those which measured patient centredness as perspective taking and those which measured patient centredness in terms of patient empowerment. Two of nine studies in the former group found a positive association between patient centredness and better physical health while nine of ten studies in the latter group found such an association. Thus, perspective taking, while important, and perhaps especially important to patients with long term illness, may not be enough to render consultations more effective in terms of health outcomes. Patient empowerment appears to be crucial.

Patient empowerment

Can we help to empower patients in their interactions with healthcare professionals? Evidence suggests that we can. Robinson and Whitfield (1985) gave patients written information before their consultation reminding them that people may regret not asking questions after the consultation, advising them to check their understanding of instructions and the feasibility of those instructions and advising patients to ask about any discrepancies between recommendations made by the doctor and what they had expected. Compared to controls, these patients asked more questions in the consultation and gave more complete and accurate accounts of the recommended treatments after the consultation. Similarly, Cegala, McClure, Marinelli and Post (2000) found that patients receiving a training booklet designed to enhance patients' communication skills engaged in more effective information seeking, provided more detailed information about their condition to their doctor, and used more summarising statements to check information provided by their doctor. Less encouraging results were reported by Kidd, Marteau, Robinson, Ukoumunne and Tydeman (2004) who found that an intervention in which patients talked to a researcher about three or more questions they wanted to ask and were encouraged to rehearse these questions did not increase question asking in the consultation. However, the researchers noted that question asking was higher than usual amongst their control group patients. The intervention did enhance self-efficacy to ask questions but had no impact on health outcomes. In a systematic review of 20 evaluations of interventions designed to increase patients' participation in medical consultations Harrington, Noble and Newman (2004) found that half of the interventions resulted in increased patient participation with greater effects being observed for clarification seeking rather than question-asking. They also noted that a variety of other positive outcomes were observed including perceptions of control over health, preferences for an active healthcare role, greater recall of information, better adherence and improved clinical outcomes. Harrington and colleagues suggest that question asking may not be best measure of whether such consultation empowerment interventions are effective. They note, for example, that patients' perceptions of control over their health and preferences for an active role in their healthcare were found in all four studies that considered these outcomes. In a review and meta-analysis of 23 studies, Werbrouck et al. (2018) found that ensuring quality information combined with facilitation of goal-setting and action planning were key features of effective empowerment interventions. Finally, in a systematic review, Wakefield, Bayly, Selman, Firth, Higginson and Murtagh (2018) demonstrate how important empowerment is for patients facing terminal or life-limiting illnesses.

One objection to interventions designed to empower patients during consultations and to patient-centred consultations is that they are likely to be longer and doctors are already hard pressed to see patients who want consultations. Howie et al. (1999) examined nearly 26,000 randomly selected adult consultations across 53 medical practices and observed consultation times ranging from less than five minutes to more than 15 minutes with a mean of eight minutes. These researchers administered a patient enablement measure which resembles a measure of consultation-generated, health-related self-efficacy (see Chapter 8). This measured whether patients felt the consultation had made them better or worse at understanding their illness, coping with their illness, keeping themselves healthy and feeling able to help themselves. They found that patient enablement was associated with longer consultations and knowing the doctor better. They concluded that, "It may be time to reward doctors who have longer consultations, provide greater continuity of care, and enable more patients" (p. 738).

Longer consultations not only support greater patient enablement but more cost-effective healthcare provision. Reporting on a review of 14 studies Freeman et al. (2002) noted that longer consultations were associated with less prescribing, better recognition and management of psychosocial problems and better clinical care of long-term illnesses. Longer appointments may also be more likely to resolve problems and so reduce follow up visits for the same problems (Hughes, 1983). This may be especially true of patients with multiple problems in deprived areas. In two randomised controlled trials with eight general practices, Mercer et al. (2016) found that using structured longer consultations, relationship continuity, practitioner support, and self-management support led to substantial cost savings over a 12-month period. Thus, a shift to longer appointments and greater continuity of care (that is seeing the same doctor over time) could enhance effectiveness and cost effectiveness of health services.

Health psychology in practice

Much of the research into consultation management, achieving concordance and patient empowerment has focused on medical practitioners. Nonetheless, these findings are relevant to the practice of healthcare professionals generally, including nurses, physiotherapists, pharmacists and, of course, health psychologists. In this last section we examine the roles of practising health psychologists.

What do health psychologists do?

An important role for a health psychologist is to conduct research. This involves understanding and developing theory, developing behaviour-change interventions, designing high-quality studies, working within consensual research guidelines, using a variety of tested methodologies in a careful and rigorous manner, applying for research funding, collecting data and interpreting both qualitative and quantitative data and then reporting findings honestly and completely so that other researchers can fully understand what work was undertaken and what the reported data may mean. Often this involves applied research in which behaviour change interventions are evaluated in everyday settings to discover if they have the potential to deliver measurable health and wellbeing benefits and may have the potential to contribute to improved population health. Chapter 9 illustrates each of these elements of the research process.

Usually, researchers require a doctoral-level qualification to conduct independent research. Indeed, the British Psychological Society (BPS) states that "primary purpose" of doctoral examination is "to determine whether the candidate is competent as an independent researcher in the discipline (BPS, 2021, p. 5). The BPS also note that parts of a doctoral thesis should be of publishable standard so that the work has the potential to advance the research field. Consequently, to become a health psychology researcher one usually has to have been awarded a doctorate degree (a PhD) in applied or health psychology and to have submitted papers (for peer review) reporting well-conducted studies in the area. The main employers for such researchers are universities, colleges and research centres. Health psychology research is often conducted by teams of researchers, so a publication in a health-related psychology journal may involve researchers with doctorates in psychology, sociology, anthropology, epidemiology, statistics, medicine and others.

Being a researcher in health psychology *does not mean that one is a "health psychologist"*. The terms "health psychologist", "practitioner health psychologist" or "practising health psychologist" refer to someone who has a nationally or internationally recognised licence to practice. The way in which health psychologists are trained and licenced varies internationally. Here we will focus on the UK system which has provided training frameworks that have been adopted or adapted internationally. Bartram and Roe (2005), for example, build on work conducted in the UK to provide a very helpful discussion of the competencies required by practitioner health psychologists across Europe (see too Quinn et al., 2020). Bartram and Roe identify 20 primary competences that any practising psychologist should be able to demonstrate. They group these into six categories; (i) goal specification, (ii) assessment, (iii) development, (iv) intervention, (v) evaluation and (vi) communication. Even a brief consideration of these high-level categories clarifies that the research discussed in this book, especially in Chapters 8–11, is directly relevant to these practitioner competences. For example, practitioner health psychologists need to be able to demonstrate that they can communicate effectively with patients and clients in a manner that will promote health (see above) and that they can design and evaluate potentially-effective interventions to promote health motivation (Chapter 8) and health-enhancing behaviour change (Chapter 9).

In the UK, health psychologists are licenced, or registered, to practice by the Health and Care Professions Council (HCPC). The HCPC is a statutory regulator of over 280,000 professionals from 15 health and care professions. The Council states that its main purpose is to protect the public. The HCPC (2022) identifies 12 core competences that all healthcare practitioners need to be able to demonstrate and take action to maintain during their practice. These are broken down into many precisely-specified sub-competences. The 12 core competencies are being able to; (1) practise safely and effectively within the scope of one's work, (2) practise within the legal and ethical boundaries of one's profession, (3) maintain fitness to practise, including one's own health, wellbeing and mental health and seeking support when needed, (4) practise as an autonomous professional, exercising one's own professional judgement (5) recognise the impact of culture, equality and diversity on practice and practise in a non-discriminatory manner, (6) understand the importance of confidentially and act to maintain confidentiality, (7) communicate effectively, (8) work appropriately with others, (9) maintain records appropriately, (10) reflect on and review practice, (11) assure the quality of one's practice, (12) understand and apply the key concepts of the knowledge base (that is the research base) relevant to one's profession. These practising competencies that are not necessarily needed by researchers working on health-related cognition and behaviour but they are all required to practice as a competent psychologist who offers services to the public. Such competency standards need to be reviewed and updated regularly and the core competencies listed above represent the revised set of standards implemented by the HCPC in 2023. The most recent revisions emphasise the importance of active implementation of standards in order to promote health and prevent illness, providing leadership within one's profession and ensuring that one's digital skills are up-to-date to facilitate relating to clients using eHealth technologies (see Chapter 11).

The HCPC (2022; 2023) also specifies competencies that apply only to practising health psychologists. These include being able to (i) develop appropriate psychological assessments based on appraisal of the influence of the biological, social and environmental contexts on health (this is, know how to undertake an evidence-based assessment of a client or patient in relation to their needs), (ii) develop psychological formulations using the outcomes of assessment, drawing on theory, research and explanatory models (that is, drawing on evidence and individual assessments to offer individual needs-based advice), (iii) carry out and analyse large-scale data gathering, including questionnaire surveys (that is being a competent, quantitative researcher), (iv) draw on knowledge of developmental, social and biological processes across the lifespan to facilitate adaptability and change in individuals, groups, families, organisations and communities (that is understand research into the complexity of behaviour change and be able to apply this in practice), (v) contrast, compare and critically evaluate a range of models of behaviour change (that is, be able to assess whether a proposed model of behaviour change is evidence-based and applicable to any particular practice challenge), (vi) understand change processes and change techniques when working with individuals who experience difficulties (that is, to be able to assess when evidence-based techniques, such as motivational and behaviour-change techniques are appropriate to a client's needs), (vii) develop and apply effective interventions to promote psychological wellbeing, social, emotional and behavioural change and to raise educational standards (that is, to select, and then apply in practice, effective, evidence-based cognitive and behavioural interventions that can change people's beliefs and behaviour patterns to promote health), (viii) to evaluate and respond to change in health psychology and in consultancy and service-delivery contexts (that is to be able to tell when an intervention has worked and to change practice as research evidence develops), (ix) to be able to implement evidence-based interventions and therapies to meet individual clients' needs drawing upon a range evidence-based interventions. This is a demanding set of competencies that requires high-level training.

Below we describe how the British Psychological Society (BPS) and the HCPC register health psychologists. The first step (in the UK) is to gain an undergraduate (or bachelor) level degree accredited by the BPS. Sometimes this may involve a degree in another discipline and a one-year conversion degree. This allows a candidate to acquire a BPS-approved "Graduate Basis for Chartership". Beyond this a candidate will need to sit and pass a BPS-accredited, Health Psychology MSc (which may take two years). Then the candidate can enrol in a university-based, stage-two Health Psychology practitioner training course which will include some research at doctoral level. These professional doctorates in Health Psychology (known as DHealthPsych's) are stage 2 qualifications that allow candidates to apply for registration by the HCPC but they are not PhDs. Of course, those with PhDs can also apply for BPS stage 2 recognition. Alternatively, having a Graduate Basis for Chartership, candidates can undertake independent study with supervisors and be assessed by the BPS for stage 2 competencies (BPS, 2021). Whatever route a candidate health psychologist takes, this training is likely to take around seven years. This is not surprising, recognising the competencies that a health psychologist needs to develop and the responsibilities involved in evidence-based practice with clients needing healthcare advice and interventions.

Two important future challenges face regulatory bodies that licence and register practising health psychologists (such as the UK HCPC). First, how can these bodies ensure evidence-based practice? The HCPC (2023) specify very particular evidence-based competencies. For example, they require practising health psychologists to be able to "contrast, compare and critically evaluate a range of models of behaviour change". This is a worthy standard but how is this assessed, and by whom? If it is self-assessed by the practising psychologist then what if that person misunderstands current scientific evidence? Consider an example. If one searches online for "stages of change" or the "transtheoretical model" then one can find many sites that explain the model and how to apply it. Such sites may make statements such as, "the stages of change are … " suggesting that the model describes known cognition patterns relevant to health behaviour change. Yet we have known for 20 years that evidence does not support this model (see West, 2005 for a useful summary). If a health psychologist bases their practice on a model that is not supported by evidence should this be grounds for de-registration? The public may expect bodies such as HCPC to ensure evidence-based practice but how can they fulfil this expectation? Should registered health psychologists sit periodic evidence-based practice examinations? If so, how long should the interval be (e.g. every five years)? Should such examinations assess understanding of how to apply current accumulated evidence reported in reviews, systematic reviews, meta-analyses and qualitative syntheses (Flemming, Booth Garside, Tunçalp & Noyes, 2019)? Who would set and examine these registration checks? While challenging, these questions need to be addressed if health psychology practice is to be, and be seen to be, evidence-based.

A second challenge is the internationalisation of practice in the context of eHealth. The HCPC has appropriately revised their competencies to include current digital skills so that health psychologists can offer remote consultations and interventions (see Chapter 11). Digital services are not contained within national borders. So, a HCPC-registered health psychologist could potentially use their digital skills to offer consultations outside the UK while practising within the HCPC guidelines. This may not be problematic if clients have full access to the qualifications and registration competencies of that health psychologist. Nonetheless, as eHealth practices become internationalised, issues arise concerning health psychologists being registered in one country while offering services to clients in another. International harmonisation of competency standards is needed to resolve this challenge.

Health psychologists work for a range of employers. The BPS Division of Health Psychology (2023) website lists a variety of current employers including; (i) multi-disciplinary healthcare teams in hospitals and clinics (public or private) in which health psychologists help people prevent illness or manage long-term illnesses, (ii) public health and health promotion teams in which health psychologists design and evaluate population-level interventions to keep people healthy; (iii) social care and local government teams in which health psychologists assess psychological needs based on data analyses and then commission tailored health and social care services, (iv) ehealth companies and services in which health psychologists design, co-create and implement digital interventions to empower people to better manage their health and wellbeing, (v) personnel departments, within organisations, in which health psychologists design and evaluate interventions to enhance employee health and practice and (vi) government agencies in which health psychologists provide evidence-based advice to improve healthcare policies grounded in psychological science in order to optimise psychological, social and environmental influences on health.

Key terms introduced in Chapter 10 (in order of appearance)

- Perceived symptom seriousness.
- Perceived effectiveness of treatment.
- Symptom detection.
- Identity.
- Cause.
- Consequences.
- Timeline and control.
- Adherence.
- Patient satisfaction.
- Understanding.
- Recall.
- Event-based recall.
- Time-based recall.
- Compliance.
- Concordance.
- Calgary–Cambridge consultation model.
- Pendleton et al.'s seven tasks.

- Doctor-centred.
- Patient-centred.
- Direct and positive consultation style.
- Perspective taking.
- Patient empowerment.
- Consultation duration.
- Continuity of care.
- UK Health and Care Professions Council.
- Practitioner competencies.

Summary of main points addressed in Chapter 10

Patients are often unable to reliably assess their symptoms. Consequently, beliefs about what symptoms mean and emotional responses to their detection are crucial to the effect they have on health behaviour including consulting healthcare professionals. Beliefs about symptoms such as perceived seriousness and perceived effectiveness of available treatment mediate the effects of personality (e.g., neuroticism and conscientiousness) on health behaviour including adherence. Most medical interventions rely on patient adherence. Yet non-adherence is high. Patients are non-adherent for different reasons but patients' understanding, recall and satisfaction with healthcare all predict adherence. Key aspects of relating to patients determine patient satisfaction. Medical practitioners' own satisfaction with their work and patient social support (especially practical support) predicts patient adherence. In general, studies suggest that we can improve adherence although it may be challenging to do so for longer-term treatments to an extent that enhanced health outcomes follow.

Patient satisfaction, adherence and health outcomes are related to consultation management. Reaching an agreed plan with patients is important and referred to as concordance. The Calgary–Cambridge consultation model identifies six key stages while Pendleton et al. (1984) identified seven key tasks to be completed in consultations with patients. Patient centeredness and especially listening to patients' concerns is crucial to patient satisfaction. However, a positive direct style communicating expertise is also important, especially for patients with a physical problem that can be treated with medication. For patients with long-term illnesses, perspective taking may need to be combined with empowering strategies which help patients take more control of the consultation and their health. Evidence suggests that interventions can be successful in empowering patients' involvement in consultations.

Professional health psychologists work in a variety of multidisciplinary settings, including healthcare settings, organisational settings and government departments. They are trained in a number of key roles and develop a range of competencies through many years of training. Competencies for health psychology practice have been defined by a number of regulatory bodies including the UK Health and Care Professionals Council. Future challenges in training and practitioner competence regulation include guaranteeing that training delivers evidence-based practice and that international practitioner regulation recognises cross-border practice delivered through digital platforms.

Recommendations for further reading

Journal articles

Little, P., Everitt, H., Williamson, I., Warner, G., Moore, M., Gould, C., Ferrier, K. & Payne, S. (2001). Observational study of effect of patient centredness and positive approach on outcomes of general practice consultations. *BMJ, 323*(7318), 908–911. https://doi.org/10.1136/bmj.323.7318.908

Osterberg, L. & Blaschke, T. (2005). Adherence to medication. *The New England Journal of Medicine, 353*(5), 487–497. https://doi.org/10.1056/NEJMra050100

Wakefield, D., Bayly, J., Selman, L. E., Firth, A. M., Higginson, I. J. & Murtagh, F. E. (2018). Patient empowerment, what does it mean for adults in the advanced stages of a life-limiting illness: A systematic review using critical interpretive synthesis. *Palliative Medicine, 32*(8), 1288–1304. doi:10.1177/0269216318783919

Websites

HCPC (2022). Revisions to the standards of proficiency. *Health and Care Professions Council*. https://www.hcpc-uk.org/standards/standards-of-proficiency/reviewing-the-standards-of-proficiency/ [accessed on 19/04/2023]

HCPC (2023). Standards of proficiency for practitioner psychologists. *Health and Care Professions Council*. https://www.hcpc-uk.org/globalassets/standards/standards-of-proficiency/reviewing/practitioner-psychologists---sop-changes.pdf [accessed on 19/04/2023]

Illustrative essay titles

How can the effectiveness of doctor–patient consultations be maximised? Discuss with reference to relevant research.

Poor adherence to health promotion and medical advice reduces the effectiveness of health services. How can we improve adherence?

What is meant by patient-centred consultations and are they effective?

How can health psychologists contribute to the improvement of healthcare services?

How can health psychology training ensure that health psychology practice is evidence based?

11 Applying psychology to improve health services

Applying psychology to improve health services

This chapter is divided into five sections.

1. Managing long term illness.
2. Using groups in healthcare.
3. Complementary therapies.
4. Placebo effects and psychological models of recovery.
5. From telemedicine to digital delivery of healthcare services.

Learning outcomes

When you have completed this chapter you should be able to:

1. Explain the needs of patients with long term illnesses and illustrate the contribution that psychological interventions can make to caring for these patients.
2. Discuss the advantages and limitations of group consultations in healthcare delivery.
3. Discuss the role of complementary therapies in healthcare.
4. Define "placebo effects" and explain how they could help us optimise healthcare delivery.
5. Describe advances in digital healthcare delivery and discuss what research is needed to create optimal digital services.

Managing long-term illness

In England, 15.4 million people have a long-term physical illness (LTI) and this is likely to rise to 18 million by 2025. About 60% of those older than 65 have a LTI compared to 17% of people under 40. People with LTIs are intensive healthcare users accounting for more than half of general practice appointments and nearly three quarters of inpatient days in hospital. LTIs include hypertension, asthma, diabetes, coronary heart disease, stroke, chronic obstructive pulmonary disease (COPD), cancer, heart failure, chronic pain and epilepsy (Department of Health, 2012).

DOI: 10.4324/9781003171096-16

LTIs affect people's lives in many ways. Sufferers are less likely to be employed, more likely to be poor, and more likely to need additional care and support from family members and others. With no medical cure in sight it is unsurprising that people with LTIs are also more likely to use complementary or alternative medical services. We have noted that people with LTIs may benefit from self-management interventions (see Chapter 8). Longer consultations focusing on the patients' beliefs and feelings and prompting patients to take control of illness management may be especially important for these patients.

The challenge for people with LTIs is to adapt to their illness, adopt the most effective coping strategies including social support seeking (see Chapter 4) and to maintain high self-efficacy (see Chapter 8) and the best possible quality of life (QoL). The extent to which they are able to do this and to enjoy life may predict longevity. For example, Moskowitz, Epel and Acree (2008) found that positive emotions, including measures of enjoying life was associated with mortality among people with diabetes and people over 65 and especially amongst those reporting higher levels of stress. The findings suggest that positive affect may buffer stress (see Chapter 3). Psychological support is crucial to helping this group and some complementary medicine practitioners may be able to offer this support more effectively than healthcare professionals because they employ longer consultations focusing on overall wellbeing (see Chapter 10). A UK Department of Health (2008) report noted that adherence among people with LTIs is poor and that people with LTIs want more healthcare services delivered in the community and in their homes. The report also notes that providing people with greater control over the services they use is likely to increase adherence, self-efficacy and quality of life.

Cognition and coping are critical to adaptation to LTI. For example, Scharloo, Kaptein, Weinman, Willems and Rooijmans (2000) found that the five categories of beliefs about symptoms identified by Leventhal and colleagues (see Chapter 10) predicted coping and adaptation in COPD patients, emphasising the importance of cognitive care and intervention for these patients. Qualitative research can reveal more detailed patterns of illness-related thought. Such studies often reveal the burden that LTIs place on people's self-concept, or identity. For example, Dovey-Pearce, Doherty and May (2007) show how diabetes can affect young people's self-concept, highlighting the desire to be "normal", the additional adult responsibilities that diabetes places on young people and the importance of peer support. Similarly, Smith and Osborne (2007) illustrated the crushing effect that chronic pain can have on self-concept. Interviewees described how their pain led to social behaviour that they were ashamed of and wanted to distance themselves from their public persona. They expressed nostalgia for a past normal self and were anxious about the self that others attributed to them as a result of their pain-directed behaviour. Patients with LTIs may also find engagement with traditional health services which focus on diagnosis and treatment challenging and alienating. For example, in a qualitative study of stories written by women with chronic pelvic pain, McGowan, Luker, Creed and Chew-Graham (2007) found that women found consultations unsatisfactory when medical tests failed to validate their experience of pain. The failure to find a physiological explanation left women feeling powerless and devalued and concerned that they were not believed or perceived to be neurotic or depressed. In some cases this led to complete disengagement from healthcare services, despite ongoing pain.

Behaviour change interventions for people with long-term illnesses

In Chapter 9, we discussed the theory, systematic development and implementation of behaviour change interventions in healthcare. Behaviour change interventions have much to offer people with LTIs (see Araújo-Soares, Hankonen, Presseau, Rodrigues & Sniehotta, 2019 for an overview). In a systematic review, Glazier, Bajcar, Kennie and Willson (2006) found that 11 of 17 interventions improved diabetes care with intervention effectiveness being associated with (i) delivery by community educators or lay people, (ii) one-to-one interaction with individualised assessment, (iii) a focus on behaviour change, (iv) provision of feedback, (v) use of ten or more sessions and (vi) a duration of six months or more. While such interventions are expensive, they are likely to be cost effective because it has been estimated that self-management interventions for people with LTIs could reduce visits to general practitioners by a quarter and hospitalisation by a half amongst this population, while also enhancing participants' QoL (Department of Health, 2008). Note too that behaviour change interventions can prevent some LTIs. For example, Knowler et al. (2002) found that a lifestyle change programme including weekly exercise targets was more effective than medication in preventing diabetes onset over a three-year period. Such findings strongly support the Lifestyle Medicine approach to healthcare outlined in Chapter 1.

In a classic paper, Kaplan (1990) argued that mortality and quality of life are always the most important outcome measures in healthcare. There are a variety of quality-of-life and health-related quality-of-life measures available including one developed by the World Health Organization (WHOQOL Group, 1995) and the Short-Form Health Survey (Ware, Kosinski, & Keller, 1996) which assess the degree to which illness imposes on everyday life and how patients' feel about their everyday life. Improving the quality of life of patients with long-term illnesses is a key healthcare objective.

Managing long-term pain

Long-term pain provides a powerful illustration of the importance of psychological and behaviour change interventions for patients with LTIs. In a comprehensive review, Gatchel, Bo Peng, Peters, Fuchs and Turk (2007) indicate how a biopsychosocial approach to understanding pain emphasises the role of psychological care in treatment. They note, for example, that anxiety reduction interventions can result in reduced distress and interference with daily living. They also note that enhanced self-efficacy in relation to controlling the impact pain has on everyday living affects the body's opioid and immune systems, reduces pain, improves recovery after surgical procedures and improves overall psychological adjustment. Higher levels of pain-related self-efficacy increases motivation to follow through with goals that become challenging and so reduces activity avoidance and may, thereby, increase social engagement and support. Consequently, these researchers note that, "pain cannot be treated successfully without attending to the patient's emotional state" (p. 602). Current treatment of pain focuses on multi-disciplinary programmes, which incorporate a combination of approaches including psychological interventions. Turk and Burwinkle (2005) highlighted the effectiveness and cost effectiveness of such programmes compared to traditional approaches treating chronic pain. They list commonly used measures of pain assessment and show that multidisciplinary programmes are effective, not only in reducing pain but in improving employment status and reducing medication and medical services usage. They also emphasise the role of psychologists both in designing and evaluating interventions within such multidisciplinary contexts.

Opioid drugs are powerful and can reduce pain experience. They have been used widely to help people with long-term pain. Unfortunately, these drugs are not effective in the longer term and can have debilitating side effects. An Agency for Healthcare Research and Quality (AHQR 2022) review concluded that opioids have small beneficial effects but are not more effective than non-opioid therapy and have increased risk of short and long-term harms. Yet millions of people are being prescribed these drugs; 142 million in the USA in 2020 (Centres of Disease Control, 2023). Consequently, considerable research has been devoted to biological and pharmacological innovations that could reduce pain without opioid use. Chapter 9 highlights how behaviour change interventions are helping patients with long-term pain to reduce opioid use and, thereby, enhancing their quality of life (Sandhu et al., 2023). Such interventions have to be carefully designed (see Chapter 9). de Kleijn et al. (2022) reviewed five randomised controlled trials of such interventions in primary care, including mindfulness and cognitive-behavioural techniques. Four found no significant differences between the intervention and control groups in opioid drug use. One, based on mindfulness, found a significant reduction in opioid use and in pain reporting (Garland et al., 2022). Yet the group-based I-WOTCH, intervention was found to be effective. This intervention included support from nurses and patients who had successfully reduced opioid use, as well as individual support and skill-based learning. The intervention significantly reduced patient-reported use of opioids compared to usual care, but, unfortunately, found no significant effects on pain interference with daily life activities (Sandhu et al., 2023). There is much work to do in helping patients reduce opioid drug use and find other ways to manage daily pain.

Psychological interventions may also focus directly on pain-related behaviour with a view to enhancing activity and quality of life rather than pain reduction. Application of techniques based on the principles of operant conditioning such as extinction and reinforcement were pioneered by Fordyce (1976). Central to this approach is the assumption that pain behaviours (e.g. withdrawal lying down, crying, limping, reliance on medication) are learned responses which become conditioned through reinforcement (e.g. receiving attention, sympathy and care in response to pain behaviour and avoided anticipated pain by taking analgesic medication). These approaches seek to:

1. Reinforce adaptive "well" behaviours such as walking without limping after a minor operation.
2. Encourage family and friends not to attend to or reward pain behaviours.
3. Provide analgesic medication on a fixed schedule (e.g. every four hours) and not when the patient requests it or is in pain.

Each of these approaches has been found to successfully reinforce adaptive behaviour and to extinguish previous maladaptive behaviour (Horn & Munafo, 1998). For example, patients' reliance on medication can be reduced over a short period of time. By providing the medication on a fixed schedule, receiving it becomes independent of requests, so eliminating reinforcement effects. Over a couple of weeks, the dosage of medication can be reduced by mixing it with a flavoured syrup to mask the taste and then gradually reducing the amount of the analgesic in the mixture. These interventions emphasise how pain and other symptoms may be strongly influences by psychological responses and behavioural routines. Health psychologists have much to offer patients with LTIs, in particular by delivering evidence-based interventions to change beliefs and behaviour patterns.

Using groups in healthcare

Shared medical appointments

In Chapter 8, we examined how discussions in groups can influence group members by changing their beliefs, attitudes and behaviour. Since changes in cognition and behaviour underpin adherence to health advice, it is unsurprising that groups are being used in healthcare delivery. Noffsinger (2009) advocated using groups in everyday healthcare delivery and, since then, "shared medical appointments" (SMAs) have been implemented and evaluated internationally.

SMAs are different to the self-management groups that we discussed in Chapter 8. In SMAs, patients sit together while a practitioner hears and responds to each patient's concerns in turn. SMAs are usually arranged when the patients share similar health challenges. For example, if all the patients have lifestyles which put them at high risk of developing diabetes or they are all struggling with alcohol use or if they share a LTI such as diabetes or asthma. A traditional individual consultation might involve one patient for ten minutes. A SMA might involve around 12 patients and last 90 minutes or more. A SMA may involve one or two practitioners, including, for example, a medical doctor and a nurse or two specialist nurses. One practitioner may consult with a patient in the group while the other records action points and outcomes, making notes and ordering prescriptions. While an individual consultation is in progress during a SMA, the other patients listen. This allows patients to learn from others who share their health challenges. Even if the concern of another patient is not the same as theirs, learning about symptoms, management strategies and treatments that may help them develop expertise in managing their own condition. The practitioner/s may use all the time on one-to-one consultations or take time to address the whole group by highlighting or explaining issues that may be relevant to most of the patients present. SMAs are only useful to patients who are willing to share in a group context and, of course, patients will only share what they are comfortable with.

SMAs serve multiple purposes. In a review of evaluations, Kirsh et al. (2017) highlight a series of benefits. Patients may benefit from understanding that their challenges are shared; they may feel socially validated. This may also reduce feelings of isolation in relation to health challenges. Patients may learn about illness self-management by witnessing others' illness experiences. Patients may also learn from others by understanding how they are coping and perhaps being inspired by them, so enhancing their own self-efficacy. The combination of professional advice and insights into the lived experience of others may strengthen the relevance and importance of advice offered so encouraging belief change and adherence. Patients may appreciate how much time and support practitioners are giving patients, like themselves, and learn more about their healthcare providers, so enhancing trust and appreciation of practitioners. While further work on standardisation of optimal implementation of SMAs and more quality randomised controlled trials are needed (Booth, Cantrell, Preston, Chambers & Goyder, 2015), evidence supports the use of SMAs. Combined with the opportunity for individual appointments, they can enhance patient trust, patients' reports of quality of care and quality of life, and, in some cases, lead to improvements in biological measures of health, including blood pressure (Wadsworth et al., 2019). SMAs are likely to be especially helpful to patients with LTIs, including diabetes (Menon et al., 2017; Swaithes et al., 2021). SMAs help patients become experts (see Chapter 8 on EPP interventions).

SMAs may also help healthcare providers. Practitioners may avoid having to repeat the same things across individual appointments. This may lead to greater time efficiency in providing services to those with LTIs. Practitioners may get to know their patients and colleagues better through SMAs, so enhancing rapport. Using SMAs may increase practitioner work satisfaction which could enhance communication with patients and patient adherence (DiMatteo et al., 1993 – see above; Egger et al., 2014; Kirsh et al., 2017). Thus, SMAs may enhance the experience of healthcare practitioners and patients and be especially effective for patients with LTIs. Adoption and optimisation of SMAs will involve behaviour change among patients, practitioners and health system managers (Jones et al., 2019). This is one more example of how health service efficiency can be facilitated by application of evidence-based behaviour change science (see Chapter 9).

Complementary therapies

Poor patient satisfaction and uncertainty about the effectiveness of traditional medicine fosters demand for complementary or alternative medicine (CAM). Complementary therapies include a wide range of interventions based on various models of mind and body that are not necessarily based on evidence-based models of physiological systems (see Chapter 1). Complementary therapies may also differ from traditional medical healthcare by focusing on the client's overall wellbeing rather than specific physical problems.

CAM use is widespread. Estimates of population usage vary widely. Use is especially high among those with LTIs. For example, a survey of nearly 1500 cancer patients indicated that most (96%) used CAM (Yalcin, Hurmuz McQuinn & Naing, 2017). More broadly, it has been estimated that 42% of the USA population have used CAM spending more than $21 billion annually (White, 2000) and two thirds of those receiving treatment for anxiety or depression report using CAM in the USA (Bassman & Uellendahl, 2003). In Europe, 75% of the French population and 50% of the UK population reported having used CAM (Murcott, 2006). A Norwegian survey found that 67% of respondents had used CAM, mainly for treatment of LTIs and that users had high satisfaction (Krokstad et al., 2017). CAM has varying levels of support among healthcare practitioners (Phutrakool & Pongpirul, 2022). Yet such therapies play an important role in healthcare, internationally.

The UK House of Lords Select Committee on Science and Technology (House of Lords, 2000) published a landmark report on CAM which distinguished between therapies which do and do not provide diagnoses. Those that do provide diagnoses include osteopathy, chiropractic (which are regulated by UK Acts of Parliament), acupuncture, herbal medicine and homeopathy. Those that do not, include aromatherapy, hypnotherapy, reflexology and shiatsu. The Select Committee made a series of recommendations including: (1) therapies which claim to treat specific conditions should have evidence of being more effective than placebo effects (see below); (2) if a therapy does gain a critical mass of evidence to support its efficacy the UK National Health Service should provide access to it; (3) training in anatomy, physiology, biochemistry and pharmacology should be included within the education of CAM practitioners likely to offer diagnostic information; (4) CAM therapists should be trained in research methodology and have a clear understanding of the principles of evidence-based medicine, including evaluation (see Chapter 9); and (6) CAM therapists should encourage patients to see traditional healthcare professionals. These recommendations highlight the challenges of, on the one hand, providing access to effective treatments based on alternative models of health and, on the other, ensuring that such treatments are effective. Applying these recommendations could help integration of CAM with traditional healthcare delivery.

Evaluating complementary therapies

The models underpinning many complementary therapies are not supported by scientific findings. For example, some homeopathic liquid treatments are diluted so many times that not even a single molecule of the original substance is likely to remain. While homeopaths claim that water somehow "remembers" the original active ingredient, this makes no sense in terms of our understanding of the chemistry of water (Murcott, 2006). Similarly, as a UK NHS (2023) website explains, acupuncture is based on the assumption (first made 2,000 years ago in China) that health depends on a life force called Qi which flows along 12 bodily meridians. Needles are inserted into the meridians to restore health by unblocking Qi flow. Yet no anatomical evidence of these meridians has been found.

Considerable efforts are devoted to testing the effectiveness of complementary therapies and acupuncture is especially well researched (see Vickers & Zollman, 1999, for a useful introduction to osteopathy and chiropractic). For example, Vas et al. (2004) found that combining acupuncture with pharmacological treatment for osteoarthritis of the knee led to greater pain reduction and increased physical functioning one week after treatment, controlling for placebo effects. However, Foster et al. (2007) found that adding acupuncture to advice and exercise for osteoarthritis of the knee did *not* enhance effectiveness. Interestingly, the acupuncture placebo condition involved use of blunt needles which collapse into their handles to give the appearance of penetration to control for contextual effects. The question here is whether this is a realistic control condition. The NHS website states that acupuncture "can be helpful in relieving pain" but also that "research into the effectiveness of acupuncture treatment for chronic pain has not produced consistent results". Studies have found that acupuncture enhances the effectiveness of traditional treatment for some conditions but the evidence is less than clear cut and evaluations of this evidence vary in their conclusions. For example, White (2000) and Bassman and Uellendahl (2003) present a fairly positive review, citing evidence for the effectiveness of acupuncture in treating depression and substance abuse. Murcott (2006) is more pessimistic about the evidence on pain relief noting that that there are few studies of longer-term effectiveness. He compares the evidence for the analgesic effects of aspirin and acupuncture and concludes that evidence for the latter is clearly weaker. This pessimism about acupuncture effectiveness is supported by a systematic review (Ezzo et al., 2000).

Many people find CAM services helpful. Yet there are serious questions about the evidence-basis of what is offered, especially by non-diagnostic CAM services. This raises an important question about the appropriate health outcome measures for people with LTIs. If there is no cure, then what should healthcare services be providing and what role do CAM services provide?

Placebo effects and psychological models of recovery

Placebo effects refer to health or wellbeing gains observed following administration of pharmacologically inert interventions such as saline injections or sugar pills. In 1955, Beecher found that, across 15 clinical trials, 35% of patients showed health gains in placebo conditions. In contrast, across 114 trails, Hro´bjartsson and Gøtzsche (2001) found that when improvement was measured using a binary outcome (e.g. cured not cured) placebo treatments had *no* significant effect on outcome. Placebo conditions also showed no benefit when evaluated using objective clinical outcomes. A separate review of 27 trials, assessing pain, found that average placebo pain reduction was equivalent a 6.5-millimetre reduction on a self-report visual-analogue scale, measured on a 100-millimetre line; not a big effect. One weakness of such a review is that, if placebo effects are limited to particular types of health gain (such as reduced pain), these effects may not be evident when trials are pooled across conditions (Stewart-Wiliams, 2004).

Effects on adherence have also been found in placebo conditions (Epstein 1984). For example, in a trial of beta blockers for women who had had a heart attack, Gallagher, Viscoli and Horwitz (1993) found that 5.6% of those who took 75% of the medication died within 26 months but 13.6% of those who took less than 75% died in the same period. Remarkably, this difference was not noticeably diminished in the placebo condition. In this study, taking beta blockers was *not* effective above and beyond the placebo effect. From a psychological perspective, the interesting observation is that taking an apparently ineffective (placebo) drug improved health and worked as well as a tested drug treatment.

In trials which only compare treatments with a placebo condition, numerous factors contribute to an observed "placebo effect". Natural fluctuations in physiological functioning mean that, for many conditions, some people spontaneously improve (referred to as spontaneous remission). This is especially true of LTIs because people are likely to seek medical help when their symptoms are most severe. People involved in intervention trials may also change how they assess their symptoms (cf. Norman & Parker, 1996). In addition, they may engage in new behaviours relevant to their treatment. Controlling for such effects necessitates a three-condition design in which treatment is compared to both placebo and a no-treatment control group (e.g. people randomly assigned to a waiting list for trial inclusion). The true placebo effect can then be defined as the additional gain seen in the placebo group over and above the no-treatment condition (Ernst & Resch, 1995). Placebo conditions need to mimic the context in which treatment is administered (see the acupuncture example above). These so called "non-specific effects" include context and communication. This is why healthcare professionals involved in trials should, ideally, be blind to which condition a patient has been allocated to. Yet such three-arm placebo trials are relatively rare in the research literature. This means that two-arm trials may confuse placebo effects and other non-treatment effects such as spontaneous remission.

Explaining placebo effects: patient expectations and anxiety reduction

Many explanations of placebo effects have been tested and it is likely that multiple processes are involved (see Stewart-Williams, 2004, for a clear summary). For example, placebo analgesic effects have been shown to be mediated by the release of endogenous opioids (Levine et al., 1978) demonstrating that some placebo effects have measurable effects on the brain and endocrine system. However, such observations do not explain *how* placebo administration affects physiological systems. This may operate through patient expectations and anxiety reduction. When a healthcare professional (perceived to be competent) communicates to a patient that her problem is understood and that she (the patient) is being advised to take an effective, manageable treatment, the patient will expect her condition to improve. Such expectations may have cognitive, physiological and behavioural effects. For example, believing that the worst is over could liberate the patient to devote time and energy to other life-enhancing pursuits. It could alter coping strategies, perhaps leading to more social support seeking. It is also likely to reduce stress and anxiety. Secondary appraisals (see Chapter 3) will be altered because patients believe they have an important new resource, namely, a treatment that will cure or alleviate adverse symptoms. Anxiety reduction is known to have physiological effects. For example, it is likely to affect endocrine functioning, reducing levels of cortisol and adrenalin in the blood stream. This, in turn, may have positive effects on blood pressure, inflammation and immune functioning (see Chapter 2) as well as on cognitive functioning (e.g. memory). Anxiety reduction is also associated with reduced pain because downward neural pathways from the brain can cut off or "gate" incoming pain signals from peripheral nerves (Melzack & Wall, 1965). Thus, a stress reduction explanation based on expectations of treatment efficacy provides a powerful explanation for some placebo effects. This explanation corresponds to Little et al.'s (2001) observation that patients reported fewer symptoms after consultations in which doctors adopted a positive and definite approach including providing guidance on when the problem would be resolved (see too Howick et al., 2018). Moreover, an expectation-based explanation could account for the direct effects of adherence because the more consciously one adheres to the apparently effective (placebo) treatment the stronger one's expectation of relief or recovery should be. Nonetheless, this explanation does not account for all placebo effects. For example, an objectively assessed bronchodilation placebo effect findings observed by Butler and Steptoe (1986) could not be explained by changes in expectations or anxiety.

Explaining placebo effects: classical conditioning

Classical conditioning theory may account for some placebo effects. The "real" drug can be regarded as the unconditioned stimulus and beneficial physiological changes as unconditioned responses. Similarity, in administration of the placebo treatment (e.g. context, nature of treatment etc.) leads to an association between the placebo treatment (the conditioned stimulus) and the unconditional stimulus. Such effects have been observed in people and animals. For example, Benedetti, Pollo, and Colloca (2007) examined the effect of repeated administrations of injected morphine during athletes' training sessions on placebo response. They found that athletes who had had morphine injections during training and who then received a saline injection (which they thought was morphine) showed greater pain endurance and physical performance during competition. This has interesting implications for drug testing in sport because it suggests that after appropriate drug conditioning it may be enough for an athlete to believe she is taking a performance-enhancing drug to improve her performance!

The placebo effect literature strongly emphasises how important it is to provide patients with expectations of recovery (where it is reasonable and ethical to do so) and to encourage commitment to adherence. The psychological consequences of these processes may greatly enhance the pharmacological processes generated by available drugs. This is an important echo of Hippurates' emphasis on the importance of the healer-client relationship. Practitioners, whether medically trained, nurses or health psychologists, who are able to harness and deliver the psychological and physiological effects evident in placebo responding will optimise the health impact of their consultations and interventions. This was confirmed by a review of 19 trials. Di Blasi et al. (2001) concluded that contextual factors affected treatment effectiveness and that, in particular, there was evidence suggesting that cognitive care (that is managing beliefs and expectations positively) and emotional care (communicating concern for the patient's problems) optimised treatment effectiveness. Healthcare professionals need to be able to deliver high-quality cognitive and emotional care to maximise their effectiveness.

Placebo effects have raised doubts about a range of treatments. For example, although the UK National Institute for Health and Clinical Excellence (2007) recommended selective serotonin reuptake inhibitors (SSRIs such as Prozac) as the preferred treatment for mild to severe depression, their effectiveness has been questioned because depressed patients in placebo conditions show good levels of recovery (Kirsch & Sapirstein, 1998; Quitkin, 2000). Kirsch et al. (2008) found that the difference in outcomes between taking antidepressants and taking placebo drugs was generally small but greater for those with severe depression because those with serious depression showed very little placebo response. Cipriani et al. (2018) reviewed 522 of 21 antidepressants and concluded that, overall, antidepressants were more effective than placebo drugs for adults with major or severe depressive disorders. However, importantly, smaller differences between antidepressants and placebo drugs were found in trials using placebo conditions (only 58% of those included). Interestingly, one of the most effective antidepressants was found to be Amitriptyline, discovered in the 1950's and approved by the USA Food and Drug Administration in 1961. Amitriptyline has many known side effects. Sadly, these findings suggest that little progress has been made in the development of pharmacological treatments for depression over more than 70 years.

A psychological approach to recovery from mental health problems

When differences between treatments and placebo effects are small, we should question whether better causal models, than those underpinning proposed treatments, are needed. In the case of depression, rather than focusing on neural mechanisms (such the lack of particular neurotransmitters in the brain, including Serotonin), another approach is to consider personal and social experiences that might create the neural states that are correlated with reported depressive symptoms. We might ask why has the brain ceased to retain neurotransmitters? What has led to this neural problem?

In 1978, Brown and Harris interviewed 458 women in London, England. Brown and Harris identified four "vulnerability factors" for depression. These were having three or more children under the age of 14 at home, not having an intimate relationship with a partner, being unemployed and having experienced the loss of their mother before the age of 11. Women who had these vulnerability factors were more likely to become depressed when they experienced stressful life events. Statistical support for this model was reported by Patten (1991). This model poses the question of whether social and psychological processes, rather than neurological processes, are the best way of understanding and, therefore, treating depression.

Acknowledging antidepressant trials results, Hari (2018) developed a model of psychological causation and intervention for depression. Hari describes how, when someone close to us dies, grief can make us feel that life is meaningless. This can make us want to withdraw and cry for what we have lost. This is not an illness. Grief is a normal part of being a person and adapting to loss. We feel bereft because we have lost someone who made our lives meaningful. We want to keep talking to that person and sharing life with them. Recovering from grief is *not* best understood as brain chemistry but as psychological adaptation to loss. Mental health services do not describe people who are grieving as "depressed" or suggest they take antidepressants. Hari asks whether depression can be better understood as loses, or disconnections, that affect our psychology and, consequently, our brain function. Hari suggests seven sources of disconnection; (i) from meaningful relationships with others, (ii) from childhood trauma, (iii) from meaningful values, (iv) from meaningful work, (v) from respect, (vi) from a hopeful and secure future and (vii) from nature. In this model, like recovery from grief, psychological adaption and reconnection the path to recovery. Just as we help others recovery from grief through reconnection so we can help people who are depressed to identify and address sources of disconnection. The proposal is that as reconnection progresses, our brains begin to regenerate neurotransmitters (such as serotonin) that we need to reengage with our social reality. The argument is that while we have had limited success in directly influencing brain function using antidepressants, it may be possible to use psychological and social interventions to indirectly improve brain function, in a very similar way to how we support grieving people to adapt to their loss. This relates directly to placebo effects. Sometimes recovery, including brain recovery, depends of psychological and social change rather than drug treatments. When drug treatments are not clearly superior to placebos then the causal model underpinning the treatments need to be re-examined.

From telemedicine to digital delivery of healthcare services

Remote consultations have been used since the early days of the telephone and two-way radio communication. For example, if someone lives in a remote area and cannot access a health centre, a telephone consultation may be crucial to effective healthcare. If the person also has monitoring devices available (such as a blood pressure or glucose monitor) then data generated by these devices can be interpreted by a remote healthcare professional. Such remote monitoring was advanced by the need to monitor astronauts' health by the USA-based National Aeronautics and Space Administration. During the COVID-19 pandemic health services used video consultations when healthcare professionals could not see patients face-to-face for fear of infection (Greenhalgh, Wherton, Shaw & Morrison, 2020). Many terms are used in this field including telemedicine (e.g. telephone consultations) telehealth (which usually refers to a broader range of digital services, including public health promotion) and eHealth referring to electronic health services in general (Gogia, 2020).

Wi-Fi and mobile device access, including smartphone access, is more widespread in richer countries such as the USA, Australia, Japan and European countries, but, globally, access is increasing rapidly towards universal access. This facilitates access to eHealth, including digital (e.g. video) consultations for ever-larger patient populations. The key questions for healthcare professionals and researchers are what kind of healthcare delivery can be facilitated by our growing capacity for digital communication and remote monitoring and how acceptable and effective will such digital services be?

Telephone calls reduce communication channels because facial expressions are not seen and even changes in tone of voice may be less recognisable. Of course, physical examinations are impossible in telephone and video consultations. Nonetheless, telephone consultations have been evaluated positively for particular patients and problems (Greenhalgh et al., 2020). Advantages for patients include being able consult from their home, or even their bed, so saving time and costs and, depending on the availability of professionals, increasing access to expert advice. This is especially helpful to patients living in remote locations, those who are working or have mobility problems (Downes, Mervin, Byrnes & Scuffham, 2017). Moreover, for some anxious patients it may be easier to manage a telephone conversation than a video or face-to-face consultation. Telemedicine can be a safe and acceptable way of delivering care, especially when in-person care is not accessible (Verma. Buch, Taralekar & Acharya, 2023).

Video consultations have the advantage that the professional and patient can see one another and learn from facial expressions. They can also share information using screen-share options. Again, although the number of evaluations, and especially quality evaluations are limited (Greenhalgh et al., 2020), early evaluations have been encouraging. For example, general practitioners in the UK judged video consultations to be better than telephone consultations in relation to building a relationship with the patient, providing reassurance, recognition of visual cues and improving communication generally (Donaghy et al., 2019). In addition, there is some evidence that video consultations (compared to telephone consultations) may improve diagnostic accuracy and reduce hospital readmission rates, perhaps particularly for those with LTIs, including those recovering from strokes (Rush, Howlett, Munro & Burton, 2018). So, it is possible that optimal use of digital services could reduce emergency admissions and increase longevity among patients with LTIs (Steventon et al., 2012).

Video consultations may not work if patients do not have access to good Wi-Fi or lack the technological training to manage video conferencing software (Donaghy et al., 2019; Greenhalgh et al., 2020). Moreover, if patients do not want video consultations, perhaps because they regard their problem as personal or sensitive or they have complex, multi-morbidity problems then face-to-face consultations may have better outcomes (Donaghy et al., 2019).

Optimising telephone and video consultations will depend of providing good training for healthcare professionals. This likely to include guidance on how to optimise communication and build trust as well as taking account to privacy issues and individual differences between patients (Zhang, Luximon & Li, 2022). Such guidance can help healthcare professionals ensure completion of the seven tasks highlighted by the Pendleton model during their telephone or video consultations (see Chapter 10). For example, Bakhai, Croney, Waller, Henshall & Felstead (2020) provide guidance to general practitioners in the UK on how to implement and deploy online consultations and the UK Royal College of General Practitioners (2020) have provided ten "top tips". Further research is needed on implementation so that practitioners understand which patients, with which conditions, under which circumstances will benefit most from telephone and video consultations and how they (healthcare professionals) can best manage such consultations (see Chapters 9 and 10).

The use of wearable monitoring devices has potential to optimise eHealth. For example, if you have a Smartphone you may be able to access information about your blood pressure, your physical activity levels and your sleep patterns. Could this data be useful to healthcare professionals? This depends on how accurate the data is. Unfortunately, there are questions about the accuracy of smartphone monitoring of physical activity and other physical functions but this does not mean that wearable devices cannot provide reliable data (e.g. Piccinini, Martinelli & Carbonaro, 2020). There are many wearable devices on the market including those that monitor (1) health and safety, (2) chronic disease management, (3) disease diagnosis and treatment and (4) rehabilitation (Lu et al., 2020). The challenge is to produce affordable monitoring devices that have been demonstrated to provide reliable data, that patients can use easily. In future, such live data could greatly facilitate healthcare practitioners' understanding of patients' health and health problems. Reliable wearable devices may be especially useful when monitoring people with reduced mobility and elderly populations over time (Kekade et al., 2018). Of course, even if wearable devices generate somewhat unreliable data they may motivate wearers. Self-monitoring of gradual but successful behaviour change can be a critical foundation for self-efficacy enhancement, practice and, therefore, behaviour change (see Chapter 8). This can be rewarded by observation of data on wearable devices, including meeting steps-per-day targets, better sleep scores or reduced blood pressure. So, we can distinguish between wearable monitoring devices that may be less accurate but, nonetheless, motivating for users (e.g. smartphones) and those that provide reliable clinical data, useful to healthcare professionals.

eHealth refers to much more than the use of video conferencing platforms to facilitate remote consultations. Digital delivery may involve use of interactive public health information sites that can deliver personalised assessments and advice on the basis of patient data entry. There are many such assessments available online and these are likely to improve in future. For example, one such health assessment included questions on: (1) biological assessments, including weight, height and blood test results, (2) physical activity levels, (3) wellbeing, social cohesion, and functional independence, (4) nutrition, (5) mental health, (6) smoking, drinking, and use of illicit substances, (7) sleep habits and quality, and (8) health and disease, as well as a summary using traffic light feedback (Reis et al., 2019). Such assessments have the advantage of building a comprehensive picture of the user's health. In this case, for example, all six pillars of the Lifestyle Medicine approach are assessed (see Chapter 1). Interactive online assessments represent an important advance over static information sheets or websites or the wall commissioned by Diogenes (see Chapter 1)!

Digital resources have the potential to empower users to understand their personal health needs and make decisions about what aspects of their health they need to prioritise in terms of health behaviour change. Such assessments could be shared with healthcare practitioners, if desired. Despite this potential, caution is warranted on two counts. First, as we have seen self-reports may be inaccurate. If someone reports their weight, alcohol usage or mental health status inaccurately, perhaps because they were rushed or did not have the necessary information at the time of assessment, then the advice they receive may be inappropriate. Second, such assessments may create unnecessary health concerns. This may increase numbers of "worried well" patients who seek health services when they do not really need them and this might be especially likely for users high in neuroticism (Chapter 6). Nonetheless, with careful supervision, digital tools of this kind could be very helpful in guiding health self-management, goal setting and goal prioritisation for users (see Chapter 9). Moreover, in future, these tools are likely to be able to draw on increasingly greater data sources, including, with permission, patients' medical records. They may facilitate the development of evolving records and goal setting priorities. For example, if patients were to complete assessment updates prior to consultations (and the data was deemed to be reliable) this could help practitioners understand changes in patients' health over time. So, empowering patients (see Chapter 10). Digital assessments may also employ novel approaches. For example, assessing a user's diet by presentation of pictures of foods and groups of foods rather than using long self-report questionnaires (Turner-McGrievy, Hutto, Bernhart & Wilson. 2022).

The development of digital resources to assist people managing their health has been dramatic. It has been estimated that between 165,000 and 325,000 health and wellness apps' are now available (Carlo, Hosseini Ghomi, Renn, & Areán, 2019) and that this market is worth more than US$200 billion. This expansion has created a quality control problem. It is increasingly challenging for practitioners or members of the public to know which digital resources are useful and can effectively help them manage their health. Few apps are evaluated and evaluations have not been encouraging. For example, a meta-analysis of 156 rigorous evaluations of health apps' found that they conferred only a weak advantage over standard care with high heterogeneity of findings, meaning some delivered slight positive effects while others did not (Iribarren et al., 2021). This is disappointing given the expense of developing such digital resources. Even effective apps tend to be underutilised, and, consequently, may have little impact on population health, because users cannot sift through the myriad of available resources to find those they most need (Ramakrishnan et al., 2021). So, a critical future development will be national identification of digital resources that are validated or "kite-marked" as useful; for patients' use. Considerable evaluation research (see Chapter 9) is needed to facilitate identification of effective digital resources. Moreover, improved development of digital resources that meet people's health assessment and advice needs is required. This may be especially useful to people with LTIs and co-development of resources is likely to optimise attractiveness, engagement and effectiveness for users (Tighe et al., 2020).

The development of digital resources is likely to transform healthcare delivery and relationships between patients and practitioners. For example, the UK government envisages complete digitalisation and integration of all citizens' health and social care records and the use of evolving records so that authorised practitioners could easily access complete patient histories. In addition, the UK government foresees much greater use of digital health self-help, diagnostics and therapies through apps and websites. The ambition is to put health services in people's pockets and to allow patients' greater control over management of their health through endorsed apps and websites (Department of Health and Social Care, 2022). Digital health services could also revolutionise communication between patients and providers with appointment-making and appointment agendas being managed by intelligent systems that respond to patients' online assessments and requests and also select and prioritise patients for practitioners.

An important element in the development of future digital health services will be the deployment of artificial intelligence (AI) (Department of Health and Social Care, 2022). The capacity of AI systems has increased rapidly because of advances in machine learning which have, for example, improved performance in image classification with implications for the accuracy and delivery of radiological services (El Naqa, 2020). Deployment of AI across other areas of healthcare is ongoing and likely to accelerate over time (see Ahuja, 2019 for an interesting overview). Current challenges include building reliable large-scale datasets and training of healthcare professionals to interact with AIs and interpret their outputs (Balagurunathan, Mitchell & Naqa, 2021). The evolution of routine healthcare into systems that are partially managed by intelligent digital systems will be transformative.

The technological expertise to develop personalised health coaches that people could interact on their Smartphones already exists and this may be the future of digital healthcare (Abraham, Borland & McNeill, 2023). Imagine a coach on your smartphone that could take you through reliable assessments (see Reis et al., 2019) and then recommend particular health goals which, of course, you could amend. Your "coach" would monitor progress with inputs from you and provide weekly feedback. Such a coach could be based on the six pillars of Lifestyle Medicine (see Chapter 1). Selection of an avatar would personalise the coach. User responses to assessments could also prompt use of health services, e.g. "I think you need to see your asthma nurse". The coach could then make the appointment with the user's permission, "Do you want me to make an appointment?". In addition the coach could share data with a trusted healthcare professional with the user's permission; a health coach in your pocket!

ACTIVITY BOX 11.1

Psychological contributions to patient care

Imagine you joined a multidisciplinary clinic for people with LTIs and were asked to draw up a brief report on how application of psychological theory and research could help improve the care the clinic was offering. Make notes for your report. See e.g. Araújo-Soares et al., 2019.

Key terms introduced in Chapter 11 (in order of appearance)

- Long term illness (LTI).
- Asthma.
- Diabetes,
- Chronic obstructive pulmonary disease (COPD).
- Chronic pain.
- Quality of life.
- Shared medical appointments.
- Complementary or alternative medicine (CAM).
- Acupuncture.
- Homeopathy.
- Placebo effect.
- Visual-analogue scale.
- Adherence main effect.
- Selective serotonin reuptake inhibitors.
- Endogenous opioids.
- Patient expectations.
- Anxiety reduction.
- Classical conditioning.
- Cognitive care.
- Emotional care.
- Psychological reconnection.
- Telemedicine.
- Telehealth.
- eHealth.
- Video consultations.
- Apps.
- AI.
- Digital health coach.

Summary of main points addressed in Chapter 11

People with long-term physical illness tend to be older and to be more intensive users of healthcare services. The challenge for people with LTIs is to adapt to their illness, adopt the most effective coping strategies and to maintain high self-efficacy and a good quality of life. Emotional responses to the illness are likely to affect quality of life and, in some cases longevity. Consequently, cognitive and emotional care is critical to efficacious and cost-effective services. Psychological interventions have much to offer. For example, cognitive interventions focusing on cognition and emotion and behavioural interventions focusing on behaviours and quality of life have been found to be effective in pain management.

Use of complementary or alternative medicine (CAM) is widespread but doubts remain about the effectiveness of such therapies, especially when placebo effects are controlled for and clinical outcomes are used. Large placebo effects have been observed but the impact of placebo respond-ing on clinical outcomes may be limited to certain health problems including pain relief. A variety of processes underpin observed placebo effects including classical conditioning of drug responses. Patient expectations and stress reduction are likely to play an important role in the psychological and physiological benefits observed in placebo conditions. Adhering to treatment can bolster such expectations which may account for the beneficial effects of adherence to placebo treatments.

The development of digital resources is transforming healthcare delivery and relationships between patients and practitioners. Integrated digital records that evolve over time and are easily available to patients and practitioners will be a useful first step. More advanced use of intelligent systems that respond to patients' online assessments and requests and also select and prioritise patients for practitioners could enhance the accessibility of services. This may involve increased use of digital apps and online video or audio consultations. The challenge will be to ensure that consultation quality and the relationships between patients and practitioners are retained. Use of AI may create entirely new roles for healthcare practitioners over time. Digital health coaches that can be used on Smartphones can already be developed and could make important contributions to effective health promotion and population-level health maintenance.

Recommendations for further reading

Journal articles

Abraham, C., Borland, R. & McNeill, I. (2023). The need for a personalized, core digital resource to facilitate health self-management. *Preventive Medicine*, *173*, 107569. doi: 10.1016/j.ypmed.2023.107569

Araújo-Soares, V., Hankonen, N., Presseau, J., Rodrigues, A. & Sniehotta F. F. (2018) Developing behavior change interventions for self-management in chronic illness: An integrative overview. *European Psychologist*, *24*(1), 7–25.

Stewart-Williams, S. (2004). The placebo puzzle: Putting together the pieces. *Health Psychology*, *23*, 198–206.

Illustrative essay titles

How can psychologists help people with long term illnesses?

Should health services increase the use group meetings and group consultations?

What are placebo effects and can they be used to improve health?

Discuss the potential benefits and potential pitfalls of the development of digital intervention health services.

REFERENCES

Aaron, R.V., Fisher, E.A., De La Vega, R., Lumley, M.A., & Palermo, T.M. (2019). Alexithymia in individuals with chronic pain and its relation to pain intensity, physical interference, depression, and anxiety: A systematic review and meta-analysis. *Pain, 160*, 994–1006. https://doi.org/10.1097/j.pain.0000000000001487

Abhyankar, P., O'Connor, D.B., & Lawton, R. (2008). The role of message framing in promoting MMR vaccination· Evidence of a loss-frame advantage. *Psychology, Health & Medicine, 13*(1), 1–16. https://doi.org/10.1080/13548500701235732

Abraham, C. (2004). Theory in health psychology research. In S. Michie & C. Abraham (Eds.), *Health psychology in practice* (pp. 65–82). Oxford: Blackwell.

Abraham, C. (2008). Beyond stages of change: Multi determinant continuum models of action readiness and menu-based interventions. *Applied Psychology: An International Review, 57*, 30–41. https://doi.org/10.1111/j.1464-0597.2007.00320.x

Abraham, C., Borland, R., & McNeill, I. (2023). The need for a personalized, core digital resource to facilitate health self-management. *Preventive Medicine, 173*, 107569. doi: 10.1016/j.ypmed.2023.107569

Abraham, C., Costa-Pereira, A., Du V Florey, C., & Ogston, S. (1999). Cognitions associated with initial medical consultations concerning recurrent breathing difficulties: A community-based study. *Psychology & Health, 14*(5), 913–925. https://doi.org/10.1080/08870449908407356

Abraham, C., & Denford, S. (2020). Design, implementation, and evaluation of behavior change interventions: A ten-task guide. In M. Hagger, L. Cameron, K. Hamilton, N. Hankonen, & T. Lintunen (Eds.), *The handbook of behavior change* (Cambridge Handbooks in Psychology, pp. 269–284). Cambridge: Cambridge University Press. https://doi.org/10.1017/9781108677318.019

Abraham, C., & Gardner, B. (2009). What psychological and behaviour changes are initiated by 'expert patient' training and what training techniques are most helpful? *Psychology & Health, 24*(10), 1153–1165. https://doi.org/10.1080/08870440802521110.

Abraham, C., & Graham-Rowe, E. (2009). Are worksite interventions effective in increasing physical activity? A systematic review and meta-analysis. *Health Psychology Review, 3*(1), 108–144. https://doi.org/10.1080/17437190903151096

Abraham, C., Johnson, B.T., de Bruin, M., & Luszczynska, A. (2014). Enhancing reporting of behavior change intervention evaluations. *Journal of Acquired Immune Deficiency Syndromes, 66*(Suppl 3), 293–299. https://doi.org/10.1097/QAI.0000000000000231

Abraham, C., Krahé, B., Dominic, R., & Fritsche, I. (2002). Do health promotion messages target cognitive and behavioural correlates of condom use? A content analysis of safer sex promotion leaflets in two countries. *British Journal of Health Psychology, 7*(Pt 2), 227–246. doi: 10.1348/135910702169466.

Abraham, C., & Michie, S. (2008). A taxonomy of behavior change techniques used in interventions. *Health Psychology, 27*(3), 379–387. https://doi.org/10.1037/0278-6133.27.3.379

Abraham, C., Norman, P., & Conner, M. (2000). Towards a psychology of health-related behaviour change. In P. Norman, C. Abraham, & M. Conner (Eds.), *Understanding and changing health behaviour: From health beliefs to self-regulation* (pp. 343–369). Switzerland: Harwood Academic.

Abraham, C., & Sheeran, P. (2003). Acting on intentions: The role of anticipated regret. *The British Journal of Social Psychology, 42*(Pt 4), 495–511. https://doi.org/10.1348/014466603322595248

Abraham, C., & Sheeran, P. (2015). Health belief model. In M. Conner & P. Norman (Eds.), *Predicting and changing health behaviour: Research and practice with social cognition models* (3rd Edn.; pp. 30–69). Maidenhead: Open University Press.

Abraham, C., Sheeran, P., & Johnston, M. (1998). From health beliefs to self-regulation: Theoretical advances in the psychology of action control. *Psychology & Health*, *13*(4), 569–591. https://doi.org/10.1080/0887044 9808407420

Abraham, C., Southby, L., Quandte, S., Krahé, B., & van der Sluijs, W. (2007). What's in a leaflet? Identifying research-based persuasive messages in European alcohol-education leaflets. *Psychology & Health*, *22*(1), 31–60. https://doi.org/10.1080/14768320600774405

Ader, R., & Cohen, N. (1975). Behaviorally conditioned immunosuppression. *Psychosomatic Medicine*, *37*, 333–340. https://doi.org/10.1097/00006842-197507000-00007

Adler, N.E., Boyce, T., Chesney, M.A., Cohen, S., Folkman, S., Kahn, R.L., & Syme, S.L. (1994). Socio-economic status and health. The challenge of the gradient. *American Psychologist*, *49*, 15–24. https://doi.org/10.1037//0003-066x.49.1.15

Affleck, G., Tennen, H., Croog, S., & Levine, S. (1987). Causal attribution, perceived benefits and morbidity following a heart attack: An 8-year study. *Journal of Consulting and Clinical Psychology*, *55*, 29–35. https://doi.org/10.1037//0022-006x.55.1.29

Affleck, G., Tennen, H., Uroows, S., & Higgins, P. (1992). Neuroticism and the pain-mood relation in rheuma-toid arthritis: Insights from a prospective daily study. *Journal of Consulting and Clinical Psychology*, *60*, 119–126. https://doi.org/10.1037//0022-006x.60.1.119

Affleck, G., Zautra, A., Tennen, H., & Armeli, S. (1999). Multilevel daily process designs for consulting and clinical psychology: A preface for the perplexed. *Journal of Consulting and Clinical Psychology*, *67*(5), 746–754. https://doi.org/10.1037//0022-006x.67.5.746

AHQR (2022). Opioid treatments for chronic pain. https://effectivehealthcare.ahrq.gov/products/opioids-chronic-pain/research

Ahuja, A.S. (2019). The impact of artificial intelligence in medicine on the future role of the physician. *PeerJ*, *4*(7), e7702. doi: 10.7717/peerj.7702

Ajzen, I. (1991). The theory of planned behavior. *Organizational Behavior and Human Decision Processes*, *50*, 179–211. https://doi.org/10.1016/0749-5978(91)90020-T

Ajzen, I. (2001). Nature and operation of attitudes. *Annual Review of Psychology*, *52*, 27–58. https://doi.org/10.1146/annurev.psych.52.1.27

Ajzen, I. (2015). The theory of planned behaviour is alive and well, and not ready to retire: A commentary on Sniehotta, Presseau, and Araújo-Soares. *Health Psychology Review*, *9*(2), 131–137. https://doi.org/10.1080/17437199.2014.883474

Ajzen, I., & Fishbein, M. (1980). *Understanding attitudes and predicting social behavior*. Englewood Cliffs, NJ: Prentice Hall.

Ajzen, I., & Fishbein, M. (2004). Questions raised by a reasoned action approach: Reply on Ogden (2003). *Health Psychology*, *23*, 431–434. https://doi.org/10.1037/0278-6133.23.4.431

Albarracín, D., Johnson, B.T., Fishbein, M., & Muellerleile, P.A. (2001). Theories of reasoned action and planned behavior as models of condom use: A meta-analysis. *Psychol Bull.* *127*(1), 142–161. doi: 10.1037/0033-2909.127.1.142. PMID: 11271752; PMCID: PMC4780418

Albrecht, L., Archibald, M., Arseneau, D., & Scott, S.D. (2013). Development of a checklist to assess the quality of reporting of knowledge translation interventions using the Workgroup for Intervention Development and Evaluation Research (WIDER) recommendations. *Implementation Science*, *8*(1), 52. https://doi.org/10.1186/1748-5908-8-52

Alloy, L.B., Abrahamson, L.Y., & Francis, E.L. (1999). Do negative cognitive styles confer vulnerability to depression? *Current Directions in Psychological Science*, *8*, 128–132. https://doi.org/10.1111/1467-8721.00030

Allport, F.H. (1924). *Social psychology*. Boston, MA: Houghton Mifflin.

Aluja, A., Malas, O., Urieta, P., Worner, F., & Balada, F. (2020). Biological correlates of the Toronto Alexithymia Scale (TAS-20) in cardiovascular disease and healthy community subjects. *Physiology & Behavior*, *227*, 113151. https://doi.org/10.1016/j.physbeh.2020.113151

Ambady, N., Laplante, D., Nguyen, T., Rosenthal, R., Chaumeton, N., & Levinson, W. (2002). Surgeons' tone of voice: A clue to malpractice history. *Surgery*, *132*(1), 5–9. https://doi.org/10.1067/msy.2002.124733

American Psychological Association (2014). The road to resilience: 10 ways to build resilience. Retrieved on April 14, 2014 from http://www.apa.org/helpcenter/road-resilience.aspx

American Psychological Association (2022). Stress in America™ 2022. https://www.apa.org/news/press/releases/stress/2022/concerned-future-inflation

Amiri, S., & Behnezhad, S. (2020). Job strain and mortality ratio: A systematic review and meta-analysis of cohort studies. *Public Health*, *181*, 24–33. https://doi.org/10.1016/j.puhe.2019.10.030

Andhi, N., Pravalika, J., Surya Teja, M., Thulasi Prasanna, V., & Sai Suma, C.H. (2023). Assessment of medication complexity and adherence in geriatric patients. *Indian Journal of Pharmacy Practice*, *16*(1), 33–40. doi:10.5530/097483261391

Andrasik, F., & Schwartz, M.S. (2006). Behavioral assessment and treatment of pediatric headache. *Behavior Modification*, *30*(1), 93–113. https://doi.org/10.1177/0145445505282164

Antoni, M.H., & Dhabhar, F.S. (2019). Impact of psychosocial stress and stress management on immune responses in cancer patients. *Cancer*, *125*, 1417–1431. https://doi.org/10.1002%2Fcncr.31943

Apanovitch, A.M., McCarthy, D., & Salovey, P. (2003). Using message framing to motivate HIV testing among low-income, ethnic minority women. *Health Psychology*, *22*(1), 60–67. https://doi.org/10.1037//0278-6133.22.1.60

Araújo-Soares, V., Hankonen, N., Presseau, J., Rodrigues, A., & Sniehotta, F.F. (2019). Developing behavior change interventions for self-management in chronic illness: An integrative overview. *European Psychologist*, *24*(1), 7–25. https://doi.org/10.1027/1016-9040/a000330

Armitage, C.J., & Conner, M. (2001). Efficacy of the theory of planned behaviour: A meta-analytic review. *British Journal of Social Psychology*, *40*, 471–499. https://doi.org/10.1348/014466601164939

Asch, S. (1952). *Social psychology*. Prentice Hall.

Aspinwall, L.G., & Taylor, S.E. (1997). A stitch in time: Self-regulation and proactive coping. *Psychological Bulletin*, *121*(3), 417–436. https://doi.org/10.1037/0033-2909.121.3.417

Austin, J.T., & Vancouver, J.B. (1996). Goal constructs in psychology: Structure, process, and content. *Psychological Review*, *120*, 338–375. https://doi.org/10.1037/0033-2909.120.3.338

Avisha, A., Conner, M., & Sheeran, P. (2019). Setting realistic health goals: Antecedents and consequences. *Annals of Behavioral Medicine*, *53*, 1020–1031. https://doi.org/10.1093/abm/kaz012

Ayling, K., Ru, J., Coupland, C., Chalder, T., Massey, A., Broadbent, E., & Vedhara, E. (2022). Psychological predictors of self-reported COVID-19 outcomes: Results from a prospective cohort study. *Annals of Behavioral Medicine*, *56*, 484–497. https://doi.org/10.1093/abm/kaab106

Bagby, M.R., Taylor, G.J., & Parker, J.D.A. (1994). The twenty-item Toronto Alexithymia Scale–II. Convergent, discriminant, and concurrent validity. *Journal of Psychosomatic Research*, *38*, 33–40. https://doi.org/10.1016/0022-3999(94)90006-x

Bagozzi, R.P. (1993). On the neglect of volition in consumer research: A critique and proposal. *Psychology and Marketing*, *10*, 215–237. https://doi.org/10.1002/mar.4220100305

Baird, G., Pickles, A., Simonoff, E., Charman, T., Sullivan, P., Chandler, S., Loucas, T., Meldrum, D., Afzal, M., Thomas, B., Jin, L., & Brown, D. (2008). Measles vaccination and antibody response in autism spectrum disorders. *Archives of Disease in Childhood*, *93*(10), 832–837. https://doi.org/10.1136/adc.2007.122937

Ball, P. (2021). The lightning-fast quest for COVID vaccines – and what it means for other diseases. *Nature*, *589*(7840), 16–18. https://doi.org/10.1038/d41586-020-03626-1

Baker, C. (2023). *Obesity statistics*. House of Commons Library. https://researchbriefings.files.parliament.uk/documents/SN03336/SN03336.pdf

Bakhai, M., Croney, L., Waller, O., Henshall, N., & Felstead. C. (2020). Using online consultations in primary care: Implementation toolkit. *NHS England*. https://www.england.nhs.uk/wp-content/uploads/2020/01/online-consultations-implementation-toolkit-v1.1-updated.pdf

Bakker, A.B., & Demerouti, E. (2007). The Job Demands-Resources model: State of the art. *Journal of Managerial Psychology*, *22*, 309–328. https://doi.org/10.1108/02683940710733115

Bakker, A.B., ten Brummelhuis, L.L, Prins, J.T., & van der Heijden, F.M.M.A. (2011). Applying the job demands-resources model to the work-home interface: A study among medical residents and their partners. *Journal of Vocational Behavior*, *79*, 170–180. https://doi.org/10.1016/j.jvb.2010.12.004

Bakker, A.B., Westman, M., & van Emmerik, I. J.H., (2009). Advancements in crossover theory. *Journal of Managerial Psychology*, *24*, 206–219. https://doi.org/10.1108/02683940910939304

Balagurunathan, Y., Mitchell, R., & El Naqa I. (2021). Requirements and reliability of AI in the medical context. *Physica Medica*, *83*, 72–78. doi: 10.1016/j.ejmp.2021.02.024

Bambra, C., Egan, M., Thomas, S., Petticrew, M., & Whitehead, M. (2007). The psychosocial and health effects of workplace reorganisation: 2. A systematic review of task restructuring interventions. *Journal of Epidemiology and Community Health*, *61*, 1028–1037. https://doi.org/10.1136/jech.2006.054999

Bandura, A. (1982). Self-efficacy mechanism in human agency. *American Psychologist*, *37*, 122–147. https://doi.org/10.1037/0003-066x.37.2.122

Bandura, A. (1997). *Self-efficacy: The exercise of control*. Freeman.

Bandura, A. (2000). Health promotion from the perspective of social cognitive theory. In: P. Norman, C. Abraham & M. Conner (Eds.), *Understanding and changing health behaviour: From health beliefs to self-regulation.* (pp. 229–242). Switzerland: Harwood Academic.

Bardone-Cone, A.M., & Cass, K.M. (2007). What does viewing a pro-anorexia website do? An experimental examination of website exposure and moderating effects. *International Journal of Eating Disorders, 40*, 537–548. https://doi.org/10.1002/eat.20396

Barlow, J., Wright, C., Sheasby, J., Turner, A., & Hainsworth, J. (2002). Self-management approaches for people with chronic conditions: A review. *Patient Education and Counseling, 48*(2), 177–187. https://doi.org/10.1016/s0738-3991(02)00032-0

Bartholomew, L.K., Parcel, G.S., Kok, G., & Gottlieb, N.H. (2006). *Intervention mapping: Designing theory- and evidence-based health promotion programs. Mayfield.*

Bartholomew Eldredge, L.K., Markham, C.M., Ruiter, R.A.C., Fernàndez, M.E., Kok, G., & Parcel, G.S. (2016). *Planning health promotion programs: An intervention mapping approach* (4th ed.). Wiley.

Bartley, M., Martikainen, P., Shipley, M., & Marmot, M. (2004). Gender differences in the relationship of partner's social class to behavioural risk factors and social support in the Whitehall II study. *Social Science and Medicine, 59*, 1925–1936. https://doi.org/10.1016/j.socscimed.2004.03.002

Bartram, D., & Roe, R.A. (2005). Definition and assessment of competences in the context of the European Diploma in Psychology. *European Psychologist, 10*(2), 93–102. https://doi.org/10.1027/1016-9040.10.2.93

Bassman, L.E., & Uellendahl, G. (2003). Complementary/alternative medicine: Ethical, professional, and practical challenges for psychologists. *Professional Psychology: Research and Practice, 34*(3), 264–270. https://doi.org/10.1037/0735-7028.34.3.264

Baum, A., & Posluszny, D.M. (1999). Health psychology: Mapping biobehavioral contributions to health and illness. *Annual Review of Psychology, 50*, 137–163. https://doi.org/10.1146/annurev.psych.50.1.137

Becker, M.H., Drachman, R.H., & Kirscht, J.P. (1974). A new approach to explaining sick-role behavior in low-income populations. *American Journal of Public Health, 64*(3), 205–216. https://doi.org/10.2105/ajph.64.3.205

Beecher, H.K. (1955). The powerful placebo. *Journal of the American Medical Association, 159*(17), 1602–1606. https://doi.org/10.1001/jama.1955.02960340022006

Beecher, H. K. (1956). Relationship of significance of wound to pain experienced. *Journal of the American Medical Association, 161*, 1609–1613. https://doi.org/10.1001/jama.1956.02970170005002

Beehr, T.A., and Newman, J.E. (1978). Job stress, employee health and organizational effectiveness: A facet analysis, model and literature review. *Personnel Psychology, 31*, 665–699. https://doi.org/10.1111/j.1744-6570.1978.tb02118.x

Beller, J., & Wagner, A. (2018). Loneliness, social isolation, their synergistic interaction and mortality. *Health Psychology, 37*, 808–813. https://doi.org/10.1037/hea0000605

Belloc, N.B., & Breslow, L. (1972). Relationship of physical health status and health practices. *Preventive Medicine, 9*, 469–421. https://doi.org/10.1016/0091-7435(72)90014-x.

Benedetti, F., Pollo, A., & Colloca, L. (2007). Opioid-mediated placebo responses boost pain endurance and physical performance: Is it doping in sport competitions? *The Journal of Neuroscience, 27*(44), 11934–11939. https://doi.org/10.1523/JNEUROSCI.3330-07.2007

Benjamin, R.M. (2012). Medication adherence: Helping patients take their medicines as directed. *Public Health Reports, 127*(1), 2–3. https://doi.org/10.1177/003335491212700102

Berkanovic, E., Telesky, C., & Reeder, S. (1981). Structural and social psychological factors in the decision to seek medical care for symptoms. *Medical Care, 19*(7), 693–709. https://doi.org/10.1097/00005650-19810 7000-00001

Berkman, L.F., & Syme, S.L. (1979). Social networks, host resistance, and mortality: A nine-year follow-up study of Alameda County residents. *American Journal of Epidemiology, 109*, 186–204. https://doi.org/10.1093/oxfordjournals.aje.a112674

Bissell, P., May, C.R., & Noyce, P.R. (2004). From compliance to concordance: Barriers to accomplishing a re-framed model of health care interactions. *Social Science & Medicine, 58*(4), 851–862. https://doi.org/10.1016/s0277-9536(03)00259-4

Blaxter, M. (1990). *Health and lifestyles.* London: Tavistock.

Bogg, T., & Roberts, B.W. (2004). Conscientiousness and health-related behaviors: A meta-analysis of the leading behavioral contributors to mortality. *Psychological Bulletin, 130*(6), 887–919. https://doi.org/10.1037/0033-2909.130.6.887

Bogg, T., & Roberts, B.W. (2013). The case for conscientiousness: Evidence and implications for a personality trait marker of health and longevity. *Annals of Behavioral Medicine, 45*, 278–288. https://doi.org/10.1007/s12160-012-9454-6

Bolger, N. (1990). Coping as a personality process: A prospective study. *Journal of Personality and Social Psychology, 59*, 525–537. https://doi.org/10.1037//0022-3514.59.3.525

Bolger, N., & Laurenceau, J.-P. (2013). *Intensive longitudinal methods: An introduction to diary and experience sampling research*. Guilford Press.

Bonanno, G.A. (2012). Uses and abuses of the resilience construct: Loss, trauma and health-related adversities. *Social Science & Medicine, 74*, 753–756. https://doi.org/10.1016/j.socscimed.2011.11.022

Bonanno, G.A. (2021). The resilience paradox. *European Journal of Psychotraumatology, 12*.1. https://doi.org /10.1080/20008198.2021.1942642

Bonanno, G.A., Galea, S., Bucciarelli, A., & Vlahov, D. (2007). What predicts psychological resilience after disaster? The role of demographics, resources, and life stress. *Journal of Consulting and Clinical Psychology, 75*, 671–682. https://doi.org/10.1037/0022-006x.75.5.671

Bonanno, G.A., Kennedy, P. Galatzer-Levy, I.R., Lude, P., & Elfström. M.L. (2012). Trajectories of resilience, depression, and anxiety following spinal cord injury. *Rehabilitation Psychology, 57*, 236–247. https://doi.org/10.1037/a0029256

Bond, F.W., & Bunce, D. (2001). Job control mediates change in a work reorganization intervention for stress reduction. *Journal of Occupational Health Psychology, 6*, 290–302. https://psycnet.apa.org/doi/10.1037/1076-8998.6.4.290

Bond, F.W., Flaxman, P.E., & Bunce, D. (2008). The influence of psychological flexibility on work redesign: Mediated moderation of a work reorganization intervention. *Journal of Applied Psychology, 93*, 645–654. https://doi.org/10.1037/0021-9010.93.3.645

Boneva, B., Kraut, R., & Frohlich, D. (2001). Using e-mail for personal relationships: The difference gender makes. *American Behavioral Scientist, 45*, 530–549. https://doi.org/10.1177/00027640121957204

Booth, A., Cantrell, A., Preston, L., Chambers, D., & Goyder, E. (2015). What is the evidence for the effectiveness, appropriateness and feasibility of group clinics for patients with chronic conditions? A systematic review. *Health Services and Delivery Research, 3*(46). https://doi.org/10.3310/hsdr03460

Booth, T., Mottus, R., Corley, J., Gow, A.J., Henderson, R.D., Munoz, S., et al. (2014). Personality, health, and brain integrity: The Lothian birth cohort study 1936. *Health Psychology, 33*, 1477–1486. https://doi.org/10.1037/hea0000012

Booth-Kewley, S., & Friedman, H. (1987). Psychological predictors of heart disease: A quantitative review. *Psychological Bulletin, 101*, 343–362. https://doi.org/10.1037/0033-2909.101.3.343

Booth-Kewley, S., & Vickers, R.R. (1994). Associations between major domains of personality and health behavior. *Journal of Personality, 62*, 281–298. https://doi.org/10.1111/j.1467-6494.1994.tb00298.x

Borek, A.J., & Abraham, C. (2018). How do small groups promote behaviour change? An integrative conceptual review of explanatory mechanisms. *Applied Psychology. Health and Well-being, 10*(1), 30–61. https://doi.org/10.1111/aphw.12120

Borek, A.J., Smith, J.R., Greaves, C.J., Gillison, F., Tarrant, M., Morgan-Trimmer, S., McCabe, R., & Abraham, C. (2019a). *Developing and applying a framework to understand mechanisms of action in group-based, behaviour change interventions: The MAGI mixed-methods study*. NIHR Journals Library.

Borek, A.J., Abraham, C., Greaves, C.J., Gillison, F., Tarrant, M., Morgan-Trimmer, S., McCabe, R., & Smith, J.R. (2019b). Identifying change processes in group-based health behaviour-change interventions: Development of the mechanisms of action in group-based interventions (MAGI) framework. *Health Psychology Review, 13*(3), 227–247. https://doi.org/10.1080/17437199.2019.1625282

Borek, A.J., Abraham, C., Greaves, C.J., Tarrant, M., Garner, N., & Pascale, M. (2019). 'We're all in the same boat': A qualitative study on how groups work in a diabetes prevention and management programme. *British Journal of Health Psychology, 24*(4), 787–805. https://doi.org/10.1111/bjhp.12379

Bower, J.E., Moskowitz, J.T., & Epel, E. (2009). Is benefit finding good for your health. *Current Directions in Psychological Science, 18*, 337–341. https://doi.org/10.1111/j.1467-8721.2009.01663.x

Boyce, J.M., & Pittet, D. (2002). Guideline for hand hygiene in health-care settings. Recommendations of the Healthcare Infection Control Practices Advisory Committee and the HICPAC/SHEA/APIC/IDSA Hand Hygiene Task Force. Society for Healthcare Epidemiology of America/Association for Professionals in Infection Control/Infectious Diseases Society of America. *MMWR. Recommendations and reports: Morbidity and Mortality Weekly Report. Recommendations and reports, 51*(RR-16), 1–45.

BPS (2007). *Qualification in Health Psychology (Stage 2): Candidate handbook*. The British Psychological Society: Leicester UK. (http://www.bps.org.uk/careers/society_qual/qual_downloads$/health_download$.cfm)

BPS (2021). *Qualification in Health Psychology (Stage 2)*. https://www.bps.org.uk/qualification-health-psychology-stage-2

Braesco, V., & Drewnowski, A. (2023). Are front-of-pack nutrition labels influencing food choices and purchases, diet quality, and modeled health outcomes? A narrative review of four systems. *Nutrients, 15*(1), 205. https://doi.org/10.3390/nu15010205

Brehm, J. (1966). *A theory of psychological reactance*. Academic Press.

Breslow, L., & Enstrom, J.E. (1980). Persistence of health habits and their relationship to mortality. *Preventive Medicine, 9*, 469–483. https://doi.org/10.1016/0091-7435(80)90042-0

Briñol, P., & Petty, R.E. (2005). Individual differences in attitude change. In: D. Albarracín, B.T. Johnson & M. Zanna (Eds.), *The handbook of attitudes* (pp. 575–616). Lawrence Erlbaum.

Brosschot, J.F., & van der Doef, M. (2006). Daily worrying and somatic health complaints: Testing the effectiveness of a simple worry reduction intervention. *Psychology and Health, 21*, 19–31. https://psycnet.apa.org/doi/10.1080/14768320500105346

Brosschot, J.F., Gerin, W., & Thayer, J.F. (2006). The perserverative cognition hypothesis: A review of worry, prolonged stress-related physiological activation, and health. *Journal of Psychosomatic Research, 60*, 113–124. https://doi.org/10.1016/j.jpsychores.2005.06.074

Brough, P., & Kelling, A. (2002). Women, work and well-being family-work conflict. *New Zealand Journal of Psychology, 31*, 29–38. [NO DOI available]

Brough, P., Timms, C., Siu, O., Kalliath, T., O'Driscoll, M., Sit, C.H.P., Lo, D., & Lu, C. (2013). Validation of the Job Demands-Resources model in cross-national samples: Cross sectional and longitudinal predictions of psychological strain and work engagement. *Human Relations, 66*, 1312–1315. https://doi.org/10.1177/0018726712472915

Brown, G.W. (1974). Meaning, measurement and stress of life events. In B.S. Dohrenwend & B.P. Dohrenwend (Eds.), *Stressful life events: Their nature and effects* (pp. 217–243). John Wiley & Sons.

Brown, G.W., & Harris, T.O. (1978). *Social origins of depression: A study of psychiatric disorder in women*. Tavistock Publications.

Burke, R.J., Weir, T., & DuWors, R.E. (1980). Perceived type A behavior of husbands and wives' satisfaction and well being. *Journal of Occupational Behavior, 1*, 139–150. https://www.jstor.org/stable/3000062

Butler, A.B., Grzywacz, J., Ettner, S.L., & Liu, B. (2009). Work flexibility, self-reported health, and health care utilisation. *Work and Stress, 23*, 45–59. https://doi.org/10.1080/02678370902833932

Butler, C., & Steptoe, A. (1986). Placebo responses: An experimental study of psychophysiological processes in asthmatic volunteers. *The British Journal of Clinical Psychology, 25*(3), 173–183. https://doi.org/10.1111/j.2044-8260.1986.tb00693.x

Byrne, D. (1961). The repression-sensitization scale: Rationale, reliability and validity. *Journal of Personality, 29*, 334–349. https://doi.org/10.1111/j.1467-6494.1961.tb01666.x

Byrne, P.S., & Long, B.E. (1976). *Doctors talking to patients: A study of the verbal behavior of general practitioners consulting in their surgeries*. Her Majesty's Stationery Office

Caldwell, G. (2019). The process of clinical consultation is crucial to patient outcomes and safety: 10 quality indicators. *Clinical Medicine, 19*(6), 503–506. https://doi.org/10.7861/clinmed.2019-0263

Canals, J., Bladé, J., & Domènech, E. (1997). Smoking and personality predictors in young Spanish people. *Personality and Individual Differences, 23*, 905–908. https://doi.org/10.1016/S0191-8869(97)00096-2

Cannon, W. (1932). *The wisdom of the body*. New York: Norton.

Cantillon, P., Morgan, M., Dundas, R., Simpson, J., Bartholomew, J., & Shaw, A. (1997). Patients' perceptions of changes in their blood pressure. *Journal of Human Hypertension, 11*(4), 221–225. https://doi.org/10.1038/sj.jhh.1000432

Capasso, M., Caso, D., & Conner, M. (2021). Anticipating pride or regret? Effects of anticipated affect focused persuasive messages on intention to get vaccinated against COVID-19. *Social Science and Medicine, 289*, 114416. https://doi.org/10.1016/j.socscimed.2021.114416

Carlo, A.D., Hosseini Ghomi, R., Renn, B., N. et al. (2019). By the numbers: Ratings and utilization of behavioral health mobile applications. *npj Digit. Med. 2*, 54. https://doi.org/10.1038/s41746-019-0129-6

Carmody, T.P., Crossen, J.R., & Wiens, A.N. (1989). Hostility as a health risk factor: Relationships with neuroticism, type A behavior, attentional focus, and interpersonal style. *Journal of Clinical Psychology, 45*, 754–762. https://doi.org/10.1002/1097-4679(198909)45:5<754::AID-JCLP2270450510>3.0.CO;2-C

Carroll, D., Bennett, P., & Davey Smith, G. (1993). Socio-economic health inequalities: Their origins and implications. *Psychology and Health, 8*, 295–316. https://doi.org/10.1080/08870449308401924

Carroll, D., Ebrahim, S., Tilling, K., Macleod, J., & Davey Smith, G. (2002). Admissions for myocardial infarction and World Cup football: Database survey. *British Medical Journal, 325*, 1439–1442. https://doi.org/10.1136/bmj.325.7378.1439

Carver, C.S., & Scheier, M.F. (1994). Situational coping and coping dispositions in a stressful transaction. *Journal of Personality and Social Psychology, 66*, 184–195. https://doi.org/10.1037//0022-3514.66.1.184

Carver, C.S., Pozo, C., Harris, S.D., et al. (1993). How coping mediates the effects of optimism on distress: A study of women with early stage breast cancer. *Journal of Personality and Social Psychology, 65*, 375–390. https://doi.org/10.1037//0022-3514.65.2.375

Carver, C.S., Scheier, M.F., & Segerstrom, S.C. (2010). Optimism. *Clinical Psychology Review, 30*, 879–889. https://doi.org/10.1016/j.cpr.2010.01.006

Carver, C.S., Scheier, M.F., & Weintraub, J.K. (1989). Assessing coping strategies: A theoretically based approach. *Journal of Personality and Social Psychology, 56*, 267–283. https://doi.org/10.1037//0022-3514.56.2.267

Carver, C.S., Smith, R.G., Antoni, M.H, Petronis, V.M., Weiss, S., & Derhagopian, R.P. (2005). Optimistic personality and psychosocial well-being during treatment predict psychosocial well-being among long-term survivors of breast cancer. *Health Psychology, 24*, 508–516. https://doi.org/10.1037/0278-6133.24.5.508

Caspi, A., Begg, D., Dickson, N., Harrington, H., Langley, J., Moffitt, T.E. & Silva, P.A. (1997). Personality differences predict health-risk behaviour in young adulthood: Evidence from a longitudinal study. *Journal of Personality and Social Psychology, 73*, 1052–1062. https://doi.org/10.1037//0022-3514.73.5.1052

Caspi, A., Roberts, B.W., & Shiner, R.L. (2005). Personality development: Stability and change. *Annual Review of Psychology, 56*, 453–484. https://doi.org/10.1146/annurev.psych.55.090902.141913

Cassidy, T., Giles, M., & McLaughlin, M. (2014) Benefit finding and resilience in child caregivers. *British Journal of Health Psychology, 19*, 606–618. https://doi.org/10.1111/bjhp.12059

Cegala, D.J., McClure, L., Marinelli, T.M., & Post, D.M. (2000). The effects of communication skills training on patients' participation during medical interviews. *Patient Education and Counseling, 41*(2), 209–222. https://doi.org/10.1016/s0738-3991(00)00093-8

Centers of Disease Control (2023). *U.S. Opioid Dispensing Rate Maps.* https://www.cdc.gov/drugoverdose/rxrate-maps/index.html

Cha, S.E., Ku, X., & Choi, I. (2023). Post COVID-19, still wear a face mask? Self-perceived facial attractiveness reduces mask-wearing intention. *Frontiers Psychology, 24*(14), 1084941. doi: 10.3389/fpsyg.2023.1084941.

Chang, S.J., Choi, S., Kim, S.-A., & Song, M. (2014). Intervention strategies based on information-motivation-behavioral skills model for health behavior change: A systematic review. *Asian Nursing Research, 8*(3), 172–181. https://doi.org/10.1016/j.anr.2014.08.002

Chaiken, S. (1980). Heuristic versus systematic information processing and the use of source versus message cues in persuasion. *Journal of Personality and Social Psychology, 39*(5), 752–766. https://doi.org/10.1037/0022-3514.39.5.752

Chaudhry, R., Dranitsaris, G., Mubashir, T., Bartoszko, J., & Riazi, S. (2020). A country level analysis measuring the impact of government actions, country preparedness and socioeconomic factors on COVID-19 mortality and related health outcomes. *EclinicalMedicine, 25*, 100464. https://doi.org/10.1016/j.eclinm.2020.100464

Chen, C.C., David, A.S., Nunnerley, H., Mitchell, M., Dawson, J.L., Berry, H., Dobbs, J., & Fahy, T. (1995). Adverse life events and breast cancer: Case-control study. *British Medical Journal, 311*, 1527–1530. https://doi.org/10.1136/bmj.311.7019.1527

Cheng, C., Ebrahimi, O.V., & Lau, Y-C (2021). Maladaptive coping with the infodemic and sleep disturbance in the COVID-19 pandemic. *Journal of Sleep Research, 30*, e13235. https://doi.org/10.1111/jsr.13235

Chesney, M.A., Eagleston, J.R., & Rosenman, R.H. (1980) The type A structured interview: A behavioral assessment in the rough. *Journal of Behavioral Assessment, 2*, 255–272. https://doi.org/10.1007/BF01666785

Chiang, J.J., Turiano, N.A., Mroczek, D.K., & Miller, G.E. (2018). Affective reactivity of daily stress and 20 year mortality risk in adults with chronic illness: Findings from the national study of daily experiences. *Health Psychology, 37*, 170–178. https://doi.org/10.1037%2Fhea0000567

Chida, Y., & Steptoe, A. (2010). Greater cardiovascular responses to laboratory mental stress are associated with poor subsequent cardiovascular risk status: A meta-analysis of prospective evidence. *Hypertension, 55*, 1026–1032. https://doi.org/10.1161/HYPERTENSIONAHA.109.146621

Christensen, A.J., Moran, P.J., & Wiebe, J.S. (1999). Assessment of irrational health beliefs: Relation to health practices and medical regimen adherence. *Health Psychology, 18*, 169–176. https://doi.org/10.1037/0278-6133.18.2.169

Christiansen, A.J., & Smith, T.W. (1995). Personality and patient adherence: Correlates of the five-factor model in renal dialysis. *Journal of Behavioral Medicine, 18*, 305–313. https://doi.org/10.1007/BF01857875

Cialdini, R.B., & Sagarin, B.J. (2005). Principles of interpersonal influence. In T.C. Brock & M.C. Green (Eds.), *Persuasion: Psychological insights and perspectives* (pp. 143–169). Sage Publications, Inc.

Cipriani, A., Furukawa, T.A., Salanti, G., Chaimani, A., Atkinson, L.Z., Ogawa, Y., Leucht, S., Ruhe, H.G., Turner, E.H., Higgins, J.P.T., Egger, M., Takeshima, N., Hayasaka, Y., Imai, H., Shinohara, K., Tajika, A., Ioannidis, J.P.A., & Geddes, J.R. (2018). Comparative efficacy and acceptability of 21 antidepressant drugs for the acute treatment of adults with major depressive disorder: A systematic review and network meta-analysis. *The Lancet, 391*(10128), 1357–1366. https://doi.org/10.1016/S0140-6736(17)32802-7

Clancy, F., Prestwich, A., Caperon, L., & O'Connor, D.B. (2016). Perseverative cognition and health behaviours. A systematic review and meta-analysis. *Frontiers in Human Neuroscience, 10,* 534. https://doi.org/10.3389/fnhum.2016.00534

Clancy, F., Prestwich, A., Caperon, L., Tsipa, A., & O'Connor, D.B. (2020). The association between worry and rumination with sleep in non-clinical populations. A systematic review and meta-analysis. *Health Psychology Review, 14,* 427–448. https://doi.org/10.1080/17437199.2019.1700819

Clemow, L.P., Pickering, T.G., Davidson, K.W., Schwartz, J.E., Williams, V.P., Shaffer, J.A., Williams, R.B., & Gerin, W. (2018). Stress management in the workplace for employees with hypertension: A randomised controlled trial. *Translational Behavioral Medicine, 8,* 761–770. https://doi.org/10.1093/tbm/iby018

Clow, A. (2001). *The physiology of stress.* In F. Jones & J. Bright (Eds). *Stress: Myth, theory and research* (pp. 47–61). England: Pearson Education Limited. ISBN-13: 978–0130411891.

Cockcroft, E.J. (2019). "Power to the people": The need for more public involvement in Sports Science for Health. *Sport Sciences for Health, 16*(1), 189–192. https://doi.org/10.1007/s11332-019-00548-y

Cohen, J. (1992) A power primer. *Psychological Bulletin, 112,* 155–159. https://doi.org/10.1037//0033-2909.112.1.155

Cohen, S. (2005). The Pittsburgh common cold studies: Psychosocial predictors of susceptibility to respiratory infectious illness. *International Journal of Behavioral Medicine, 12,* 123–131. https://doi.org/10.1207/s15327558ijbm1203_1

Cohen, S. (2021). Psychosocial vulnerabilities to upper respiratory infectious illness: Implications for susceptibility to coronavirus disease 2019 (COVID-19). *Perspectives on Psychological Science, 16,* 161–174. https://doi.org/10.1177/1745691620942516

Cohen, S., Doyle, W.J., & Baum, A. (2006). Socio-economic status is associated with stress hormones. *Psychosomatic Medicine, 68,* 414–420. https://doi.org/10.1097/01.psy.0000221236.37158.b9

Cohen, S., Doyle, W. J., & Skoner, D. P. (1999). Psychological stress, cytokine production, and severity of upper respiratory illness. *Psychological Medicine, 61,* 175–180. https://doi.org/10.1097/00006842-199903000-00009

Cohen, S., Frank, E., Doyle, W. J., Skoner, D. P., Rabin, B. S., & Gwaltney, J. M., Jr. (1998). Types of stressors that increase susceptibility to the common cold in adults. *Health Psychology, 17,* 214–223. https://doi.org/10.1037//0278-6133.17.3.214

Cohen, S., Janicki-Deverts, D., Turner, R. B., Casselbrant, M. L., Li-Korotky, H., Epel, E. S., & Doyle, W. J. (2013a). Association between telomere length and experimentally induced upper respiratory viral infection in healthy adults. *Journal of the American Medical Association, 309,* 699–705. https://doi.org/10.1001/jama.2013.613

Cohen, S., Janicki-Deverts, D., Turner, R.B., Marsland, A.L., Casselbrant, M.L., Li-Korotky, H-S, Epel, E.S., & Doyle, W.J. (2013b). Childhood socioeconomic status, telomere length and susceptibility to upper respiratory infection. *Brain, Behavior and Immunity, 34,* 31–38. https://doi.org/10.1016%2Fj.bbi.2013.06.009

Cohen, S., Kamarck, T., & Mermelstein, R. (1983). A global measure of perceived stress. *Journal of Health & Social Behavior, 24,* 386–396. https://doi.org/10.2307/2136404

Cohen, S., Murphy, M.L.M. & Prather, A.A. (2019).Ten surprising facts about stressful life events and disease risk. *Annual Review of Psychology, 70,* 577–597. https://doi.org/10.1146/annurev-psych-010418-102857

Cohen, S., Tyrrell, D.A.J., & Smith, A.P. (1991). Psychological stress and susceptibility to the common cold. *New England Journal of Medicine, 325,* 606–612. https://doi.org/10.1056/nejm199108293250903

Cohen, S., & Wills, T.A. (1985). Stress, social support and the buffering hypothesis. *Psychological Bulletin, 98,* 310–357. https://psycnet.apa.org/doi/10.1037/0033-2909.98.2.310

Conner, M., & Abraham, C. (2001). Conscientiousness and the Theory of Planned Behavior: Towards a more complete model of the antecedents of intentions and behavior. *Personality and Social Psychology Bulletin, 27,* 1547–1561. https://doi.org/10.1177/01461672012711014

Conner, M., Abraham, C., Prestwich, A., Hutter, R., Hallam, J., Sykes-Muskett, B., Morris, B., & Hurling, R. (2016). Impact of goal priority and goal conflict on the intention-health behavior relationship: Tests on physical activity and other health behaviors. *Health Psychology, 35,* 1017–1026. https://doi.org/10.137/hea0000340.

Conner, M., Fitter, M., & Fletcher, W. (1999). Stress and snacking: A diary study of daily hassles and between meal snacking. *Psychology and Health, 14,* 51–63. https://doi.org/10.1080/08870449908407313

Conner, M., Godin, G., Norman, P., & Sheeran, P. (2011). Using the question-behavior effect to promote disease prevention behaviors: Two randomized controlled trials. *Health Psychology, 30,* 300–309. https://doi.org/10.1037/a0023036

Conner, M., Grogan, S., Fry, G., Gough, B., & Higgins, A.R. (2009). Direct, mediated and moderated impacts of personality variables on smoking initiation in adolescents. *Psychology & Health*, 24, 1085–1104. https://doi.org/10.1080/08870440802239192

Conner, M., Grogan, S., West, R., Simms-Ellis, R., Scholtens, K., Sykes-Muskett, B., Cowap, L., Lawton, R., Armitage, C.J., Meads, D., Schmitt, L., Torgerson, C., & Siddiqi, K. (2019). Effectiveness and cost-effectiveness of repeated implementation intention formation plus anti-smoking messages on adolescent smoking initiation: A cluster randomized controlled trial. *Journal of Consulting and Clinical Psychology*, 87, 422–432. https:/doi.org/10.1037/ccp0000387

Conner, M., & Higgins, A. (2010). Long-term effects of implementation intentions on prevention of smoking uptake among adolescents: A cluster randomized controlled trial. *Health Psychology*, 29, 529–538. https://doi.org/10.1037/a0020317

Conner, M., McEachan, R., Jackson, C., McMillan, B., Woolridge, M., & Lawton, R. (2013). Moderating effect of socioeconomic status on the relationship between health cognitions and behaviors. *Annals of Behavioral Medicine*, 46, 19–30. https://doi.org/10.1007/s12160-013-9481-y

Conner, M., McEachan, R., Lawton, J., & Gardner, P. (2017). Applying the reasoned action approach to understanding health protection and health risk behaviors. *Social Science and Medicine*, 195, 140–148. https:/doi.org/10.1016/j.socscimed.2017.10.022

Conner, M. & Norman, P. (2005) (Eds.). *Predicting health behaviour: Research and practice with social cognition models* (2nd Edn.). Maidenhead: Open University Press.

Conner, M., & Norman, P. (2015). (Eds.). *Predicting and changing health behaviour: Research and practice with social cognition models* (3rd Edn.; pp. 252–278). Maidenhead: Open University Press.

Conner, M., & Norman, P. (2015). Predicting and changing health behaviour: A social cognition approach. In M. Conner & P. Norman (Eds.), *Predicting and changing health behaviour: Research and practice with social cognition models* (3rd Edn.; pp. 1–29). Maidenhead: Open University Press.

Conner, M., & Norman, P. (2022). Understanding the intention-behavior gap: The role of intention strength. *Frontiers in Psychology*, 13, 923464. https://doi.org/10.3389/fpsyg.2022.

Conner, M., & Norman, P. (2023). Models of health behavior: Revisiting Ajzen (1998). In M. Hagger & M. Tarrant (Eds.) *Health Psychology: Revisiting the classics*. Sage.

Conner, M., Norman, P., & Bell, R. (2002). The theory of planned behavior and healthy eating. *Health Psychology*, 21, 194–201. https://doi.org/10.1037/0278-6133.21.2.194

Conner, M., Rodgers, W., & Murray, T. (2007). Conscientiousness and the intention-behavior relationship: Predicting exercise behavior. *Journal of Sports and Exercise Psychology*, 29, 518–533. https://doi.org/10.1123/jsep.29.4.518

Conner, M., & Sparks, P. (2005). The theory of planned behavior. In M. Conner, & P. Norman (Eds.), *Predicting health behaviour: Research and practice with social cognition models* (pp. 121–162). Open University Press.

Conner, M., & Sparks, P. (2015). Theory of planned behaviour. In M. Conner & P. Norman (Eds.), *Predicting and changing health behaviour: Research and practice with social cognition models* (3rd Edn.; pp. 142–188). Maidenhead: Open University Press.

Conner, M., van Harreveld F., & Norman, P. (2020). Attitude stability as a moderator of the relationships between cognitive and affective attitudes and behaviour. *British Journal of Social Psychology*, 61(1), 121–142. https://doi.org/10.1111/bjso.12473

Conner, M., Wilding, S., & Norman, P. (2022). Testing predictors of attitude strength as determinants of attitude stability and attitude-behavior relationships: A multi-behavior study. *European Journal of Social Psychology*, 52(4), 656–668. https://doi.org/10.1002/ejsp2844

Conner, M., Wilding, S., Prestwich, A., Hutter, R., Hurling, R., van Harreveld, F., Abraham, C., & Sheeran, P. (2022). Goal prioritization and behavior change: Evaluation of an intervention for multiple behaviors. *Health Psychology*, 41(5), 356–365. https://doi.org/10.1037/hea0001149

Conner, M., Wilding, S., Wright, C.A., & Sheeran, P. (2023). How does self-control promote health behaviors? A multi-behavior test of five potential pathways. *Annals of Behavioral Medicine*, 57(4), 313–322. https://doi.org/10.1093/abm/kaac053

Conner, M., Williams, D., & Rhodes, R. (2020). Affect-based interventions. In M. Hagger, L. Cameron, K. Hamilton, N. Hankonen, & T. Lintunen (Eds.), *The handbook of behavior change* (Cambridge Handbooks in Psychology, pp. 495–509). Cambridge: Cambridge University Press. https://doi.org/10.1017/9781108677318.034

Conrad, P. (1985). The meaning of medications: Another look at compliance. *Social Science & Medicine*, 20(1), 29–37. https://doi.org/10.1016/0277-9536(85)90308-9

Cook, W.W., & Medley, D.M. (1954). Proposed hostility and pharisaic-virtue scores for the MMPI. *Journal of Applied Psychology, 38*, 414–418. https://doi.org/10.1037/H0060667

Cooke, R., & Sheeran, P. (2004). Moderation of cognition-intention and cognition-behaviour relations: A meta-analysis of properties of variables from the theory of planned behaviour. *British Journal of Social Psychology, 43*, 159–186. https://doi.org/10.1348/0144666041501688

Cooper, C.L., Sloan, S.J., & Williams, S. (1988). *The occupational stress indicator*. Windsor: NFER-Nelson.

Cooper, M.L., Wood, P.K., Orcutt, H.K., & Albino, A.W. (2003). Personality and the predisposition to engage in risky or problem behaviors during adolescence. *Journal of Personality and Social Psychology, 84*, 390–410. https://doi.org/10.1037//0022-3514.84.2.390

Cornwell, E.Y., & Waite, L.J. (2009). Social disconnectedness, perceived isolation, and health among older adults. *Journal of Health and Social Behavior, 50*, 31–48. https://doi.org/10.1177%2F002214650905000103

Costa, P.T. Jr., & McCrae, R.R. (1980). Influence of extraversion and neuroticism on subjective well-being: Happy and unhappy people. *Journal of Personality and Social Psychology, 40*, 19–28. https://doi.org/10.1037/0022-3514.38.4.668

Costa, P.T. Jr., & McCrae, R.R. (1987). Neuroticism, somatic complaints, and disease: Is the bark worse than the bite? *Journal of Personality, 55*, 299–316. https://doi.org/10.1111/j.1467-6494.1987.tb00438.x

Costa, P.T. Jr., & McCrae, R.R. (1990). Personality: Another 'hidden factor' in stress research. *Psychological Inquiry, 1*, 22–24. https://doi.org/10.1207/s15327965pli0101_5

Costa, P.T. Jr., & McCrae, R.R. (1992). Four ways five factors are basic. *Personality and Individual Differences, 13*, 653–665. https://doi.org/10.1016/0191-8869(92)90236-I

Coulson, N.S. (2013). How do online patient support communities affect the experience of inflammatory bowel disease? An online survey. *Journal of the Royal Society of Social Medicine Short Reports, 4*, 1–8. https://doi.org/10.1177/2042533313478004

Coulson, N.S., & Buchanan, H. (2022). The role of online support groups in helping individuals affected by HIV and AIDS: Scoping review of the literature. *Journal of Medical Internet Research, 24*, e27648. https://doi.org/10.2196%2F27648

Coulson, N.S., Buchanan, H., & Aubeeluck, A. (2007). Social support in cyberspace: A content analysis of communication within a Huntington's disease online support group. *Patient Education and Counseling, 68*, 173–178. https://doi.org/10.1016/j.pec.2007.06.002

Coulter, A., Entwistle, V., & Gilbert, D. (1999). Sharing decisions with patients: Is the information good enough?. *BMJ, 318*(7179), 318–322. https://doi.org/10.1136/bmj.318.7179.318

Courneya, K.S., & Hellsten, L.M. (1998). Personality correlates of exercise behavior, motives, barriers and preferences: An application of the five-factor model. *Personality and Individual Differences, 24*, 625–633. https://doi.org/10.1016/S0191-8869(97)00231-6

Cox, T., & Mackay, C. (1985). The measurement of self-reported stress and arousal. *British Journal of Psychology, 76*, 183–186. https://doi.org/10.1111/j.2044-8295.1985.tb01941.x

Cramer S. (2016). Food should be labelled with the exercise needed to expend its calories. *BMJ, 353*, i1856. https://doi.org/10.1136/bmj.i1856

Creswell, J.D., Lam, S., Stanton, A.L., Taylor, S.E., Bower, J.E., & Sherman, D.K. (2007). Does self-affirmation, cognitive processing, or discovery of meaning explain cancer-related health benefits of expressive writing? *Personality and Social Psychology Bulletin, 33*, 238–250. https://doi.org/10.1177/0146167206294412

Crowley, A.E., & Hoyer, W.D. (1994). An integrative framework for understanding two-sided persuasion. *Journal of Consumer Research, 20*(4), 561–574. https://doi.org/10.1086/209370

Crowne, D.P., & Marlowe, D. (1960). A new scale of social desirability independent of psychopathology. *Journal of Consulting Psychology, 24*, 349–354. https://doi.org/10.1037/h0047358

Csiernik, R. (2011). The glass is filling: An examination of employee assistance program evaluations in the first decade of the new millennium. *Journal of Workplace Behavioral Health, 26*, 334–335. https://psycnet.apa.org/doi/10.1080/15555240.2011.618438

Cummings, M.K., Becker, M.H., & Maile, M.C. (1980). Bringing models together: An Empirical approach to combining variables used to explain health actions. *Journal of Behavioral Medicine, 3*, 123–145. https://doi.org/10.1007/BF00844986

Cunningham, A.J. (1985). The influence of mind on cancer. *Canadian Psychology, 26*, 13–29. https://doi.org/10.1037/h0080019

Dahlén, A.D., Miguet, M., Schiöth, H.B., & Rukh. (2022). The influence of personality on the risk of myocardial infarction in UK Biobank cohort. *Scientific Reports, 12*, 6706. https://doi.org/10.1038/s41598-022-10573-6

Daley, A.J., McGee, E., Bayliss, S., Coombe, A., & Parretti, H.M. (2020). Effects of physical activity calorie equivalent food labelling to reduce food selection and consumption: Systematic review and meta-analysis of randomised controlled studies. *Journal of Epidemiology and Community Health*, *74*(3), 269–275. https://doi.org/10.1136/jech-2019-213216

Dancey, C.P., Taghavi, M., &, Fox, R.J. (1998). The relationship between daily stress and symptoms of irritable bowel: A time-series approach. *Journal of Psychosomatic Research*, *44*, 537–545. https://doi.org/10.1016/s0022-3999(97)00255-9

Danner, D.D., Snowdon, D.A. & Friesen, W.V. (2001). Positive emotions in early life and longevity: Findings from the Nun Study. *Journal of Personality and Social Psychology*, *80*, 804–813. https://doi.org/10.1037/0022-3514.80.5.804

Das, E.H.H.J., de Wit, J.B.F., & Stroebe, W. (2003). Fear appeals motivate acceptance of action recommendations: Evidence for a positive bias in the processing of persuasive messages. *Personality and Social Psychology Bulletin*, *29*(5), 650–664. https://doi.org/10.1177/0146167203029005009

Davidson, K.W., Gidron, Y., Mostofsky, E., & Trudeau, K.J. (2007). Hospitalization cost offset of a hostility intervention for coronary heart disease patients. *Journal of Consulting and Clinical Psychology*, *75*, 657–662. https://doi.org/10.1037/0022-006X.75.4.657

Davidson, K.W., Goldstein, M., Kaplan, R.M., Kaufmann, P.G., Knatterud, G.L., Orleans, C.T., Spring, B., Trudeau, K.J., & Whitlock, E.P. (2003). Evidence-based behavioral medicine: What is it and how do we achieve it?. *Annals of Behavioral Medicine*, *26*(3), 161–171. https://doi.org/10.1207/S15324796ABM2603_01

de Kleijn, L., Pedersen, J.R., Rijkels-Otters, H., Chiarotto, A., & Koes, B. (2022). Opioid reduction for patients with chronic pain in primary care: Systematic review. *The British Journal of General Practice*, *72*(717), e293–e300. https://doi.org/10.3399/BJGP.2021.0537

de Lange, A.H., Taris, T.W., Kompier, M.A.J., Houtman, I.L.D., & Bongers, P.M. (2003). 'The very best of the millennium': Longitudinal research and the demand-control-(support) model. *Journal of Occupational Health Psychology*, *8*, 282–305. https://doi.org/10.1037/1076-8998.8.4.282

de Ridder, D., Kroese, F., Evers, C., Adriaanse, M., & Gillebaart, M. (2017). Healthy diet: Health impact, prevalence, correlates, and interventions. *Psychology & Health*, *32*, 907–941. https://doi.org/10.1080/08870446.2017.1316849

de Ridder, D.T.D., Lensvelt-Mulders, G., Finkenauer, C., Stok, F.M., & Baumeister, R.F. (2012). Taking stock of self-control: A meta-analysis of how trait self-control relates to a wide range of behaviors. *Personality and Social Psychology Review*, *16*, 76–99. https://doi.org/10.1177/1088868311418749

de Rijk, A.E., Le Blance, P.M., Schaufeli, W.B., & de Jonge, J. (1998). Active coping and need for control as moderators of the job demand-control model: Effects on burnout. *Journal of Occupational and Organizational Psychology*, *71*, 1–18. https://doi.org/10.1111/j.2044-8325.1998.tb00658.x

de Wit, J. B. F., Adam, P. C. G., den Daas, C., & Jonas, K. (2023). Sexually transmitted infection prevention behaviours: health impact, prevalence, correlates, and interventions. *Psychology & Health*, *38*(6), 675–700. https://doi.org/10.1080/08870446.2022.2090560

Deaton, A., & Cartwright, N. (2018). Understanding and misunderstanding randomized controlled trials. *Social Science & Medicine*, *210*, 2–21. https://doi.org/10.1016/j.socscimed.2017.12.005.

Deelstra, J.T., Peeters, M.C.W., Zijlstra, F.R.H., & van Doornen, L.P. (2003). Receiving instrumental support at work: When help is not welcome. *Journal of Applied Psychology*, *88*, 324–331. https://doi.org/10.1037/0021-9010.88.2.324

Deery, C.B., Hales, D., Viera, L., Lin, F.C., Liu, Z., Olsson, E., Gras-Najjar, J., Linnan, L., Noar, S.M., Ammerman, A.S., & Viera, A.J. (2019). Physical activity calorie expenditure (PACE) labels in worksite cafeterias: Effects on physical activity. *BMC Public Health*, *19*(1), 1596. https://doi.org/10.1186/s12889-019-7960-1

DeLongis, A., Coyne, J.C., Dakof, G., Folkman, S., & Lazarus, R. (1982). Relationships of daily hassles, uplifts and major life events to health status. *Health Psychology*, *1*, 119–136. https://psycnet.apa.org/doi/10.1037/0278-6133.1.2.119 https://psycnet.apa.org/doi/10.1037/0278-6133.1.2.119

Demerouti, E., Bakker, A.B., Nachreiner, F., & Schaufeli, W.B. (2001). The job demand-resources model of burnout. *Journal of Applied Psychology*, *86*, 499–512. https://psycnet.apa.org/doi/10.1037/0021-9010.86.3.499

Demers, R.Y., Altamore, R., Mustin, H., Kleinman, A., & Leonardi, D. (1980). An exploration of the dimensions of illness behavior. *The Journal of Family Practice*, *11*(7), 1085–1092

Denford, S., Abraham, C., Campbell, R., & Busse, H. (2017). A comprehensive review of reviews of school-based interventions to improve sexual-health. *Health Psychology Review*, *11*(1), 33–52. https://doi.org/10.1080/17437199.2016.1240625

Denollet, J., Sys, S.U., Stroobant, N., Rombouts, H., Gillebert, T.C., & Brutsaert, D.L. (1996). Personality as independent predictors of long-term mortality in patients with coronary heart disease. *Lancet*, *34*, 417–421. https://doi.org/10.1016/s0140-6736(96)90007-0

Department of Health (2008). *Raising the profile of long-term conditions care: A compendium of information.* https://www.gov.uk/government/publications

Department of Health (2012). *Long-term conditions compendium of information: 3rd edition.* https://www.gov.uk/government/publications/long-term-conditions-compendium-of-information-third-edition

Department of Health and Social Care (2022). *A plan for digital health and social care.* https://www.gov.uk/government/publications/a-plan-for-digital-health-and-social-care/a-plan-for-digital-health-and-social-care

Derakshan, N., & Eysenck, M.W. (1997). Repression and repressors: Theoretical and experimental approaches. *European Psychologist, 2*, 235–246. https://psycnet.apa.org/doi/10.1027/1016-9040.2.3.235

Detweiler, J.B., Bedell, B.T., Salovey, P., Pronin, E., & Rothman, A.J. (1999). Message framing and sunscreen use: Gain-framed messages motivate beach-goers. *Health Psychology, 18*(2), 189–196. https://doi.org/10.1037/0278-6133.18.2.189

Deutsch, M., & Gerard, H.B. (1955). A study of normative and informational social influences upon individual judgment. *The Journal of Abnormal and Social Psychology, 51*(3), 629–636. https://doi.org/10.1037/h0046408

Di Blasi, Z., Harkness, E., Ernst, E., Georgiou, A., & Kleijnen, J. (2001). Influence of context effects on health outcomes: A systematic review. *Lancet, 357*(9258), 757–762. https://doi.org/10.1016/s0140-6736(00)04169-6

DiClemente, C.C., Prochaska, J.O., Fairhurst, S.K., Velicer, W.F., Velasquez, M.M., & Rossi, J.S. (1991). The process of smoking cessation: An analysis of precontemplation, contemplation, and preparation stages of change. *Journal of Consulting and Clinical Psychology, 59*, 295–304. https://doi.org/10.1037//0022-006x.59.2.295

Diderichsen, F., Hallqvist, J., & Whitehead, M. (2019). Differential vulnerability and susceptibility: How to make use of recent development in our understanding of mediation and interaction to tackle health inequalities. *International Journal of Epidemiology, 48*, 268–274. https://doi.org/10.1093/ije/dyy167

Dienstbier, R.A. (1989). Arousal and physiological toughness: Implications for mental and physical health. *Psychological Review, 96*(1), 84–100. https://doi.org/10.1037/0033-295X.96.1.84

Digman, J.M. (1990). Personality structure: Emergence of the five-factor model. *Annual Review of Psychology, 41*, 417–440. https://doi.org/10.1146/annurev.ps.41.020190.002221

DiMatteo, M.R., Sherbourne, C.D., Hays, R.D., Ordway, L., Kravitz, R.L., McGlynn, E.A., Kaplan, S., & Rogers, W.H. (1993). Physicians' characteristics influence patients' adherence to medical treatment: Results from the Medical Outcomes Study. *Health Psychology, 12*(2), 93–102. https://doi.org/10.1037/0278-6133.12.2.93

Dohrenwend, B.P. (2006). Inventorying stressful life events as risk factors for psychopathology: Towards resolution of the problem of intracategory variability. *Psychological Bulletin, 132*, 477–495. https://doi.org/10.1037/0033-2909.132.3.477

Dohrenwend, B.P., & Shrout, P.E. (1985). 'Hassles' in the conceptualization and measurement of life stress variables. *American Psychologist, 40*, 780–785. https://psycnet.apa.org/doi/10.1037/0003-066X.40.7.780

Donaghy, E., Atherton, H., Hammersley, V., McNeilly, H., Bikker, A, Robbins, L., Campbell. J., & McKinstry, B. (2019). Acceptability, benefits, and challenges of video consulting: A qualitative study in primary care. *British Journal of General Practice, 69*(686), e586–e594. doi: 10.3399/bjgp19X704141

Doll, R., Peto, R., Wheatley, K., Gray, R., & Sutherland, I. (1994). Mortality in relation to smoking: 40 years' observations on male British doctors. *British Medical Journal, 309*, 901–911. https://doi.org/10.1136/bmj.309.6959.901

Donovan, J.L., & Blake, D.R. (1992). Patient non-compliance: Deviance or reasoned decision-making?. *Social Science & Medicine, 34*(5), 507–513. https://doi.org/10.1016/0277-9536(92)90206-6

Downes, M.J., Mervin, M.C., Byrnes, J.M., & Scuffham, P.A. (2017). Telephone consultations for general practice: A systematic review. *Systematic Reviews, 6*(1), 128. doi: 10.1186/s13643-017-0529-0

Dovey-Pearce, G., Doherty, Y., & May, C. (2007). The influence of diabetes upon adolescent and young adult development: A qualitative study. *British Journal of Health Psychology, 12*(1), 75–91. https://doi.org/10.1348/135910706X98317

Dugravot, A., Fayosse, A., Dumurgier, J., Bouillon, K., Ben Rayana, T., Schnitzler, A., Kivimaki, M., Sabia, S., & Singh-Manoux, A. (2020). Social inequalities in multimorbidity, frailty, disability, and transitions to mortality: A 24-year follow up of the Whitehall II cohort study. *The Lancet Public Health, 5*, e42–e50. https://doi.org/10.1016/s2468-2667(19)30226-9

Durantini, M.R., Albarracín, D., Mitchell, A.L., Earl, A.N., & Gillette, J.C. (2006). Conceptualizing the influence of social agents of behavior change: A meta-analysis of the effectiveness of HIV-prevention interventionists for different groups. *Psychological Bulletin, 132*(2), 212–248. https://doi.org/10.1037/0033-2909.132.2.212

Egger, G., Binns, A., Cole, M.A., Ewald, D., Davies, L., Meldrum, H., Stevens, J., & Noffsinger, E. (2014). Shared medical appointments – An adjunct for chronic disease management in Australia?. *Australian Family Physician*, *43*(3), 151–154.

Eisend, M. (2006). Two-sided advertising: A meta-analysis. *International Journal of Research in Marketing*, *23*(2), 187–198. https://doi.org/10.1016/j.ijresmar.2005.11.001

Eisend, M. (2007). Understanding two-sided persuasion: An empirical assessment of theoretical approaches. *Psychology & Marketing*, *24*(7), 615–640. https://doi.org/10.1002/mar.20176

El Naqa, I., & Das, S. (2020). The role of machine and deep learning in modern medical physics, *Medical Physics*. https://doi.org/10.1002/mp.14088

Ellis, J. (1998). Prospective memory and medicine-taking. In L.B. Myers & K. Midence (Eds.), *Adherence to treatment in medical conditions*. Harwood Academic.

Engbers, L.H., van Poppel, M.N., Chin A Paw, J. M., & van Mechelen, W. (2005). Worksite health promotion programs with environmental changes: A systematic review. *American Journal of Preventive Medicine*, *29*(1), 61–70. https://doi.org/10.1016/j.amepre.2005.03.001

Epstein, L.H. (1984). The direct effects of compliance on health outcome. *Health Psychology*, *3*(4), 385–393. https://doi.org/10.1037//0278-6133.3.4.385

Ernst, E., & Resch, K.L. (1995). Concept of true and perceived placebo effects. *BMJ*, *311*(7004), 551–553. https://doi.org/10.1136/bmj.311.7004.551

Esterling, B.A., Antoni, M.H., Kumar, M., & Schneiderman, N. (1993). Defensiveness, trait anxiety, and Epstein–Barr viral capsid antigen antibody titers in health college students. *Health Psychology*, *12*, 132–139. https://doi.org/10.1037//0278-6133.12.2.132

Everson, S.A., Goldberg, D.E., Kaplan, G.A., & Cohen, R.D. (1996). Hopelessness and risk of mortality and incidence of myocardial infarction and cancer. *Psychosomatic Medicine*, 58, 103–121. https://doi.org/10.1097/00006842-199603000-00003

Everson, S.A., Kaplan, G.A., Goldberg, D.E., & Salonen, J.T. (1996). Anticipatory blood pressure response to exercise predicts future high blood pressure in middle-aged men. *Hypertension*, *27*(5), 1059–1064. https://doi.org/10.1161/01.hyp.27.5.1059

Everson, S.A., Lynch, J.W., Kaplan, G.A., Lakka, T.A., Sivenius, J., & Salonen, J.T. (2001). Stress-induced blood pressure reactivity and incident stroke in middle-aged men. *Stroke*, *32*(6), 1263–1270. https://doi.org/10.1161/01.str.32.6.1263

Eysenck, H.J. (1967). *The biological basis of personality*. Springfield, IL: Charles Thomas.

Eysenck, H.J., & Eysenck, S.B.G. (1964). *Eysenck personality inventory*. San Diego, CA: Education and Industry Testing Service.

Eysenck, M.W., & Matthews, A. (1987). Trait anxiety and cognition (pp. 197–216). In H.J. Eysenck & M. Martin (Eds.), *Theoretical foundations of behavior therapy*. Dordrecht: Kluwer Academic/Plenum.

Ezzo, J., Berman, B., Hadhazy, V.A., Jadad, A.R., Lao, L., & Singh, B.B. (2000). Is acupuncture effective for the treatment of chronic pain? A systematic review. *Pain*, *86*(3), 217–225. https://doi.org/10.1016/S0304-3959(99)00304-8

Falco, A., Girardi, D., Dal Corso, L., Yildirim, M, & Converso, D. (2021). The perceived risk of being infected at work: An application of the job demands-resources model to workplace safety during the COVID-19 outbreak. *PloS ONE*, *16*(9): e0257197. https://doi.org/10.1371/journal.pone.0257197

Falk, E.B., O'Donnell, M.B., Cascio, C.N., Tinney, F., Kang, Y., Lieberman, M.D., Taylor, S.E., An, L., Resnicow, K., & Strecher, V.J. (2015). Self-affirmation alters the brain's response to health messages and subsequent behavior change. *Proceedings of the National Academy of Sciences of the United States of America*, *112*(7), 1977–1982. https://doi.org/10.1073/pnas.1500247112

Feldman, P.J., Cohen, S., Doyle, W.J., Skoner, D.P., & Gwaltney, J.M., Jr (1999). The impact of personality on the reporting of unfounded symptoms and illness. *Journal of Personality and Social Psychology*, *77*(2), 370–378. https://doi.org/10.1037//0022-3514.77.2.370

Ferguson, E. (2013). Personality is of central concern to understand health: Towards a theoretical model for health psychology. *Health Psychology Review*, 7, S32–S70. https://doi.org/10.1080/17437199.2010.547985

Ferguson, E. Williams, L., O'Connor, R.C., Howard, S., Hughes, B., Johnston, D.W., Hay, J., O'Connor, D.B., Lewis, C.A., Grealy, M.A., & O'Carroll, R.E (2009). A taxometric analysis of Type-D personality. *Psychosomatic Medicine*, *71*, 981–986. https://doi.org/10.1097/PSY.0b013e3181bd888b

Ferguson, E., Matthews, G., & Cox, T. (1999). The appraisal of life events (ALE) scale: Reliability, and validity. *British Journal of Health Psychology*, *4*, 97–11. https://doi/10.1348/135910799168506

Fernandez-Lazaro, C.I., García-González, J.M., Adams, D.P., Fernandez-Lazaro, D., Mielgo-Ayuso, J., Caballero-Garcia, A., Moreno Racionero, F., Córdova, A., & Miron-Canelo, J.A. (2019). Adherence to treatment and related factors among patients with chronic conditions in primary care: A cross-sectional study. *BMC Family Practice*, *20*(1), 132. https://doi.org/10.1186/s12875-019-1019-3

Fernandez, E., & Turk, D.C. (1989). The utility of cognitive coping strategies for altering pain perception: A meta-analysis. *Pain*, *38*(2), 123–135. https://doi.org/10.1016/0304-3959(89)90230-3

Festinger, L. (1957). *A theory of cognitive dissonance.* Stanford University Press.

Figueroa, W.S., Zoccola, P.M., Manigault, A.W., Hamilton, K.R., Scanlin, M.C., & Johnson, R.C. (2021). Daily stressors and diurnal cortisol among sexual and gender minority young adults. *Health Psychology*, *40*, 145–154. https://doi.org/10.1037/hea0001054

Filluková, P., Ayton, P., Rand, K., & Langguth, J. (2021). What should I trust? Individual differences in attitudes to conflicting information and misinformation on COVID-19. *Frontiers in Psychology*, *12*, 588478. https://doi.org/10.3389/fpsyg.2021.588478

Finlay, S., Rudd, D., McDermott, B., & Sarnyai, Z. (2022). Allostatic load and systemic comorbidities in psychiatric disorders. *Psychoneuroendocrinology*, *140*, 105726. https://doi.org/10.1016/j.psyneuen.2022.105726

Fishbein, M., & Ajzen, I. (2010). *Predicting and changing behaviour: The reasoned action approach.* New York: Psychology Press.

Fishbein, M., Triandis, H.C., Kanfer, F.H., Becker, M., Middlestadt, S.E., & Eichler, A. (2001). Factors influencing behavior and behavior change. In: A. Baum, T.A. Revenson & J.E. Singer (Eds.), *Handbook of health psychology* (pp. 3–17). Mahwah, NJ: Lawrence Erlbaum.

Fishbein, M., von Haeften, I., & Appleyard, J. (2001). The role of theory in developing effective interventions: Implications from Project SAFER. *Psychology, Health & Medicine*, *6*(2), 223–238. https://doi.org/10.1080/13548500120035463

Fisher, W.A., & Fisher, J.D. (1992). Understanding and promoting AIDS preventive behaviour: A conceptual model and educational tools. *Canadian Journal of Human Sexuality*, *1*(3), 99–106.

Fisher, J.D., Fisher, W.A., Bryan, A.D., & Misovich, S.J. (2002). Information-motivation-behavioral skills model-based HIV risk behavior change intervention for inner-city high school youth. *Health Psychology*, *21*(2), 177–186.

Fisher, J.D., Fisher, W.A., Misovich, S.J., Kimble, D.L., & Malloy, T.E. (1996). Changing AIDS risk behavior: Effects of an intervention emphasizing AIDS risk reduction information, motivation, and behavioral skills in a college student population. *Health Psychology*, *15*(2), 114–123. https://doi.org/10.1037//0278-6133.15.2.114

Fiske, S.T., & Taylor, S.E. (1991). *Social cognition*, (2nd Edn). New York: McGraw-Hill.

Flaxman, P.E., & Bond, F.W. (2010) Worksite stress management training: Moderated effects and clinical significance. *Journal of Occupational Health Psychology*, *14*, 347–358. https://doi.org/10.1037/a0020522

Flemming, K., Booth, A., Garside, R., Tunçalp, O., & Noyes, J. (2019). Qualitative evidence synthesis for complex interventions and guideline development: Clarification of the purpose, designs and relevant methods. *BMJ Global Health*, *4*, e000882. doi: 10.1136/bmjgh-2018–000882.

Flesch, R. (1948). A new readability yardstick. *The Journal of Applied Psychology*, *32*(3), 221–233. https://doi.org/10.1037/h0057532

Floyd, D.L., Prentice-Dunn, S., & Rogers, R.W. (2000). A meta-analysis of research on protection motivation theory. *Journal of Applied Social Psychology*, *30*(2), 407–429. https://doi.org/10.1111/j.1559-1816.2000.tb02323.x

Fogel, J., Albert, S.M., Schnabel, F., Ditkoff, B.A., & Neugut, A.I. (2002). Internet use and social support in women with breast cancer. *Health Psychology*, *21*, 398–404. https://psycnet.apa.org/doi/10.1037/0278-6133.21.4.398

Folkman, S. (1997). Positive psychological states and coping with severe stress. *Social Science and Medicine*, *45*, 1207–1221. https://doi.org/10.1016/s0277-9536(97)00040-3

Folkman, S., & Lazarus, R.S. (1985). If it changes it must be a process: Study of emotion and coping during three stages of a college examination. *Journal of Personality and Social Psychology*, *48*, 150–170. https://doi.org/10.1037//0022-3514.48.1.150

Folkman, S., & Lazarus, R.S. (1988). *Ways of coping questionnaire sampler set: manual, test booklet, scoring key.* Palo Alto, CA: Consulting Psychologists Press.

Folkman, S., & Moskowitz, J.T. (2000). Positive affect and the other side of coping. *American Psychologist*, *55*, 647–654. https://doi.org/10.1037//0003-066x.55.6.647

Fonk, G.E., Sant'Ana, S.J., Kaye, J.T., & Curtin, J.J. (2020). Stress allostasis in substance use disorders: Promise, progress and emerging priorities in clinical research. *Annual Review of Clinical Psychology*, *16*, 401–430. https://doi.org/10.1146%2Fannurev-clinpsy-102419-125016

Fordyce, W.E. (1976). *Behavioural methods for chronic pain and illness.* Mosby.

Foster, N.E., Thomas, E., Barlas, P., Hill, J.C., Young, J., Mason, E., & Hay, E.M. (2007). Acupuncture as an adjunct to exercise based physiotherapy for osteoarthritis of the knee: Randomised controlled trial. *BMJ*, *335*(7617), 436. https://doi.org/10.1136/bmj.39280.509803.BE

Frattaroli, J. (2006). Experimental disclosure and its moderators: A meta-analysis. *Psychological Bulletin*, *132*, 823–865. https://doi.org/10.1037/0033-2909.132.6.823

Freeman, G.K., Horder, J.P., Howie, J.G., Hungin, A.P., Hill, A.P., Shah, N.C., & Wilson, A. (2002). Evolving general practice consultation in Britain: Issues of length and context. *BMJ*, *324*(7342), 880–882. https://doi.org/10.1136/bmj.324.7342.880

French, J.P.R. Jr., & Raven, B. (1960). The bases of social power. In D. Cartwright & A. Zander (Eds.), *Group dynamics* (pp. 607–623). Harper and Row.

Friedman, H.S. (2000). Long-term relations of personality and health: Dynamisms, mechanisms, tropisms. *Journal of Personality*, *68*, 1089–1108. 10.1111/1467-6494.00127

Friedman, H.S., & Booth-Kewley, S. (1987). The disease-prone personality. *American Psychologist*, *42*, 539–555. https://doi.org/10.1037/0003-066X.42.6.539

Friedman, H.S., & Hampson, S.E. (2021). Personality and health: A lifespan perspective. In O.P. John & R.W. Robins (Eds.), *Handbook of personality: Theory and research* (pp. 773–790). The Guilford Press.

Friedman, H.S., Tucker, J.S., Schwartz, J.E., et al. (1995). Childhood conscientiousness and longevity: Health behaviors and cause of death. *Journal of Personality and Social Psychology*, *68*, 696–703. https://doi.org/10.1037/0022-3514.68.4.696

Friedman, H.S., Tucker, J.S., Tomlinson-Keasay, C., Schwartz, J.E., Wingard, D.L., & Criqui, M.H. (1993). Does childhood personality predict longevity? *Journal of Personality and Social Psychology*, *65*, 176–185. 10.1037//0022-3514.65.1.176

Friedman, M., & Rosenman, R.H. (1974). *Type A behavior and your heart*. New York: Knopf.

Friedman, R., Sobel, D., Myers, P., Caudill, M., & Benson, H. (1995). Behavioral medicine, clinical health psychology, and cost offset. *Health Psychology*, *14*(6), 509–518. https://doi.org/10.1037//0278-6133.14.6.509

Frisina, P.G., Borod, J.C., & Lepore, S.J. (2004). A meta analysis of the effects of written emotional disclosure on the health outcomes of clinical populations. *Journal of Nervous and Mental Disease*, *192*, 629–634. https://doi.org/10.1097/01.nmd.0000138317.30764.63

Gallagher, E.J., Viscoli, C.M., & Horwitz, R.I. (1993). The relationship of treatment adherence to the risk of death after myocardial infarction in women. *JAMA*, *270*(6), 742–744.

Gallo, L.C., & Matthews, K.A. (2003). Understanding the association between socioeconomic status and physical health: Do negative emotions play a role? *Psychological Bulletin*, *129*, 10–51. https://doi.org/10.1037/0033-2909.129.1.10

Ganster, D.C., Mayes, B.T., Sime, W.E., & Tharp, G.D. (1982). Managing organizational stress: A field experiment. *Journal of Applied Psychology*, *67*, 533–542. https://psycnet.apa.org/doi/10.1037/0021-9010.67.5.533

Gardner, B. (2015). A review and analysis of the use of 'habit' in understanding, predicting and influencing health-related behaviour. *Health Psychology Review*, *9*(3), 277–295. https://doi.org/10.1080/17437199.2013.876238

Garland, E.L., Hanley, A.W., Nakamura, Y., Barrett, J.W., Baker, A.K., Reese, S.E., Riquino, M.R., Froeliger, B., & Donaldson, G.W. (2022). Mindfulness-oriented recovery enhancement vs supportive group therapy for co-occurring opioid misuse and chronic pain in primary care: A randomized clinical trial. *JAMA Internal Medicine*, *182*(4), 407–417. https://doi.org/10.1001/jamainternmed.2022.0033

Gartland, N., O'Connor, D., Lawton, R., & Ferguson, E. (2014). Investigating the effects of conscientiousness on daily stress, affect and physical symptom processes: A daily diary study. *British Journal of Health Psychology*, *19*. 311–328. https://doi.org/10.1111/bjhp.12077

Gartland, N., O'Connor, D.B., & Lawton, R. (2012). Effects of conscientiousness on the appraisals of daily stressors. *Stress & Health*, *28*, 80–86. https://doi.org/10.1002/smi.1404

Gartland, N., Wilson, A., Lawton, R., & O'Connor, D.B. (2021). Conscientiousness and engagement with national health behaviour guidelines. *Psychology, Health & Medicine*, *26*(4), 421–432. https://doi.org/10.1080/13548506.2020.1814961

Gast, A., & Mathes, T. (2019). Medication adherence influencing factors–An (updated) overview of systematic reviews. *Systematic Reviews*, *8*(1), 112. https://doi.org/10.1186/s13643-019-1014-8

Gatchel, R.J., Peng, Y.B., Peters, M.L., Fuchs, P.N., & Turk, D.C. (2007). The biopsychosocial approach to chronic pain: Scientific advances and future directions. *Psychological Bulletin*, *133*(4), 581–624. https://doi.org/10.1037/0033-2909.133.4.581

GBD 2017 Diet Collaborators (2019). Health effects of dietary risks in 195 countries, 1990–2017: A systematic analysis for the Global Burden of Disease Study 2017. *Lancet, 393*(10184), 1958–1972. https://doi.org/10.1016/S0140-6736(19)30041-8

Ghazi, C., Nyland, J., Whaley, R., Rogers, T., Wera, J., & Henzman, C. (2018). Social cognitive or learning theory use to improve self-efficacy in musculoskeletal rehabilitation: A systematic review and meta-analysis. *Physiotherapy Theory & Practice, 34*, 495–504. https://doi.org/10.1080/09593985.2017.1422204

Gidron, Y., Davidson, K., & Bata, I. (1999). The short-term effects of a hostility-reduction intervention on male coronary heart disease patients. *Health Psychology, 18*, 416–420. https://doi.org/10.1037/0278-6133.18.4.416

Glasgow, R.E., Bull, S.S., Gillette, C., Klesges, L.M., & Dzewaltowski, D.A. (2002). Behavior change intervention research in healthcare settings: A review of recent reports with emphasis on external validity. *American Journal of Preventive Medicine, 23*(1), 62–69. https://doi.org/10.1016/s0749-3797(02)00437-3

Glazier, R.H., Bajcar, J., Kennie, N.R., & Willson, K. (2006). A systematic review of interventions to improve diabetes care in socially disadvantaged populations. *Diabetes Care, 29*(7), 1675–1688. https://doi.org/10.2337/dc05-1942

Godin, G., & Conner, M. (2008). Intention-behavior relationship based on epidemiological indices: An application to physical activity. *American Journal of Health Promotion, 22*, 180–182. https://doi.org/10.4278/ajhp.22.3.180

Godin, G., Sheeran, P., Conner, M., & Germain, M. (2008). Asking questions changes behavior: Mere measurement effects on frequency of blood donation. *Health Psychology, 27*, 179–184. https://doi.org/10.1037/0278-6133.27.2.179.

Godin, G., Sheeran, P., Conner, M., Germain, M., Blondeau, D., Gagné, C., Beaulieu, D., & Naccache, H. (2005). Factors explaining the intention to give blood among the general population. *Vox Sanguinis, 89*, 140–149. https://doi.org/10.1111/j.1423-0410.2005.00674.x

Gogia, S. (2020). Chapter 2—Rationale, history, and basics of telehealth. In S. Gogia (Ed.), *Fundamentals of telemedicine and telehealth* (pp. 11–34). Academic Press. https://doi.org/10.1016/B978-0-12-814309-4.00002-1

Gollwitzer, P.M. (1990). Action phases and mind-sets. In: E.T. Higgins & R.M. Sorrentino (Eds.), *Handbook of motivation and cognition: Foundations of social behavior* (Vol. 2, pp. 53–92). New York: Guilford Press.

Gollwitzer, P.M. (1993). Goal achievement: I role of intentions. *European Review of Social Psychology, 4*, 142–185. https://doi.org/10.1080/14792779343000059

Gollwitzer, P.M., & Sheeran, P. (2006). Implementation intentions and goal achievement: A meta analysis of effects and processes. *Advances in Experimental Social Psychology, 38*, 69–121. https://doi.org/10.1016/S0065-2601(06)38002-1

González-Yubero, S., Lázaro-Visa, S., & Palomera, R. (2021). Personal variables of protection against cannabis use in adolescence: The roles of emotional intelligence, coping styles, and assertiveness as associated factors. *International Journal of Environmental Research and Public Health, 18*(11), 5576. https://doi.org/10.3390/ijerph18115576

Good, A., Harris, P.R., Jessop, D., & Abraham, C. (2015). Open-mindedness can decrease persuasion amongst adolescents: The role of self-affirmation. *British Journal of Health Psychology, 20*(2), 228–242. https://doi.org/10.1111/bjhp.12090

Grande, G., Romppel, M., & Barth, J. (2012). Association between type D personality and prognosis in patients with cardiovascular diseases: A systematic review and meta-analysis. *Annals of Behavioral Medicine, 43*, 299–310. https://doi.org/10.1007/s12160-011-9339-0

Grandey, A.A., & Cropanzano, R. (1999). The conservation of resources model applied to work-family conflict and strain. *Journal of Vocational Behavior, 54*, 350–370. https://doi.org/10.1006/jvbe.1998.1666

Gray, P., Senabe, S., Naicker, N., Kgalamono, S., Yassi, A., & Spiegel, J.M. (2019). Workplace-based organizational interventions promoting mental health and happiness among healthcare workers: A realist review. *International Journal of Environmental Research and Public Health, 16*, 4396. https://doi.org/10.3390/ijerph16224396

Green, L.W., & Glasgow, R.E. (2006). Evaluating the relevance, generalization, and applicability of research: Issues in external validation and translation methodology. *Evaluation & The Health Professions, 29*(1), 126–153. https://doi.org/10.1177/0163278705284445

Greenhalgh, T., Wherton, J., Shaw, S., Morrison, C. (2020). Video consultations for covid-19. *BMJ. 12*(368), m998. doi: 10.1136/bmj.m998.

Greenhaus, J.H., & Beutell, N.J. (1985). Sources of conflict between work and family roles. *Academy of Management Review, 10*, 76–80. https://www.jstor.org/stable/258214

Greve, W. (2001). Traps and gaps in action explanation: Theoretical problems of a psychology of human action. *Psychological Bulletin, 108*, 435–451. https://doi.org/10.1037/0033-295X.108.2.435

Grzywacz, J.G., Casey, P.R., & Jones, F. (2007). The effects of workplace flexibility on health behaviors: A cross-sectional and longitudinal analysis. *Journal of Occupational and Environmental Medicine, 49*, 1302–1309. https://doi.org/10.1097/jom.0b013e31815ae9bc

Hadlow, J., & Pitts, M. (1991). The understanding of common health terms by doctors, nurses and patients. *Social Science & Medicine (1982), 32*(2), 193–196. https://doi.org/10.1016/0277-9536(91)90059-l

Haefner, D.P., & Kirscht, J.P. (1970). Motivational and behavioural effects of modifying health beliefs. *Public Health Reports, 85*, 478–484. https://doi.org/10.1016/s0738-3991(79)80003-8.

Hagger, M.S., Cameron, L.D., Hamilton, K. Hankonen, N., & Lintunen, T. (2020). Changing behavior: A theory- and evidence-based approach. In M.S. Hagger, L.D. Cameron, K. Hamilton, N. Hankonen, & T. Lintunen (Eds.), *The handbook of behavior change* (pp. 1–14). Cambridge University Press. https://doi.org/10.1017/9781108677318.001

Hagger, M.S. & Hamilton K. (2020). Changing behaviour using integrated theories. In M.S. Hagger, L.D. Cameron, K. Hamilton, N. Hankonen, & T. Lintunen (Eds.), *The handbook of behaviour change* (pp. 208–224). Cambridge: Cambridge University Press.

Hagger, M.S. & Orbell, S. (2022) The common sense model of illness self-regulation: A conceptual review and proposed extended model, *Health Psychology Review, 16*(3), 347–377, DOI: 10.1080/17437199.2021.1878050

Hagger-Johnson, G., Bell, S., Britton, A., Cable, N., Conner, M., O'Connor, D.B., Shickle, D., Shelton, N., & Bewick, B.M. (2013). Cigarette smoking and alcohol drinking in a representative sample of English school pupils: Cross-sectional and longitudinal associations. *Preventive Medicine*, 56, 304–308. https://doi.org/10.1016/j.ypmed.2013.02.004

Hahn, V.C., Binneweis, C., Sonnentag, S., & Mojza, E.J. (2011). Learning how to recover from job stress: Effects of a recovery training program on recovery, recovery-related self-efficacy, and wellbeing. *Journal of Occupational Health Psychology, 16*, 202–216. https://doi.org/10.1037/a0022169

Hahn, V.C., & Dormann, C. (2013). The role of partners and children for employees' psychological detachment from work and well-being. *Journal of Applied Psychology, 98*, 26–36. https://doi.org/10.1037/1076-8998.11.4.305

Haines, V.Y., III, Marchand, A., & Harvey, S. (2006). Crossover of workplace aggression experiences in dual-earner couples. *Journal of Occupational Health Psychology, 11*, 305–314.

Hampson, S., Goldberg, L.R., Vogt, T.M., & Dubanoski, J.P. (2006). Forty years on: Teachers' assessment of children's personality traits predict self-reported health behaviors and outcomes at midlife health. *Health Psychology, 25*, 57–64. https://doi.org/10.1037/0278-6133.25.1.57

Hampson, S.E. (2012). Personality processes: Mechanisms by which personality traits "Get Outside the Skin". *Annual Review of Psychology, 63*, 315–339. https://doi.org/10.1146/annurev-psych-120710-100419

Hampson, S.E., Andrews, J.A., Barckley, M., Lichtenstein, E., & Lee, M.E. (2000). Conscientiousness, perceived risk, and risk-reduction behaviors: A preliminary study. *Health Psychology, 19*(5), 496–500. https://doi.org/10.1037/0278-6133.19.5.496

Hampson, S.E., Edmonds, G.W., Goldberg, L.R., Dubanoski, J.P., & Hillier, T.A. (2013). Childhood conscientiousness relates to objectively measured adult physical health four decades later. *Health Psychology, 32*, 925–928. https://doi.org/10.1037/a0031655

Hanson, E.K., Maas, C.J., Meijman, T.F., & Godaert, G.L. (2000). Cortisol secretion throughout the day, perceptions of the work environment, and negative affect. *Annals of Behavioral Medicine, 22*, 316–324. https://doi.org/10.1007/BF02895668

Hari, J. (2018). *Lost connections: Uncovering the real causes of depression – And the unexpected solutions.* Bloomsbury USA.

Hanusch, B.C., O'Connor, D.B., Scott, A., Ions, P., Ions, K., & Gregg, P.J. (2014). Effects of psychological distress and illness perceptions on recovery from total knee replacement. *Bone and Joint Journal, 96-B*, 210–216. https://doi.org/10.1302/0301-620x.96b2.31136

Harden, K.P. (2021). "Reports of my death were greatly exaggerated": Behavior genetics in a postgenomic era. *Annual Review of Psychology, 72*, 37–60. https://doi.org/10.1146/annurev-psych-052220-103822

Harrington, J., Noble, L.M., & Newman, S.P. (2004). Improving patients' communication with doctors: A systematic review of intervention studies. *Patient Education and Counseling, 52*(1), 7–16. https://doi.org/10.1016/s0738-3991(03)00017-x

Harris, P.R., & Napper, L. (2005). Self-affirmation and the biased processing of threatening health-risk information. *Personality and Social Psychology Bulletin, 31*(9), 1250–1263. https://doi.org/10.1177/0146167205274694

Harvey, S.B., Sellahewa, D.A., Wang, M-J., Milligan-Saville, J., Bryan, B.T., Henderson, M., Hatch, S.L., & Mykletun, A. (2018). The role of job strain in understanding midlife common mental disorder: A national birth cohort study. *The Lancet Psychiatry, 5*, 498–506. https://doi.org/10.1016/s2215-0366(18)30137-8

Hausser, J.A., Mojzisch, A., Niesel, M., & Schulz-Hardt, S. (2010) Ten years on: A review of recent research on the Job Demand — Control (-Support) model and psychological wellbeing. *Work and Stress, 24*, 1–35. https://doi.org/10.1080/02678371003683747

Hawkley, L.C., & Cacioppo, J.T. (2010). Loneliness matters: A theoretical and empirical review of consequences and mechanisms. *Annals of Behavioral Medicine, 40*, 218–227. https://doi.org/10.1007%2Fs12160-010-9210-8

Hay, J.L., Ford, J.S., Klein, D., et al. (2003). Adherence to colorectal cancer screening in mammography-adherent older women. *Journal of Behavioral Medicine, 26*, 553–576. https://doi.org/10.1023/a:1026253802962

Haynes, R.B., Yao, X., Degani, A., Kripalani, S., Garg, A., & McDonald, H.P. (2005). Interventions to enhance medication adherence. *The Cochrane Database of Systematic Reviews*, (4), CD000011. https://doi.org/10.1002/14651858.CD000011.pub2

Health and Safety Executive (2022). *Work-related stress, anxiety and depression statistics in Great Britain.* London: Crown Copyright.

Heatherton, T.F., Herman, C.P., & Polivy, J. (1992). Effects of distress on eating: The importance of ego-involvement. *Journal of Personality and Social Psychology, 62*, 801–803. https://psycnet.apa.org/doi/10.1037/0022-3514.62.5.801

Hedges, L.V., & Olkin, I. (1985). *Statistical methods for meta-analysis.* San Diego, CA: Academic Press.

Hegel, M. T., Ayllon, T., Thiel, G., & Oulton, B. (1992). Improving adherence to fluid restrictions in male hemodialysis patients: a comparison of cognitive and behavioral approaches. *Health Psychology, 11*(5), 324–330. https://doi.org/10.1037//0278-6133.11.5.324

Heikkila, K. et al. (2013). Job strain and health-related lifestyle: Findings from an individual-participant meta-analysis of 118,000 working adults. *American Journal of Public Health, 103*, 2090–2097. https://doi.org/10.2105/ajph.2012.301090

Helgeson, V.S., Reynolds, K.A., & Tomich, P.L. (2006). A meta-analytic review of benefit finding and growth. *Journal of Consulting and Clinical Psychology, 74*, 797–816. https://doi.org/10.1037/0022-006x.74.5.797

Herbert, T.B., & Cohen, S. (1993). Depression and immunity: A meta-analytic review. *Psychological Bulletin, 113*, 472–486. https://doi.org/10.1037/0033-2909.113.3.472

Hewitt, P.L., & Flett, G.L. (1996). Personality traits and the coping process (pp. 410–433). In M. Zeidner & N.S. Endler (Eds.), *Handbook of coping: Theory, research, applications.* New York: Wiley.

Hill, C., Abraham, C., & Wright, D.B. (2007). Can theory-based messages in combination with cognitive prompts promote exercise in classroom settings? *Social Science & Medicine, 65*(5), 1049–1058. https://doi.org/10.1016/j.socscimed.2007.04.024

Hill, D., Conner, M., Clancy, F., Moss, R., Bristow, M., & O'Connor, D.B. (2022). Stress and eating behaviours in adults: A systematic review and meta-analysis. *Health Psychology Review, 16*, 280–304. https://doi.org/10.1080/17437199.2021.1923406

Hill, D.C., Moss, R.H., Sykes-Muskett, B., Conner, M., & O'Connor, D.B. (2018). Stress and eating behaviors in children and adolescents: Systematic review and meta-analysis. *Appetite, 123*, 14–22. https://doi.org/10.1016/j.appet.2017.11.109

Hillier-Brown, F.C., Summerbell, C.D., Moore, H.J., Routen, A., Lake, A.A., Adams, J., White, M., Araujo-Soares, V., Abraham, C., Adamson, A.J., & Brown, T.J. (2017). The impact of interventions to promote healthier ready-to-eat meals (to eat in, to take away or to be delivered) sold by specific food outlets open to the general public: A systematic review. *Obesity Reviews, 18*(2), 227–246. https://doi.org/10.1111/obr.12479

Hingson, R.W., & Howland, J. (2002). Comprehensive community interventions to promote health: Implications for college-age drinking problems. *Journal of Studies on Alcohol. Supplement*, (14), 226–240. https://doi.org/10.15288/jsas.2002.s14.226

Hobfoll, S.E. (1989). Conservation of resources: A new attempt at conceptualizing stress. *American Psychologist, 44*, 513–524. https://doi.org/10.1037//0003-066x.44.3.513

Hobfoll, S.E. (2001). The influence of culture, community, and the nested-self in the stress process: Advancing conservation of resources theory. *Applied Psychology: An International Review, 50*, 337–421. https://psycnet.apa.org/doi/10.1111/1464-0597.00062

Hobfoll, S.E. (2011). Conservation of Resources Theory: Its implications for stress, health and resiliency (pp. 127–147). In S. Folkman (Ed.), *Oxford handbook of stress health and coping.* Oxford University Press.

Hobfoll, S.E., Halbesleben, J., Neveu, J-P., & Westman, M. (2018). Conservation of resources in the organizational context: The reality of resources and their consequences. *Annual Review of Organizational Psychology and Organizational Behavior, 5*, 103–128. https://doi.org/10.1146/annurev-orgpsych-032117-104640

Hochbaum, G.M. (1958). *Public participation in medical screening programs: A socio-psychological study*. Public Health Service Publication No. 572. Washington, DC: United States Government Printing Office.

Holman, D., Johnson, S., & O'Connor, E. (2018). Stress management interventions: Improving subjective psychological well-being in the workplace. In E. Diener, S. Oishi & L. Tay (Eds.), *Handbook of well-being* (pp. 101–121). Salt Lake City, UT: DEF Publishers.

Holmes, T. H., & Masuda, M. (1974). Life change and illness susceptibility. In: B. S. Dohrenwend & B. P. Dohrenwend (Eds), *Stressful life events: Their nature and effects* (pp. 45–72). John Wiley & Sons.

Holmes, T. H., & Rahe, R. H. (1967). The social readjustment rating scale. *Journal of Psychosomatic Research*, *11*, 213–218. https://psycnet.apa.org/doi/10.1016/0022-3999(67)90010-4

Holroyd, K.A., Nash, J.M., Pingel, J.D., Cordingley, G.E., & Jerome, A. (1991). A comparison of pharmacological (amitriptyline HCL) and nonpharmacological (cognitive-behavioral) therapies for chronic tension headaches. *Journal of Consulting and Clinical Psychology*, *59*(3), 387–393. https://doi.org/10.1037//0022-006x.59.3.387

Holroyd, K.A., O'Donnell, F.J., Stensland, M., Lipchik, G.L., Cordingley, G.E., & Carlson, B.W. (2001). Management of chronic tension-type headache with tricyclic antidepressant medication, stress management therapy, and their combination: A randomized controlled trial. *JAMA*, *285*(17), 2208–2215. https://doi.org/10.1001/jama.285.17.2208

Holtman, G.A., Burger, H., Verheij, R.A., Wouters, H., Berger, M.Y., Rosmalen, J.G., & Verhaak, P.F. (2021). Developing a clinical prediction rule for repeated consultations with functional somatic symptoms in primary care: A cohort study. *BMJ Open*, *11*(1), e040730. https://doi.org/10.1136/bmjopen-2020-040730

Holt-Lunstad, J., & Steptoe, A. (2022). Social isolation: An underappreciated determinant of physical health. *Current Opinion in Psychology*, *43*, 232–237. https://doi.org/10.1016/j.copsyc.2021.07.012

Horn, S., & Munafo, M. (1998). *Pain: Theory, research and intervention*. Open University Press.

Horne, A. M., & Rosenthal, R. (1997). Research in group work: How did we get where we are? *Journal for Specialists in Group Work*, *22*(4), 228–240. https://doi.org/10.1080/01933929708415527

House, J.S., Landis, K.R., & Umberson, D. (1988). Social relationships and health. *Science*, *241*, 540–545. https://doi.org/10.1126/science.3399889

House of Lords (2000). *Select Committee on Technology and Science, Sixth Report*. http://www.publications.parliament.uk/pa/ld199900/ldselect/ldsctech/123/12301.htm

Howarth, E., O'Connor, D.B., Panagioti, M., Hodkinson, A., Wilding, S., & Johnson, J. (2020). Are stressful life events prospectively associated with increased suicidality? A systematic review and meta-analysis. *Journal of Affective Disorders*, *266*, 731–742. https://doi.org/10.1016/j.jad.2020.01.171

Howick, J., Moscrop, A., Mebius, A., et al. (2018). Effects of empathic and positive communication in healthcare consultations: A systematic review and meta-analysis. *Journal of the Royal Society of Medicine*, *111*(7), 240–252. doi:10.1177/0141076818769477

Howie, J.G., Heaney, D.J., Maxwell, M., Walker, J.J., Freeman, G.K., & Rai, H. (1999). Quality at general practice consultations: Cross sectional survey. *BMJ*, *319*(7212), 738–743. https://doi.org/10.1136/bmj.319.7212.738

Hróbjartsson, A., & Gøtzsche, P. C. (2001). Is the placebo powerless? An analysis of clinical trials comparing placebo with no treatment. *The New England Journal of Medicine*, *344*(21), 1594–1602. https://doi.org/10.1056/NEJM200105243442106

HSE (1995). *Stress at work: A guide for employers*. Suffolk: HSE Books.

HSE (2017). *Tackling work-related stress using the Management Standards approach: A step-by-step workbook*. Retrieved 1st July 2023 from https://www.hse.gov.uk/pubns/wbk01.htm

Hu, Q., Schaufeli, W.B., & Toon, T.W. (2011). The job demands-resources model: An analysis of additive and joint effects of demands and resources. *Journal of Vocational Behavior*, *79*, 181–190. https://doi.org/10.1016/j.jvb.2010.12.009

Hudson, J., Moon, Z., Hughes, L., & Moss-Morris, R. (2020). Engagement of stakeholders in the design, evaluation, and implementation of complex interventions. In M. Hagger, L. Cameron, K. Hamilton, N. Hankonen, & T. Lintunen (Eds.), *The handbook of behavior change* (Cambridge Handbooks in Psychology, pp. 349–360). Cambridge: Cambridge University Press. https://doi.org/10.1017/9781108677318.024

Hughes, D. (1983). Consultation length and outcome in two group general practices. *The Journal of the Royal College of General Practitioners*, *33*(248), 143–147.

Inagaki, T.K. (2020). Health neuroscience 2.0: Integration with social, cognitive and affective neuroscience. *Social Cognitive and Affective Neuroscience*, *15*(10), 1017–1023. https://doi.org/10.1093/scan/nsaa123

Iribarren, S.J., Akande, T.O., Kamp, K.J., Barry, D., Kader, Y.G., & Suelzer, E. (2021). Effectiveness of mobile apps to promote health and manage disease: Systematic review and meta-analysis of randomized controlled trials. *JMIR Mhealth Uhealth*. *9*(1), e21563. doi: 10.2196/21563.

Jacobs, N., Myin-Germeys, I., Derom, C., Delespaul, P., van Os, J., & Nicolson, N.A. (2007). A momentary assessment study of the relationship between affective and adrenocortical stress responses in daily life. *Biological Psychology, 74*, 60–66. https://doi.org/10.1016/j.biopsycho.2006.07.002

Janz, N.K., & Becker, M.H. (1984). The health belief model: A decade later. *Health Education Quarterly, 11*, 1–47. https://doi.org/10.1177/109019818401100101

Javaras, K.N., Williams, M., & Baskin-Sommers, A.R. (2019). Psychological interventions potentially useful for increasing conscientiousness. *Personality Disorders, 10(1)*, 13–24. https://doi.org/10.1037/per0000267

Jenkins, C.D., Zyzanski, S.J., & Rosenmann, R.H. (1971). Progress toward validation of a computer-scored test for the type A coronary-prone behavior pattern. *Psychosomatic Medicine, 33*, 193–202. https://doi.org/10.1097/00006842-197105000-00001

Jenkins, V., Fallowfield, L., & Saul, J. (2001). Information needs of patients with cancer: Results from a large study in UK cancer centres. *British Journal of Cancer, 84*(1), 48–51. https://doi.org/10.1054/bjoc.2000.1573

Jensen, M.P., & Turk, D.C. (2014). Contributions of psychology to the understanding and treatment of people with chronic pain: Why it matters to ALL psychologists. *American Psychologist, 69*, 105–118. https://doi.org/10.1037/a0035641

John, O.P., & Srivastava, S. (1999). The Big Five trait taxonomy: History, measurement, and theoretical perspectives. In L.A. Pervin and O.P. John (Eds), *Handbook of personality: Theory and research* (2nd Ed.; pp. 102–138). New York: Guilford Press.

Johnson, J.V., & Hall, E.M. (1988). Job strain, work place social support and cardiovascular disease: A cross-sectional study of a random sample of the working population. *American Journal of Public Health, 78*, 1336–1342. https://doi.org/10.2105%2Fajph.78.10.1336

Jokela, M., Batty, G.D., Nyberg, S.T., Virtanen, M., Nabi, H., Singh-Manoux, A., & Kivimaki, M. (2013b). Personality and all-cause mortality: Individual-participant meta-analysis of 3,947 deaths in 76,150 adults. *American Journal of Epidemiology, 178*, 667–675. https://doi.org/10.1093/aje/kwt170

Jokela, M., Hintsanen, M., Hakulinen, C., Batty, G.D., Nabi, H., Singh-Manoux, A., & Kivimaki, M. (2013a). Association of personality with the development and persistence of obesity: A meta-analysis based on individual-participant data. *Obesity Reviews, 14*, 315–323. https://doi.org/10.1111/obr.12007

Jonason, P.K., Talbot, D., Cunningham, M.L., & Chonody, J. (2020). Higher-order coping strategies: Who uses them and what outcomes are linked to them. *Personality and Individual Differences, 155*, 109755. https://doi.org/10.1016/j.paid.2019.109755

Jones, F., Bright, J.E.H., Searle, B., & Cooper, L. (1998). Modelling occupational stress and health: The impact of the demand-control model on academic research and on workplace practice. *Stress Medicine, 14*(4), 231–236. https://doi.org/10.1002/(SICI)1099-1700(1998100)14:4<231::AID-SMI802>3.0.CO;2-X

Jones, F., & Kinman, G. (2001). Approaches to studying stress. In F. Jones & J. Bright (Eds.), *Stress: Myth, theory and research* (pp. 17–45). London: Prentice Hall.

Jones, F., Kinman, G., & Payne, N. (2006). Work stress and health behaviours: A work life balance issue. In F. Jones, R.J. Burke & M. Westman (Eds), *Work-life balance: A psychological perspective* (pp. 185–215). Hove: Psychology Press.

Jones, F., O'Connor, D.B., Conner, M., McMillan, B., & Ferguson, E. (2007). Impact of daily mood, work hours, and iso-strain variables on self-reported health behaviors. *Journal of Applied Psychology, 92*, 1731–1740. https://doi.org/10.1037/0021-9010.92.6.1731

Jones, P.K., Jones, S.L., & Katz, J. (1987). Improving compliance for asthmatic patients visiting the emergency department using a health belief model intervention. *Journal of Asthma, 24*, 199–206. https://doi.org/10.3109/02770908709070940

Jones, T., Darzi, A., Egger, G., Ickovics, J., Noffsinger, E., Kamalini, R., Stevens, J., Sumego, S., & Birrell, F. (2019). A systems approach to embedding group consultations in the NHS. *Future Healthcare Journal, 6*(1), 8–16. https://www.groupconsultations.com/wp-content/uploads/2019/09/asystemapproachtoembeddinggroupconsultations.pdf

Junghaenel, D.U., & Stone, A.A. (2020). Ecological momentary assessment for the psychosocial study of health. *The Wiley encyclopedia of health psychology* (pp. 185–215). Wiley & Sons.

Kabat-Zinn, J. (2003). Mindfulness-based interventions in context: Past, present, and future. *Clinical Psychology: Science and Practice, 10*, 144–156. https://doi.org/10.1093/clipsy.bpg016

Kagan, J. (2016). An overly permissive extension. *Perspectives in Psychological Science, 11*, 442–450. https://doi.org/10.1177/1745691616635593

Kalichman, S.C., Benotsch, E.G., Weinhardt, L., Austin, J., Luke, W., & Cherry, C. (2003). Health-related internet use, coping, social support, and health indicators in people living with HIV/AIDS: Preliminary results from a community survey. *Health Psychology, 22*, 111–116. https://doi.org/10.1037//0278-6133.22.1.111

Kamarck, T.W., & Lovallo, W.R. (2003). Cardiovascular reactivity to psychological challenge: Conceptual and measurement considerations. *Psychosomatic Medicine*, *65*, 9–21. https://doi.org/10.1097/01.psy.000003 0390.34416.3e

Kanner, A.D., Coyne, J.C., Schaefer, C., & Lazarus, R.S. (1981). Comparison of two modes of stress measurement: Daily hassles and uplifts versus major life events. *Journal of Behavioral Medicine*, *4*, 1–39. https://doi.org/10.1007/bf00844845

Kaplan, R.M. (1990). Behavior as the central outcome in health care. *The American Psychologist*, *45*(11), 1211–1220. https://doi.org/10.1037//0003-066x.45.11.1211

Kaplan, R.M., & Stone, A.A. (2013). Bringing the laboratory and clinic to the community: Mobile technologies for health promotion and disease prevention. *Annual Review of Psychology*, *64*, 471–498. https://doi.org/10.1146/annurev-psych-113011-143736

Karasek, R.A. (1979). Job demands, job decision latitude and mental strain: Implications for job design. *Administrative Science Quarterly*, *24*, 285–308. https://doi.org/10.2307/2392498

Karasek, R.A. (1985). *Job Content Questionnaire and user's guide*. Lowell, MA: Department of Work Environment, University of Massachusetts.

Karasek, R.A. (1989). Control in the workplace and its health related aspects. In S.L. Sauter, J.J. Hurrell & C.L. Cooper (Eds.), *Job control and worker health* (pp. 129–160). Chichester: Wiley & Sons.

Kasl, S.V., & Cobb, S. (1966). Health behavior, illness behavior and sick role behavior. *Archives of Environmental Health*, *12*, 246–266. https://doi.org/10.1080/00039896.1966.10664421

Kekade, S., Hseieh, C.H., Islam, M.M, Atique, S, Mohammed Khalfan, A., Li, Y.C., & Abdul S.S. (2018). The usefulness and actual use of wearable devices among the elderly population. *Computer Methods Programs Biomed*, *153*, 137–159. doi: 10.1016/j.cmpb.2017.10.008

Kellogg Foundation (2004). *W.K. Kellogg Foundation logic model development guide*. W.K. Kellogg Foundation.

Kendler, K.S., Kessler, R.C., Walters, E.E., Maclean, C., Neale, M.C., Heath, A.C., & Eaves, L.J. (1995). Stressful life events, genetic liability, and onset of an episode of major depression in women. *American Journal of Psychiatry*, *152*, 833–842. https://doi.org/10.1176/ajp.152.6.833

Kendrick, A.H., Higgs, C.M., Whitfield, M.J., & Laszlo, G. (1993). Accuracy of perception of severity of asthma: Patients treated in general practice. *BMJ*, *307*(6901), 422–424. https://doi.org/10.1136/bmj.307.6901.422

Kennedy, A., Reeves, D., Bower, P., Lee, V., Middleton, E., Richardson, G., Gardner, C., Gately, C., & Rogers, A. (2007). The effectiveness and cost effectiveness of a national lay-led self care support programme for patients with long-term conditions: A pragmatic questionn controlled trial. *Journal of Epidemiology and Community Health*, *61*(3), 254–261. https://doi.org/10.1136/jech.2006.053538

Kern, M.L., & Friedman, H.S. (2008). Do conscientious individuals live longer? A quantitative review. *Health Psychology*, *27*, 505–512. https://doi.org/10.1037/0278-6133.27.5.505

Keusch, F., & Conrad, F.G. (2022). Using smartphones to capture and combine self-reports and passively measured behavior in social research. *Journal of Survey Statistics and Methodology*, 10, 863–885. https://doi.org/10.1093/jssam/smab035

Khaw, K. T., Wareham, N., Bingham, S., Welch, A., Luben, R., & Day, N. (2008). Combined impact of health behaviours and mortality in men and women: the EPIC-Norfolk prospective population study. *PloS Medicine*, *5*(1), e12. https://doi.org/10.1371/journal.pmed.0050012

Kidd, J., Marteau, T.M., Robinson, S., Ukoumunne, O.C., & Tydeman, C. (2004). Promoting patient participation in consultations: A questionn controlled trial to evaluate the effectiveness of three patient-focused interventions. *Patient Education and Counseling*, *52*(1), 107–112. https://doi.org/10.1016/s0738-3991(03)00018-1

Kiecolt-Glaser, J.K., Marucha, P.T., Malarkey, W.B., Mercado, A.M., & Glaser, R. (1995). Slowing of wound healing by psychological stress. *Lancet*, *346*, 1194–1196. https://doi.org/10.1016/s0140-6736(95)92899-5

Kiecolt-Glaser, J.K., McGuire, L., Robles, T., & Glaser, R. (2002). Emotions, morbidity, and mortality: New perspectives from psychoneuroimmunology. *Annual Review of Psychology*, *53*, 83–107. https://doi.org/10.1146/annurev.psych.53.100901.135217

Kiecolt-Glaser, J.K., Page, G.G., Marucha, P.T., MacCallum, R.C., & Glaser, R. (1998). Psychological influences on surgical recovery: Perspectives from psychoneuroimmunology. *American Psychologist*, *53*, 1209–1218. https://doi.org/10.1037//0003-066x.53.11.1209

King, A.C., Carl, F., Birkel, L., & Haskell, W.L. (1988). Increasing exercise among blue-collar employees: The tailoring of worksite programs to meet specific needs. *Preventive Medicine*, *17*(3), 357–365. https://doi.org/10.1016/0091-7435(88)90010-2

King, J.B. (1982). The impact of patients perceptions of high blood pressure on attendance at screening, An extension of the Health Belief Model. *Social Science & Medicine, 16*(10), 1079–1091. https://doi.org/10.1016/0277-9536(82)90184-8

Kini, V., & Ho, P.M. (2018). Interventions to improve medication adherence: A review. *JAMA, 320*(23), 2461–2473. https://doi.org/10.1001/jama.2018.19271

Kirsch, I., Deacon, B.J., Huedo-Medina, T.B., Scoboria, A., Moore, T.J., & Johnson, B.T. (2008). Initial severity and antidepressant benefits: A meta-analysis of data submitted to the Food and Drug Administration. *PloS Medicine, 5*(2), e45. https://doi.org/10.1371/journal.pmed.0050045

Kirsch, I., & Sapirstein, G. (1998). Listening to Prozac but hearing placebo: A meta-analysis of antidepressant medication. *Prevention & Treatment, 1*(2). https://doi.org/10.1037/1522-3736.1.1.12a

Kirschbaum, C., Pirke, K.M., & Hellhammer, D.H. (1993). The 'Trier Social Stress Test' – A tool for investigating psychobiology stress responses in a laboratory setting. *Neuropsychobiology, 28*, 76–81. https://doi.org/10.1159/000119004

Kirsh, S.R., Aron, D.C., Johnson, K.D., Santurri, L.E., Stevenson, L.D., Jones, K.R., & Jagosh, J. (2017). A realist review of shared medical appointments: How, for whom, and under what circumstances do they work? *BMC Health Services Research, 17*(1), 113. https://doi.org/10.1186/s12913-017-2064-z

Kivimaki, M., Leino-Arjas, P., Luukonen, R., Riihimaki, H., Vahtera, J., & Kirjonen, J. (2002). Work stress and risk of cardiovascular mortality: Prospective cohort study of industrial employees. *British Medical Journal, 325*, 857. https://doi.org/10.1136/bmj.325.7369.857

Kivimäki, M., Nyberg, S.T., Batty, G.D., Fransson, E.I., Heikkilä, K., Alfredsson, L., Bjorner, J.B., Borritz, M., Burr, H., Casini, A., Clays, E., De Bacquer, D., Dragano, N., Ferrie, J.E., Geuskens, G.A., Goldberg, M., Hamer, M., Hooftman, W.E., Houtman, I.L., Joensuu, M., . . . IPD-Work Consortium (2012). Job strain as a risk factor for coronary heart disease: A collaborative meta-analysis of individual participant data. *Lancet, 380*, 1491–1497. https://doi.org/10.1016/S0140-6736(12)60994-5

Kleinsinger, F. (2018). The unmet challenge of medication nonadherence. *The Permanente Journal, 22*, 18–033. https://doi.org/10.7812/TPP/18-033

Knittle, K., Heino, M., Marques, M.M., Stenius, M., Beattie, M., Ehbrecht, F., Hagger, M.S., Hardeman, W., & Hankonen, N. (2020). The compendium of self-enactable techniques to change and self-manage motivation and behaviour v.1.0. *Nature Human Behaviour, 4*(2), 215–223. https://doi.org/10.1038/s41562-019-0798-9

Knowler, W.C., Barrett-Connor, E., Fowler, S.E., Hamman, R.F., Lachin, J.M., Walker, E.A., Nathan, D.M., & Diabetes Prevention Program Research Group (2002). Reduction in the incidence of type 2 diabetes with lifestyle intervention or metformin. *The New England Journal of Medicine, 346*(6), 393–403. https://doi.org/10.1056/NEJMoa012512

Knowles, E.S., & Rinner, D.D. (2007). Omega approaches to persuasion: Overcoming resistance. In A.R. Pratkanis (Ed.), *The science of social influence: Advances and future progress* (pp. 83–114). Psychology Press.

Kola, S., Walsh, J.C., Hughes, B.M., & Howard, S. (2013). Matching intra-procedural information with coping style reduces psychophysiological arousal in women undergoing colposcopy. *Journal of Behavioural Medicine, 36*, 401–412. https://doi.org/10.1007/s10865-012-9435-z

Kolk, A.M., Hanewald, G.J., Schagen, S., & Gijsbers van Wijk, C.M. (2003). A symptom perception approach to common physical symptoms. *Social Science & Medicine, 57*(12), 2343–2354. https://doi.org/10.1016/s0277-9536(02)00451-3

Kong, J., Liu, Y., Goldberg, J., & Almeida, D.M. (2021). Adverse childhood experiences amplify the longitudinal associations of adult stress and health. *Child Abuse & Neglect, 105337*. https://doi.org/10.1016/j.chiabu.2021.105337

Kools, M., van de Wiel, M.W., Ruiter, R.A., Crüts, A., & Kok, G. (2006). The effect of graphic organizers on subjective and objective comprehension of a health education text. *Health Education & Behavior, 33*(6), 760–772. https://doi.org/10.1177/1090198106288950

Korsch, B.M., Gozzi, E.K., & Francis, V. (1968). Gaps in doctor-patient communication. 1. Doctor-patient interaction and patient satisfaction. *Pediatrics, 42*(5), 855–871.

Kowalski, R.M., & Black, K.J. (2021). Protection motivation and the COVID-19 virus. *Health Communication, 36*(1), 15–22. https://doi.org/10.1080/10410236.2020.1847448

Kraut, R., Kiesler, S., Boneva, B., Cummings, J.N., Helgeson, V., & Crawford, A.M. (2002). Internet paradox revisited. *Journal of Social Issues, 58*, 49–74. https://doi.org/10.1111/1540-4560.00248

Kraut, R., Patterson, M., Lundmark, V., Kiesler, S., Mukopadhyay, T., & Scherlis, W. (1998). Internet paradox: A social technology that reduces social involvement and psychological well-being. *American Psychologist, 53*, 1017–1031. https://doi.org/10.1037//0003-066x.53.9.1017

Kraynak, T.E., Marsland, A.L., Hanson, J.L., & Gianaros, P.J. (2019). Retrospectively reported childhood physical abuse, systematic inflammation, and resting corticolimbic connectivity in midlife adults. *Brain, Behavior and Immunity*, *82*, 203–213. https://doi.org/10.1016/j.bbi.2019.08.186

Krokstad, S., Ding, D., Grunseit, A. C., Sund, E. R., Holmen, T. L., Rangul, V., & Bauman, A. (2017). Multiple lifestyle behaviours and mortality, findings from a large population-based Norwegian cohort study – The HUNT Study. *BMC Public Health*, *17*(1), 58. https://doi.org/10.1186/s12889-016-3993-x

Kunz, S., Haasova, S., Rieß, J., & Florack, A. (2020). Beyond healthiness: The impact of traffic light labels on taste expectations and purchase intentions. *Foods (Basel, Switzerland)*, *9*(2), 134. https://doi.org/10.3390/foods9020134

Kunz-Ebrecht, S.R., Mohamed-Ali, V., Feldman, P.J., Kirschbaum, C., & Steptoe, A. (2003). Cortisol responses to mild psychological stress are inversely associated with proinflammatory cytokines. *Brain, Behavior and Immunity*, *17*, 373–383. https://doi.org/10.1016/s0889-1591(03)00029-1

Kupper, N., & Denollet, J. (2018). Type D personality as a risk factor in coronary heart disease: A review of current evidence. *Current Cardiology Reports*, *20*, 104. https://doi.org/10.1007/s11886-018-1048-x

Lai-Bao, Z., Wu, Y., Giron, M.S., Jin-Jing, P., & Hui-Xin, W (2020). Impact of effort reward imbalance at work on suicidal symptoms. *Journal of Affective Disorders*, *260*, 214–221. https://doi.org/10.1016/j.jad.2019.09.007

Lake, A.J., Browne, J.L., Abraham, C., Tumino, D., Hines, C., Rees, G., & Speight, J. (2018). A tailored intervention to promote uptake of retinal screening among young adults with type 2 diabetes—An intervention mapping approach. *BMC Health Services Research*, *18*(1), 396. https://doi.org/10.1186/s12913-018-3188-5

Lam, W.Y., & Fresco, P. (2015). Medication adherence measures: An overview. *BioMed Research International*, *2015*, 1–12. https://doi.org/10.1155/2015/217047

Lambert, J.D., Greaves, C.J., Farrand, P., Cross, R., Haase, A.M., & Taylor, A.H. (2017). Assessment of fidelity in individual level behaviour change interventions promoting physical activity among adults: A systematic review. *BMC Public Health*, *17*(1), 765. https://doi.org/10.1186/s12889-017-4778-6

Lazarus, R.S. (1966). *Psychological stress and the coping process*. New York: McGraw-Hill.

Lazarus, R.S. (1999). *Stress and emotion: A new synthesis*. London: Springer.

Lazarus, R.S. (2001). Conservation of resources theory (COR): Little more than words masquerading as a new theory. *Applied Psychology: An International Review*, *50*, 381–391. https://doi.org/10.1111/1464-0597.00063

Lazarus, R.S., & Folkman, S. (1984). *Stress, appraisal and coping*. New York: Springer.

Lazarus, R.S., Kanner, A.D., & Folkman, S. (1980). Emotions: A cognitive-phenomenological analysis. In R. Plutchik & H. Kellerman (Eds.), *Theories of emotion* (pp. 189–217). New York: Academic Press.

Lee, D.J., & Sirgy, M.J. (2019). Work-life balance in the digital workplace: The impact of schedule flexibility and telecommuting on work-life balance and overall life satisfaction. In M. Coetzee (Ed.), *Thriving in digital workspaces* (pp. 355–384). Springer.

Lesener, T., Gusy, B., & Wolter, C. (2019). The job demands-resources model: A meta-analytic review of longitudinal studies. *Work & Stress*, *33*, 76–103. https://doi.org/10.1080/02678373.2018.1529065

Lessard, J., & Holman, E.A. (2014). FKBP5 and CRHRi polymorphisms moderate the stress-physical health association in a national sample. *Health Psychology*, *33*, 1046–1056. https://doi.org/10.1037/a0033968

Leventhal, H., Benyamini, Y., Brownlee, S., Diefenbach, M., Leventhal, E.A., Parker-Miller, L., & Robitaille, C. (1997). Illness representations: Theoretical foundations. In K.J. Petrie and J. Weinman (Eds.), *Perceptions of health and illness: Current research and applications* (pp. 19–45). Harwood Academic.

Leventhal, H., Nerenz, D.R., & Steele, D.J. (1984). Illness representation and coping with health threats. In A. Baum, S.E. Taylor, & J.E. Singer (Eds.), *Handbook of psychology and health* (pp. 219–252). Lawrence Erlbaum Associates.

Levine, J.D., Gordon, N.C., & Fields, H.L. (1978). The mechanism of placebo analgesia. *Lancet*, *2*(8091), 654–657. https://doi.org/10.1016/s0140-6736(78)92762-9

Levy, B.R., Slade, M.D., Kunkel, S.R., & Kasl, S.V. (2002). Longevity increased by positive self-perceptions of aging. *Journal of Personality and Social Psychology*, *83*, 261–270. https://doi.org/10.1037//0022-3514.83.2.261

Ley, P. (1988) *Communicating with the patient*. Croom Helm.

Ley, P., Whitworth, M.A., Skilbeck, C.E., Woodward, R., Pinsent, R.J., Pike, L.A., Clarkson, M.E., & Clark, P.B. (1976). Improving doctor-patient communication in general practice. *Journal of the Royal College of General Practitioners*, *26*(171), 720–724.

Liang, J., Krause, N.M., & Bennett, J.M. (2001). Social exchange and well-being: Is giving better than receiving? *Psychology and Aging*, *16*, 511–523. https://doi.org/10.1037//0882-7974.16.3.511

Lin, J., & Epel, E. (2022). Stress and telomere shortening: Insights from cellular mechanisms. *Ageing Research Reviews*, *73*, 101507. https://doi.org/10.1016/j.arr.2021.101507

Litt, M.D., Tennen, H., Affleck, G., & Klock, S. (1992). Coping and cognitive factors in adaptation to in vitro fertilization failure. *Journal of Behavioral Medicine, 15*, 171–188. https://doi.org/10.1007/BF00848324

Littell, J.H., & Girvin, H. (2002). Stages of change. A critique. *Behavior Modification, 26*, 223–273. https://doi.org/10.1177/0145445502026002006

Little, P., Everitt, H., Williamson, I., Warner, G., Moore, M., Gould, C., Ferrier, K., & Payne, S. (2001). Observational study of effect of patient centredness and positive approach on outcomes of general practice consultations. *BMJ, 323*(7318), 908–911. https://doi.org/10.1136/bmj.323.7318.908

Lloyd, J.J., Creanor, S., Logan, S., Green, C., Dean, S., Hillsdon, M., Abraham, C., Tomlinson, R., Pearson, V., Taylor, R.S., Ryan, E., Streeter, A., & Wyatt, K. (2018). Effectiveness of the Healthy Lifestyles Programme (HeLP) to prevent obesity in UK primary-school children: A cluster randomised controlled trial. *Lancet Child and Adolescence, 2*(1), 35–45. https://doi.org/10.1016/S2352-4642(17)30151-7

Lo Martire, V., Caruso, D., Palgini, L., Zoccoli, G., & Bastianini, S. (2020). Stress and sleep: A relationship lasting a lifetime. *Neuroscience and Biobehavioral Reviews, 117*, 65–77. https://doi.org/10.1016/j.neubiorev.2019.08.024

Lockwood, P., Wong, C., McShane, K., & Dolderman, D. (2005). The impact of positive and negative fitness exemplars on motivation. *Basic & Applied Social Psychology, 27*(1), 1–13. https://doi.org/10.1207/s15324834basp2701_1

Long, B.C., & Flood, K.R. (1993). Coping with work stress: Psychological benefits of exercise. *Work and Stress, 1*, 108–119. https://doi.org/10.1080/02678379308257055

Lorig, K.R., Mazonson, P.D., & Holman, H.R. (1993). Evidence suggesting that health education for self-management in patients with chronic arthritis has sustained health benefits while reducing health care costs. *Arthritis and Rheumatism, 36*(4), 439–446. https://doi.org/10.1002/art.1780360403

Lorig, K.R., Sobel, D.S., Stewart, A.L., Brown, B.W., Jr, Bandura, A., Ritter, P., Gonzalez, V.M., Laurent, D.D., & Holman, H.R. (1999). Evidence suggesting that a chronic disease self-management program can improve health status while reducing hospitalization: A randomized trial. *Medical Care, 37*(1), 5–14. https://doi.org/10.1097/00005650-199901000-00003

Lu, L., Zhang, J., Xie, Y., Gao, F., Xu, S., Wu, X., & Ye, Z. (2020). Wearable health devices in health care: Narrative systematic review. *JMIR Mhealth Uhealth.* 8(11), e18907. doi: 10.2196/18907

Lumley, M.A., Tojek, T.M., & MacKlem, D.J. (1999). The effects of written emotional disclosure among repressive and alexithymic people. In S.L. LePore & J.M. Smyth (Eds.), *The writing cure* (pp. 75–117). Washington: American Psychological Association.

Luo, F., Guo, L., Thapa, A., & Yu, B. (2021). Social isolation and depression onset among middle-aged and older adults in China: Moderating effects of education and gender differences. *Journal of Affective Disorders, 283*, 71–76. https://doi.org/10.1016/j.jad.2021.01.022

Luo, J., Zhang, B., & Roberts, B.W. (2021). Sensitization or inoculation: Investigating the effects of early adversity on personality traits and stress experiences in adulthood. *PLoS ONE, 16*(4): e0248822. https://doi.org/10.1371%2Fjournal.pone.0248822

Luszczynska, A., Lobczowska, K., & Horodyska, K. (2020). Implementation science and translation in behavior change. In M. Hagger, L. Cameron, K. Hamilton, N. Hankonen, & T. Lintunen (Eds.), *The handbook of behavior change* (Cambridge Handbooks in Psychology, pp. 333–348). Cambridge: Cambridge University Press. https://doi.org/10.1017/9781108677318.023

Luszczynska, A., & Schwarzer, R. (2015). Social cognitive theory and the health action approach. In M. Conner & P. Norman (Eds.), *Predicting and changing health behaviour: Research and practice with social cognition models* (3rd Edn.; pp. 225–251). Maidenhead: Open University Press. https://doi.org/10.1017/9781108677318.003

Luszczynska, A., Sobczyk, A., & Abraham, C. (2007). Planning to lose weight: randomized controlled trial of an implementation intention prompt to enhance weight reduction among overweight and obese women. *Health Psychology, 26*(4), 507–512. https://doi.org/10.1037/0278-6133.26.4.507

Luszczynska, A., Szczuka, Z., Abraham, C., Baban, A., Brooks, S., Cipolletta, S., Danso, E., Dombrowski, S.U., Gan, Y., Gaspar, T., de Matos, M.G., Griva, K., Jongenelis, M.I., Keller, J., Knoll, N., Ma, J., Miah, M.A.A., Morgan, K., Peraud, W., Quintard, B., . . . Wolf, H. (2022). The interplay between strictness of policies and individuals' self-regulatory efforts: Associations with handwashing during the COVID-19 pandemic. *Annals of Behavioral Medicine, 56*(4), 368–380. https://doi.org/10.1093/abm/kaab102

Mackay, S., Burdayron, R., & Körner, A. (2021). Factor structure of the Brief COPE in patients with melanoma. *Canadian Journal of Behavioural Science/Revue canadienne des sciences du comportement, 53*, 78–83. https://psycnet.apa.org/doi/10.1037/cbs0000184

Mackenbach, J.P. (2006). *Health inequalities: Europe in profile – an independent, expert report commissioned by UK Presidency of the EU.* London: Department of Health.

Maddux, J.E., & Rogers, R.W. (1983). Protection motivation and self-efficacy: A revised theory of fear appeals and attitude change. *Journal of Experimental Social Psychology, 19*, 469–479. https://doi.org/10.1016/0022-1031(83)90023-9

Magee, C.A., Heaven, P.C.L., & Miller, L.M. (2013). Personality change predicts self-reported mental and physical health. *Journal of Personality, 81(3)*, 324–334. https://doi.org/10.1111/j.1467-6494.2012.00802.x

Major, D.A., & Germano, L.M. (2006). The changing nature of work and its impact on the work-family interface. In F. Jones, R.J. Burke, & M. Westman (Eds.), *Work-life balance: A psychological perspective* (pp. 13–38). Hove: Psychology Press.

Manuck, S.B., Kaplan, J.R., & Clarkson, T.B. (1983). Behaviourally induced heart rate reactivity and atherosclerosis in cynomolgus monkeys. *Psychosomatic Medicine, 45*, 95–108. https://doi.org/10.1097/00006842-198305000-00002

Marmot, M.G., Davey-Smith, G.M., Stansfield, S., Patel, C., North, F., Head, J., White, I., Brunner, E., & Feeney, A. (1991). Health inequalities among British civil servants: The Whitehall II study. *Lancet, 337*, 1387–1393. https://doi.org/10.1016/0140-6736(91)93068-k

Martin, R., Hewstone, M., & Martin, P.Y. (2007). Majority versus minority influence: I role of message processing in determining resistance to counter-persuasion. *European Journal of Social Psychology, 38*(1), 16–34. https://doi.org/10.1002/ejsp.426

Marucha, P.T., Kiecolt-Glaser, J.K., & Favagehi, M. (1998). Mucosal wound healing is impaired by examination stress. *Psychosomatic Medicine, 60*, 362–365. https://doi.org/10.1097/00006842-199805000-00025

Maslach, C. (1982). Understanding burnout: Definitional issues in analyzing a complex phenomenon. In W.S. Paine (Ed.), *Job Stress and burnout* (pp. 29–40). Beverley Hills, CA: Sage.

Mason, J.W. (1971). A re-evaluation of the concept of 'non-specificity' in stress theory. *Journal of Psychiatric Research, 8*, 323–353. https://doi.org/10.1016/0022-3956(71)90028-8

Matarazzo, J. D. (1982). Behavioral health's challenge to academic, scientific, and professional psychology. *The American Psychologist, 37*(1), 1–14. https://doi.org/10.1037//0003-066x.37.1.1

Matthews, K. (1988). Coronary heart disease and type A behavior: Update on and alternative to the Booth-Kewley and Friedman (1987) quantitative review. *Psychological Bulletin, 104*, 373–380. https://doi.org/10.1111/j.1467-6494.2012.00802.x

Matthews, K.A., Katholi, C.R., McCreath, H., Whooley, M.A., Williams, D.R., Zhu, S., & Markovitz, J.H. (2004). Blood pressure reactivity to psychological stress predicts hypertension in the CARDIA Study. *Circulation, 110*, 74–78. https://doi.org/10.1161/01.cir.0000133415.37578.e4

Matthews, K.A., Woodall, K.L., Kenyon, K., & Jacob, T. (1996) Negative family environment as a predictor of boys' future status on measures of hostile attitudes, interview behaviour and anger expression. *Health Psychology, 15*, 30–37. https://doi.org/10.1037//0278-6133.15.1.30

McCabe, P.M., Schneiderman, N., Field, T., & Wellens, A.R. (Eds.) (2000). *Stress, coping, and cardiovascular disease*. Mahwah, NJ: Lawrence Erlbaum.

McCrae, R.R., & Costa, P.T. (1987). Validation of the five-factor model of personality across instruments and observers. *Journal of Personality and Social Psychology, 54*, 81–90. https://doi.org/10.1037/0022-3514.52.1.81

McEachan, R., Taylor, N., Harrison, R., Lawton, R., Gardner, P., & Conner, M. (2016). Meta-analysis of the Reasoned Action Approach (RAA) to understanding health behaviors. *Annals of Behavioral Medicine, 50*, 592–612. https://doi.org/10.1007/s12160-016-9798-4

McEachan, R.R.C., Conner, M., Taylor, N.J., & Lawton, R.J. (2011). Prospective prediction of health-related behaviors with the Theory of Planned Behavior: A meta-analysis. *Health Psychology Review, 5*, 97–144. https://doi.org/10.1080/17437199.2010.521684

McEwen, B.S. (1998). Protective and damaging effects of stress mediators. *New England Journal of Medicine, 338*, 171–179. https://doi.org/10.31887%2FDCNS.2006.8.4%2Fbmcewen

McEwen, B.S., & Stellar, E. (1993). Stress and the individual: Mechanisms leading to disease. *Archives of Internal Medicine, 153*, 2093–2101. http://doi:10.1001/archinte.1993.00410180039004

McGowan, L., Luker, K., Creed, F., & Chew, G.C.A. (2007). "How do you explain a pain that can't be seen?": The narratives of women with chronic pelvic pain and their disengagement with the diagnostic cycle. *British Journal of Health Psychology, 12*(2), 261–274. https://doi.org/10.1348/135910706X104076

McLaughlin, J.A., & Jordan, G.B. (1999). Logic models: A tool for telling your programs performance story. *Evaluation and Program Planning, 22*(1), 65–72. https://doi.org/10.1016/S0149-7189(98)00042-1

McNeil, A.D., Jarvis, M.J., Stapleton, J.A., Russell, M.A.H., Eiser, J.R., Gammage, P., & Gray, E.M. (1988). Prospective study of factors predicting uptake of smoking in adolescents. *Journal of Epidemiology and Community Health, 43*, 72–78. https://doi.org/10.1136/jech.43.1.72

Meissner, M. (1971). The long arm of the job: A study of work and leisure. *Industrial Relations, 10*, 239–423. https://doi.org/10.1111/j.1468-232X.1971.tb00023.x

Melzack, R. (1999). From the gate to the neuromatrix. *Pain, Suppl. 6*, S121–S126. https://doi.org/10.1016/s0304-3959(99)00145-1

Melzack, R., & Wall, P.D. (1965). Pain mechanisms: A new theory. *Science, 50*, 971–979. https://doi.org/10.1126/science.150.3699.971

Menon, K., Mousa, A., de Courten, M.P., Soldatos, G., Egger, G., & de Courten, B. (2017). Shared medical appointments may be effective for improving clinical and behavioral outcomes in Type 2 diabetes: A narrative review. *Frontiers in Endocrinology, 8*, 263. https://doi.org/10.3389/fendo.2017.00263

Mercadante, A.R., & Law, A.V. (2021). Will they, or won't they? Examining patients' vaccine intention for flu and COVID-19 using the Health Belief Model. *Research in Social and Administrative Pharmacy, 17*, 1596–1605. https://doi.org/10.1016/j.sapharm.2020.12.012

Mercer, S.W., Fitzpatrick, B., Guthrie, B., Fenwick, E., Grieve, E., Lawson, K., Boyer, N., McConnachie, A., Lloyd, S.M., O'Brien, R., Watt, G.C., & Wyke, S. (2016). The CARE Plus study — a whole-system intervention to improve quality of life of primary care patients with multimorbidity in areas of high socioeconomic deprivation: Exploratory cluster question controlled trial and cost-utility analysis. *BMC Medicine, 14*(1), 88. https://doi.org/10.1186/s12916-016-0634-2

Merz, E.L., Fox, R.S., & Malcarne, V.L. (2014). Expressive writing interventions in cancer patients: A systematic review. *Health Psychology Review, 8*, 339–361. https://doi.org/10.1080/17437199.2014.882007

Michie, S., Miles, J., & Weinman, J. (2003). Patient-centredness in chronic illness: What is it and does it matter?. *Patient Education and Counseling, 51*(3), 197–206. https://doi.org/10.1016/s0738-3991(02)00194-5

Michie, S., & Wood, C.E. (2015). Health behaviour change techniques. In M. Conner & P. Norman (Eds.), *Predicting and changing health behaviour: Research and practice with social cognition models* (3rd Edn.; pp. 358–389). Maidenhead: Open University Press.

Mielewczyk, F., & Willig, C. (2007). Old clothes and an older look: The case for a radical makeover in health behaviour research. *Theory & Psychology, 17*, 811–837. https://doi.org/10.1177/0959354307083496

Milgram, S. (1974). *Obedience to authority: An experimental view.* Harper and Row.

Miller, G. A., Galanter, E., & Pribram, K. H. (1960). *Plans and the structure of behavior.* New York: Henry Holt and Co. https://doi.org/10.1037/10039-000

Miller, G.E., Cohen, S., & Ritchey, A.K. (2002). Chronic psychological stress and the regulation of pro-inflammatory cytokines: A glucocorticoid-resistance model. *Health Psychology, 21*, 531–541. https://doi.org/10.1037/0278-6133.21.6.531

Miller, S.M., & Mangan, C.E. (1983). Interacting effects of information and coping style in adapting to gynecologic stress: Should the doctor tell all. *Journal of Personality and Social Psychology, 45*, 223–236. https://doi.org/10.1037//0022-3514.45.1.223

Miller, S.M., Summerton, J., & Brody, D.S. (1988). Styles of coping with threat: Implications for health. *Journal of Personality and Social Psychology, 54*, 142–148. https://doi.org/10.1037//0022-3514.54.1.142

Miller, T.Q., Smith, T.W., Turner, C.W., Guijarro, M.L., & Hallet, A.J. (1996). A meta-analytic review of research on hostility and physical health. *Psychological Bulletin, 119*, 322–348. https://doi.org/10.1037/0033-2909.119.2.322

Miller, T.Q., Turner, C.W., Tindale, R.S., Posavac, E.J., & Dugoni, B.L. (1991). Reasons for the trend towards null findings in research on type A behavior. *Psychological Bulletin, 110*, 469–485. https://doi.org/10.1037/0033-2909.110.3.469

Milne, S., Orbell, S., & Sheeran, P. (2002). Combining motivational and volitional interventions to promote exercise participation: Protection motivation theory and implementation intentions. *British Journal of Health Psychology, 7*, 163–184. https://doi.org/10.1348/135910702169420

Mo, P.K.H., & Coulson, N. S. (2012). Developing a model for online support group use, empowering processes and psychosocial outcomes for individuals living with HIV/AIDS. *Psychology and Health, 27*, 445–449. https://doi.org/10.1080/08870446.2011.592981

Mokdad, A.H., Marks, J.S., Stroup, D.F., & Gerberding, J.L. (2004). Actual causes of death in the United States, 2000. *JAMA, 291*(10), 1238–1245. https://doi.org/10.1001/jama.291.10.1238

Mongkhon, P., Ashcroft, D.M., Scholfield, C.N., & Kongkaew, C. (2018). Hospital admissions associated with medication non-adherence: A systematic review of prospective observational studies. *BMJ Quality & Safety, 27*(11), 902–914. https://doi.org/10.1136/bmjqs-2017-007453

Moore, G.F., Audrey, S., Barker, M., Bond, L., Bonell, C., Hardeman, W., Moore, L., O'Cathain, A., Tinati, T., Wight, D., & Baird, J. (2015). Process evaluation of complex interventions: Medical Research Council guidance. *BMJ, 350*. https://doi.org/10.1136/bmj.h1258

Morisky, D.E., Green, L.W., & Levine, D.M. (1986). Concurrent and predictive validity of a self-reported measure of medication adherence. *Medical Care, 24*(1), 67–74. https://doi.org/10.1097/00005650-198601000-00007

Morley, S., Eccleston, C., & Williams, A. (1999). Systematic review and meta-analysis of randomized controlled trials of cognitive behaviour therapy and behaviour therapy for chronic pain in adults, excluding headache. *Pain, 80*(1–2), 1–13. https://doi.org/10.1016/s0304-3959(98)00255-3

Moscovici, S. (1976). *Social influence and social change*. Academic Press.

Moscovici, S., & Lage, E. (1976). Studies in social influence III: Majority versus minority influence in a group. *European Journal of Social Psychology, 6*(2), 149–174. https://doi.org/10.1002/ejsp.2420060202

Moskowitz J.T., Cheung E.O., Snowberg K.E., Verstaen A., Merrilees J., Salsman J.M., & Dowling G.A. (2019). Randomized controlled trial of a facilitated online positive emotion regulation intervention for dementia caregivers. *Health Psychology, 38*, 391–440. https://doi.org/10.1037%2Fhea0000680

Moskowitz, J.T., Epel, E.S., & Acree, M. (2008). Positive affect uniquely predicts lower risk of mortality in people with diabetes. *Health Psychology, 27*(1S), S73–S82. https://doi.org/10.1037/0278-6133.27.1.S73

Moss, R.H., Conner, M., & O'Connor, D.B. (2020). Exploring the effects of daily hassles on eating behaviour in children: The role of cortisol reactivity. *Psychoneuroendocrinology*, 104692. https://doi.org/10.1016/j.psyneuen.2020.104692

Mostofsky, E., Maclure, M., Sherwood, J.B., Tofler, G.H., Muller, J.E., & Mittleman, M.A. (2012). Risk of acute myocardial infarction after the death of a significant person in one's life: The Determinants of Myocardial Infarction Onset Study. *Circulation, 125*, 491–496. https://doi.org/10.1161/circulationaha.111.061770

Mullen, P.D. (1997). Compliance becomes concordance. *BMJ, 314*(7082), 691–692. https://doi.org/10.1136/bmj.314.7082.691

Mund, M., & Mitte, K. (2012). The costs of repression: A meta-analysis on the relations between repressive coping and somatic diseases. *Health Psychology, 31*, 640–649. https://doi.org/10.1037/a0026257

Murdoch, J., Salter, C., Ford, J., Lenaghan, E., Shiner, A., & Steel, N. (2020). The "unknown territory" of goal-setting: Negotiating a novel interactional activity within primary care doctor-patient consultations for patients with multiple chronic conditions. *Social Science & Medicine, 256*, 113040. https://doi.org/10.1016/j.socscimed.2020.113040

Murcott, T. (2006). *The whole story; Alternative medicine on trial?* UK Macmillan.

Murphy, L.R. (2003). Stress management at work: Secondary prevention of stress. In M.J. Schabracq, J.A.M. Winnubst, & C.L. Cooper (Eds.), *The handbook of work and health psychology* (pp. 533–548). Chichester: Wiley.

Myers, L.B., Vetere, A., & Derakshan, N. (2004). Are suppression and repressive coping related? *Personality and Individual Differences, 36*, 1009–1013. https://doi.org/10.1016/S0191-8869(03)00196-X

Myers, L.B., & Midence, K. (1998). Concepts and issues in adherence. In L.B. Myers & K. Midence (Eds.), *Adherence to treatment in medical conditions* (pp. 1–24). Harwood Academic Publishers.

Myrtek, M. (2001). Meta-analyses of prospective studies on coronary heart disease, type A personality, and hostility. *International Journal of Cardiology, 79*, 245–251. https://doi.org/10.1016/s0167-5273(01)00441-7

Nagler, R.H., Vogel, R.I., Gollust, S.E., Rothman, A.J., Fowler, E.F., & Yzer, M.C. (2020). Public perceptions of conflicting information surrounding COVID-19: Results from a nationally representative survey of U.S. adults. *PloS One, 15*(10), e0240776. https://doi.org/10.1371/journal.pone.0240776

National Institute of Health and Clinical Excellence (NICE) (2007). *Behaviour change at population, community and individual levels*. Public Health Guidance 6. London: NICE.

Neisser, U. (1967). *Cognitive psychology*. Hoboken, NJ: Prentice-Hall.

Netterstrom, B., Friebel, L., & Ladegaard, Y. (2013). Effects of a multidisciplinary stress treatment programme on patient return to work and symptom reduction: Results from a randomised, wait-list controlled trial. *Psychotherapy and Psychosomatics, 82*, 177–186. https://doi.org/10.1159/000346369

Newman, E., O'Connor, D.B., & Conner, M. (2007). Daily hassles and eating behaviour: The role of cortisol reactivity status. *Psychoneuroendocrinology, 32*, 125–132. https://doi.org/10.1016/j.psyneuen.2006.11.006

Newton, T.L., & Contrada, R.J. (1992). Repressive coping and verbal–autonomic response dissociation: The influence of social context. *Journal of Personality and Social Psychology, 62*, 159–167. https://doi.org/10.1037//0022-3514.62.1.159

Nezlek, J.B. (2001). Multilevel random coefficient analyses of event- and interval-contingent data in social and personality psychology research. *Personality and Social Psychology Bulletin, 27*, 771–785. https://doi.org/10.1177/0146167201277001

NHS (2023). *Acupuncture*. https://www.nhs.uk/conditions/acupuncture/

Nielsen, K., Randall, R., Holten, A.-L., & González, E.R. (2010). Conducting organizational-level occupational health interventions: What works? *Work & Stress, 24*(3), 234–259. https://doi.org/10.1080/02678373.2010.515393

Nielsen, M.B., Mearns, K., Matthiesen, S.B., & Eid, J. (2011). Using the Job Demands-Resources model to investigate risk perception, safety climate and job satisfaction in safety critical organizations. *Scandinavian Journal of Psychology, 52*, 465–475. https://doi.org/10.1111/j.1467-9450.2011.00885.x

Nielsen, N.R., & Brønbæk, M (2006). Stress and breast cancer: A systematic update on current knowledge. *Nature Clinical Practice Oncology, 3*, 612–620. https://doi.org/10.1038/ncponc0652

NIOSH (2013). NIOSH safety and health topic: Occupational Health Psychology, retrieved 3rd November 2022 from https://www.cdc.gov/niosh/topics/ohp/.

Noffsinger, E.B. (2009). *Running group visits in your practice*. Springer Science & Business Media.

Norman, P., & Conner, M. (2015). Predicting and changing health behaviour: Future directions. In M. Conner & P. Norman (Eds.), *Predicting and changing health behaviour: Research and practice with social cognition models* (3rd Edn.; pp. 391–430). Maidenhead: Open University Press.

Norman, P., & Parker, S. (1996). The interpretation of change in verbal reports: Implications for health psychology. *Psychology & Health, 11*(2), 301–314. https://doi.org/10.1080/08870449608400259

Norman, P., Boer, H., & Seydel, R. (2015). Protection motivation theory. In M. Conner & P. Norman (Eds.), *Predicting and changing health behaviour: Research and practice with social cognition models* (3rd Edn.; pp. 70–105). Maidenhead: Open University Press.

Norman, P., Griffin, B.L., & Conner, M. (2022). Applying an extended protection motivation theory to predict Covid-19 vaccination intentions and uptake in 50–64 year olds in the UK. *Social Science and Medicine, 298*, 114819. https://doi.org/10.1016/j.socscimed.2022.114819

Norman, P., Wilding, S., & Conner, M. (2020). Reasoned action approach and compliance with recommended behaviours to prevent the transmission of the SARS-CoV-2 virus in the UK. *British Journal of Health Psychology, 25*(4), 1006–1019. https://doi.org/10.1111/bjhp.12474

O'Brien, T.B., & DeLongis, A. (1996). The interactional context of problem-, emotion-, and relationship-focused coping: The role of the Big Five personality factors. *Journal of Personality, 64*: 775–813. https://doi.org/10.1111/j.1467-6494.1996.tb00944.x

O'Connor, D.B. (2020). The future of health behaviour change interventions: Opportunities for open science and personality research. *Health Psychology Review, 14*(1): 176–181. doi: 10.1080/17437199.2019.1707107

O'Connor, D.B., Aggleton, J.P., Chakarabati, D., Cooper, C.L., Creswell, C., Dunsmuir, S., Fiske, S.T., Gathercole, S., Gough, B., Ireland, J.L., Jones, M.V., Jowett, A., Kagan, C., Karanika-Murray, M., Kaye, L.K., Kumari, V., Lewandowsky, S., Lightman, S., Malpass, D., Meins, E., Morgan, B.P., Morrison Coulthard, L.J., Reicher, S.D., Schacter, D.L., Sherman, S.M., Simms, V., Williams, A., Wykes, T., & Armitage, C.J. (2020). Research priorities for the COVID-19 pandemic and beyond: A call to action for psychological science. *British Journal of Psychology, 111*, 603–629. https://doi.org/10.1111/bjop.12468

O'Connor, D.B., Armitage, C.J., & Ferguson, E. (2015). Randomized test of an implementation intention-based tool to reduce stress-induced eating. *Annals of Behavioral Medicine, 49*, 331–343. https://doi.org/10.1007/s12160-014-9668-x

O'Connor, D.B., Branley-Bell, D., Green, J., Ferguson, E., O'Carroll, R., & O'Connor, R.C. (2020). Effects of childhood trauma, daily stress and emotions on daily cortisol levels in individuals vulnerable to suicide. *Journal of Abnormal Psychology, 121*, 92–107. https://doi.org/10.1037/abn0000482

O'Connor, D.B., & Ashley, L. (2008). Are alexithymia and emotional characteristics of disclosure associated with blood pressure reactivity and psychological distress following written emotional disclosure? *British Journal of Health Psychology, 13*, 495–512. https://doi.org/10.1348/135910707X224496

O'Connor, D.B., Conner, M., Jones, F., McMillan, B., & Ferguson, E. (2009). Exploring the benefits of conscientiousness: An investigation of the role of daily stressors and health behaviors. *Annals of Behavioral Medicine, 37*, 184–196. https://doi.org/10.1007/s12160-009-9087-6.

O'Connor, D.B., Ferguson, E., & O'Connor, R.C. (2005). Intentions to use hormonal male contraception: I role of message framing, attitudes and stress appraisals. *British Journal of Psychology, 96*(3), 351–369. https://doi.org/10.1348/000712605X49114

O'Connor, D.B., Green, J.A., Ferguson, E., O'Carroll, R.E., & O'Connor, R.C. (2018). Effects of childhood trauma on cortisol levels in suicide attempters and ideators. *Psychoneuroendocrinology, 88*, 9–16. https://doi.org/10.1016/j.psyneuen.2017.11.004

O'Connor, D.B., Hurling, R., Hendrickx, H., Osborne, G., Hall, J., Walklet, E., Whaley, A., & Wood, H. (2011). Effects of written emotional disclosure on implicit self-esteem and body image. *British Journal of Health Psychology, 16*, 488–501. https://doi.org/10.1348/135910710x523210

O'Connor, D.B., Jones, F., Conner, M., McMillan, B., & Ferguson, E. (2008). Effects of daily hassles and eating style on eating behaviour. *Health Psychology, 27*, S20–S31. https://doi.org/10.1037/0278-6133.27.1.s20

O'Connor, R.C., & O'Connor, D.B. (2003). Predicting hopelessness and psychological distress: The role of perfectionism and coping. *Journal of Counseling Psychology*, *50*, 362–372. https://psycnet.apa.org/doi/10.1037/0022-0167.50.3.362

O'Connor, D.B., & O'Connor, R.C. (2004). Perceived changes in food intake in response to stress: The role of conscientiousness. *Stress and Health*, *20*, 279–291. https://doi.org/10.1002/smi.1028

O'Connor, D.B., O'Connor, R.C., & Marshall, R. (2007). Perfectionism and psychological distress: Evidence of the mediating effects of rumination. *European Journal of Personality*, *21*, 429–452. https://doi.org/10.1002/per.616

O'Connor, D.B., O'Connor, R.C., White, B.L., & Bundred, P.E. (2000a). Job strain and ambulatory blood pressure in British general practitioners: A preliminary study. *Psychology, Health and Medicine*, *5*, 241–250. https://doi.org/10.1080/713690191

O'Connor, D.B., O'Connor, R.C., White, B.L., & Bundred, P.E. (2000b). The effect of job strain on British general practitioners' mental health. *Journal of Mental Health*, *9*, 637–654. https://doi.org/10.1080/jmh.9.6.637.654

O'Connor, D.B., Thayer, J.F., & Vedhara, K. (2021). Stress and health: A review of psychobiological processes. *Annual Review of Psychology*, *72*, 663–688. https://doi.org/10.1146/annurev-psych-062520-122331

O'Connor, D.B., Walker, S., Hendrickx, H., Talbot, D., & Schaefer, A. (2013). Stress-related thinking predicts the cortisol awakening response and somatic symptoms in healthy adults. *Psychoneuroendocrinology*, *38*, 438–446. https://doi.org/10.1016/j.psyneuen.2012.07.004

O'Driscoll, M. Brough, P., & Kalliath, T. (2006). Work-family conflict and facilitation. In: F. Jones, R.J. Burke & M. Westman (Eds.), *Work-life balance: A psychological perspective* (pp. 117–142). Hove: Psychology Press.

Office of National Statistics (2022). The National Statistics Socioeconomic Classification (NS-SEC). Retrieved 4th November 2022 from https://www.ons.gov.uk/methodology/classificationsandstandards/otherclassifications/thenationalstatisticssocioeconomicclassificationnssecrebasedonsoc2010

Ogden, J. (2003). Some problems with social cognition models: A pragmatic and conceptual analysis. *Health Psychology*, *22*, 424–428. https://doi.org/10.1037/0278-6133.22.4.424

Okello, D.R.O., & Gilson, L. (2015). Exploring the influence of trust relationships on motivation in the health sector: A systematic review. *Human Resources for Health*, *13*(1), 1–18. https://doi.org/10.1186/s12960-015-0007-5

Ong, A.D., Bergeman, C.S., Bisconti, T.L., & Wallace, K.A. (2006). Psychological resilience, positive emotions, and successful adaptation to stress in later life. *Journal of Personality and Social Psychology*, *91*, 730–749. https://doi.org/10.1037/0022-3514.91.4.730

Ong, A.D., & Leger, K.A. (2022). Advancing the study of resilience to daily stressors. *Perspectives on Psychological Science*, *17*, 1591–1603. https://doi.org/10.1177/17456916211071092

Orbell, S., Crombie, I., & Johnston, G. (1995). Social cognition and social structure in the prediction of cervical screening uptake. *British Journal of Health Psychology*, *1*, 35–50. https://doi.org/10.1111/j.2044-8287.1996.tb00490.x

Ormell, J., & Wohlfarth, T. (1991). How neuroticism, long-term difficulties, and life situation change influence psychological distress: A longitudinal model. *Journal of Personality and Social Psychology*, *60*, 744–755. https://doi.org/10.1037/0022-3514.60.5.744

Oskis, A., Smyth, N., Flynn, M., & Clow, A. (2019). Repressors exhibit lower cortisol reactivity to group psychological stress. *Psychoneuroendocrinology*, *103*, 33–40. https://doi.org/10.1016/j.psyneuen.2018.12.220

Osterberg, L., & Blaschke, T. (2005). Adherence to medication. *The New England Journal of Medicine*, *353*(5), 487–497. https://doi.org/10.1056/NEJMra050100

Ottaviani, C., Thayer, J.F., Verkuil, B., Lonigro, A., Medea, B., Couyoumdjian, A., & Brosschot, J.F. (2016). Physiological concomitants of perseverative cognition: A systematic review and meta-analysis. *Psychological Bulletin*, *142*, 231–259. https://doi.org/10.1037/bul0000036

Ozer, D.J., & Benet-Martinez, V. (2006). Personality and the prediction of consequential outcomes. *Annual Review of Psychology*, *57*, 401–421. https://doi.org/10.1146/annurev.psych.57.102904.190127

Pacheco-Barrios, K., Meng, X., & Fregni, F. (2020). Neuromodulation techniques in phantom limb pain: A systematic review and meta-analysis. *Pain Medicine*, *21*, 2310–2322. https://doi.org/10.1093/pm/pnaa039

Parker, H.W., Abreu, A.M., Sullivan, M.C., & Vadiveloo, M.K. (2022). Allostatic load and mortality: A systematic review and meta-analysis. *American Journal of Preventive Medicine*, *63*, 131–140. https://doi.org/10.1016/j.amepre.2022.02.003

Patten, S.B. (1991). Are the Brown and Harris "vulnerability factors" risk factors for depression?. *Journal of Psychiatry & Neuroscience*, *16*(5), 267–271.

Paulussen, T., Kok, G., & Schaalma, H. (1994). Antecedents to adoption of classroom-based AIDS education in secondary schools. *Health Education Research*, *9*(4), 485–496. https://doi.org/10.1093/her/9.4.485

Payne, S., Large, S., Jarrett, N., & Turner, P. (2000). Written information given to patients and families by palliative care units: A national survey. *Lancet, 355*(9217), 1792. https://doi.org/10.1016/S0140-6736(00) 02272-8

Pearson, M., Chilton, R., Wyatt, K., Abraham, C., Ford, T., Woods, H., & Anderson, R. (2015). Implementing health promotion programmes in schools: A realist systematic review of research and experience in the United Kingdom. *Implementation Science, 10*(1), 149. https://doi.org/10.1186/s13012-015-0338-6

Pena-Gralle, A., Talbot, D., Duchaine, C.S., Lavigne-Robichaud, M., Trudel, X., Aubé, K., Gralle, M., Gilbert-Ouimet, M., Milot, A., & Brisson, C. (2022). Job strain and effort-reward imbalance as risk factors for type 2 diabetes mellitus: A systematic review and meta-analysis of prospective studies. *Scandinavian Journal of Work, Environment & Health, 48*, 5–20. https://doi.org/10.5271/sjweh.3987

Pendleton, D., Schofield, T., Tate, P., & Havelock, P. (1984). *The consultation: An approach to learning and teaching.* Oxford University Press.

Penley, J.A., & Tomaka, J. (2002). Associations among the Big Five, emotional responses and coping with acute stress. *Personality and Individual Differences, 32*, 1215–1128. https://doi.org/10.1016/S0191-8869(01) 00087-3

Pennebaker, J.W. (1997). Writing about emotional experiences as a therapeutic process. *Psychological Science, 8*, 162–166. https://doi.org/10.1111/j.1467-9280.1997.tb00403.x

Peters, G.J., Ruiter, R.A., & Kok, G. (2013). Threatening communication: A critical re-analysis and a revised meta-analytic test of fear appeal theory. *Health Psychology Review, 7*(Suppl 1), S8–S31. https://doi.org/10. 1080/17437199.2012.703527

Peterson, C. (2000). The future of optimism. *American Psychologist, 55*, 44–55. https://doi.org/10.1037/0003-066X.55.1.44

Peterson, C., & Seligman, M.E.P. (1987). Explanatory style and illness. *Journal of Personality, 55*, 237–265. https://doi.org/10.1111/j.1467-6494.1987.tb00436.x

Peterson, C., Vaillant, G.E., & Seligman, M.E.P. (1988). Pessimistic explanatory style is a risk factor for physical illness: A thirty-five-year longitudinal study. *Journal of Personality and Social Psychology, 55*, 23–27. https://doi.org/10.1037//0022-3514.55.1.23

Petrie, K.J., Fontanilla, I., Thomas, M.G., Booth, R.J., & Pennebaker, J.W. (2004). Effect of written emotional expression on immune function in patients with human immunodeficiency virus infection: A randomised trial. *Psychosomatic Medicine, 66*, 272–275. https://doi.org/10.1097/01.psy.0000116782.49850.d3

Petticrew, M.P., Lee, K., & McKee, M. (2012) Type A behavior pattern and coronary heart disease: Philip Morris's "Crown Jewel". *American Journal of Public Health, 102*, 2018–2025. https://doi.org/10.2105/ AJPH.2012.300816

Petty, R.E., Briñol, P., & Tormala, Z.L. (2002). Thought confidence as a determinant of persuasion: I self-validation hypothesis. *Journal of Personality and Social Psychology, 82*(5), 722–741. https://doi. org/10.1037//0022-3514.82.5.722

Petty, R.E., & Cacioppo, J.T. (1986). The elaboration likelihood model of persuasion. In L. Berkowitz (Ed.), *Advances in experimental social psychology* (Vol. 19, pp. 123–205). Academic Press. https://doi.org/10.1016/ S0065-2601(08)60214-2

Phutrakool, P., & Pongpirul, K. (2022). Acceptance and use of complementary and alternative medicine among medical specialists: A 15-year systematic review and data synthesis. *Systematic Reviews, 11*(1), 10. https://doi.org/10.1186/s13643-021-01882-4

Piccinini, F., Martinelli, G., & Carbonaro. A. (2020). Accuracy of mobile applications versus wearable devices in long-term step measurements. *Sensors (Basel), 5*;20(21): 6293. doi: 10.3390/s20216293

Piet, J., Wurtzen, H., & Zachariae, R. (2012). The effect of mindfulness-based training on symptoms of anxiety in adult cancer patients and survivors: a systematic review and meta-analysis. *Journal of Consulting and Clinical Psychology, 6*, 1007–1020. https://doi.org/10.1037/a0028329

Pollock, K. (1988). On the nature of social stress: Production of a modern mythology. *Social Science and Medicine, 26*, 381–391. https://doi.org/10.1016/0277-9536(88)90404-2

Pollock, K. (2002). *Concordance in medical consultations: A critical review.* CRC Press.

Popper, K. (1963). *Conjecture and refutation.* London: Routledge.

Porter, M. (2004). Deciding to consult. In B. Alder, M. Porter, C. Abraham, & E. van Teijlingen (Eds. 2nd ed.), *Psychology and sociology: Applied to medicine* (pp. 86–87). Churchill Livingstone

Pratkanis, A.R. (2007). Social influence analysis: An index of tactics. In A.R. Pratkanis (Ed.), *The science of social influence: Advances and future progress* (pp. 17–82). Psychology Press.

Presseau, J., Ivers, N.M., Newham, J.J., Knittle, K., Danko, K.J., & Grimshaw, J.M. (2015). Using a behaviour change techniques taxonomy to identify active ingredients within trials of implementation interventions for diabetes care. *Implementation Science, 10*(1), 55. https://doi.org/10.1186/s13012-015-0248-7

Pressman, S.D., & Cohen, S. (2005). Does positive affect influence health? *Psychological Bulletin, 131,* 925–971. https://doi.org/10.1037/0033-2909.131.6.925

Pressman, S.D., Jenkins, B.N., & Moskowitz, J.T. (2019). Positive affect and health: What do we know and where next should we go? *Annual Review of Psychology, 70,* 627–650. https://pubmed.ncbi.nlm.nih.gov/30260746/

Prestwich, A., Conner, M., Lawton, R., Ward, J., McEachan, R., & Ayres, K. (2012). Randomized controlled trial of collaborative implementation intentions targeting working adults' physical activity. *Health Psychology, 31,* 486–495. https://doi.org/10.1037/a0027672

Prestwich, A., Sheeran, P., Webb, T., & Gollwitzer, P. (2015). Implementation intentions. In M. Conner & P. Norman (Eds.), *Predicting and changing health behaviour: Research and practice with social cognition models* (3rd Edn.; pp. 321–357). Maidenhead: Open University Press.

Prochaska, J.O., & DiClemente, C.C. (1984). *The transtheoretical approach: Crossing traditional boundaries of therapy.* Homewood, IL: Dow Jones Irwin.

Prochaska, J.O., DiClemente, C.C., & Norcross, J.C. (1992). In search of how people change: Applications to addictive behaviors. *American Psychologist, 47,* 1102–1114. https://doi.org/10.1037//0003-066x.47.9.1102

Prochaska, J.O., Velicer, W.F., Guadagnoli, E., Rossi, J.S., & DiClemente, C.C. (1991). Patterns of change: Dynamic topology applied to smoking cessation. *Multivariate Behavioral Research, 26,* 83–107. https://doi.org/10.1207/s15327906mbr2601_5

Proper, K.I., Koning, M., van der Beek, A.J., Hildebrandt, V.H., Bosscher, R.J., & van Mechelen, W. (2003). The effectiveness of worksite physical activity programs on physical activity, physical fitness, and health. *Clinical Journal of Sport Medicine, 13*(2), 106–117. https://doi.org/10.1097/00042752-200303000-00008

Protheroe, D., Turvey, K., Horgan, K., Benson, E., Bowers, D., & House, A. (1999). Stressful life events and difficulties and onset of breast cancer: Case control study. *British Medical Journal, 319,* 1027–1030. https://doi.org/10.1136/bmj.319.7216.1027

Prudenzi, A., Graham, C.D., Clancy, F., Hill, D., O'Driscoll, R., Day, F., & O'Connor, D.B. (2021). Group-based acceptance and commitment therapy interventions for improving general distress and work-related distress in healthcare professionals: A systematic review and meta-Analysis. *Journal of Affective Disorders, 295,* 192–202. https://doi.org/10.1016/j.jad.2021.07.084

Prudenzi, A., Graham, C.D., Flaxman, P., Wilding, S., Day, F., & O'Connor, D.B. (2022). A workplace acceptance and commitment therapy (ACT) intervention for improving healthcare staff psychological distress: A randomized controlled trial. *PLoS ONE, 17,* e0266357. https://doi.org/10.1371/journal.pone.0266357

Quinn, F., Chater, A., & Morrison, V. (2020). An oral history of health psychology in the UK. *British Journal of Health Psychology, 25*(3), 502–518. https://doi.org/10.1111/bjhp.12418

Quitkin, F.M., Rabkin, J.G., Gerald, J., Davis, J.M., & Klein, D.F. (2000). Validity of clinical trials of antidepressants. *The American Journal of Psychiatry, 157*(3), 327–337. https://doi.org/10.1176/appi.ajp.157.3.327

Ragland, D.R., & Brand, R.J. (1985). Coronary heart disease mortality in the western collaborative group study: Follow-up experience of 22 years. *American Journal of Epidemiology, 127,* 462–475. https://doi.org/10.1093/oxfordjournals.aje.a114823

Ramakrishnan, P., Yan, K., Balijepalli, C. & Druyts, E. (2021). Changing face of healthcare: Digital therapeutics in the management of diabetes. *Current Medical Research Opinion, 37*(12), 2089–2091. doi: 10.1080/03007995.2021.1976737

Randall, R., Griffiths, A., & Cox, T. (2005). Evaluating organizational stress-management interventions using adapted study designs. *European Journal of Work and Organizational Psychology, 14,* 23–41. https://doi.org/10.1080/13594320444000209

Rank, S.G., & Jacobson, C.K. (1977). Hospital nurses' compliance with medication overdose orders: A failure to replicate. *Journal of Health and Social Behavior, 18*(2), 188–193.

Reed, G.M., Kemeny, M.E., Taylor, S.E., Wang, H.-Y.J., & Vissher, B.R. (1994). Realistic acceptance as a predictor of decreased survival time in gay men with AIDS. *Health Psychology, 13,* 299–307. https://doi.org/10.1037/0278-6133.13.4.299

Reid, L.D., & Christensen, D.B. (1988). A psychosocial perspective in the explanation of patients' drug-taking behaviour. *Social Science and Medicine, 27,* 277–285. https://doi.org/10.1016/0277-9536(88)90132-3

Reis, F., Sá-Moura, B., Guardado, D., Couceiro, P., Catarino, L., Mota-Pinto, A., Veríssimo, M.T., Teixeira, A.M., Ferreira. P.L., Lima, M.P., Palavra, F., Rama, L., Santos. L., van der Heijden, R.A., Gonçalves, C.E., Cunha, A., & Malva, J.O. (2019). Development of a healthy lifestyle assessment toolkit for the general public. *Frontiers Medicine (Lausanne), 27*(6), 134. doi: 10.3389/fmed.2019.00134

Repetti, R.L., & Wood, J. (1997). Effects of daily stress at work on mothers' interactions with preschoolers. *Journal of Family Psychology, 11,* 90–108. https://psycnet.apa.org/doi/10.1037/0893-3200.11.1.90

Reynolds, J.S., & Perrin, N.A. (2004). Mismatches in social support and psychosocial adjustment to breast cancer. *Health Psychology*, *23*, 425–430. https://doi.org/10.1037/0278-6133.23.4.425

Rhodes, R., Janssen, I., Bredin, S., Warburton, D., & Bauman, A. (2017). Physical activity: Health impact, prevalence, correlates and interventions. *Psychology & Health*, *32*, 942–975. https://doi.org/10.1080/088704 46.2017.1325486

Rhodes, R.E., Courneya, K.S., & Hayduk, L.A. (2002). Does personality moderate the theory of planned behavior in the exercise domain? *Journal of Sport and Exercise Psychology*, *24*, 120–132. https://doi.org/10.1123/jsep.24.2.120

Riazi, A., Pickup, J., & Bradley, C. (2004). Daily stress and glycaemic control in Type 1 diabetes: Individual differences in magnitude, direction, and timing of stress-reactivity. *Diabetes Research and Clinical Practice*, *66*, 237–244. https://doi.org/10.1016/j.diabres.2004.04.001

Richardson, K.M., & Rothstein, H.R. (2008). Effects of occupational stress management intervention programs: A meta-analysis. *Journal of Occupational Health Psychology*, *13*, 69–93. https://doi.org/10.1037/1076-8998.13.1.69

Rietveld, S., & Prins, P. J. (1998). The relationship between negative emotions and acute subjective and objective symptoms of childhood asthma. *Psychological Medicine*, *28*(2), 407–415. https://doi.org/10.1017/s0033291797006387

Rivis, A., & Sheeran, P. (2003). Descriptive norms as an additional predictor in the theory of planned behaviour: A meta-analysis. *Current Psychology*, *22*(3), 218–233. https://doi.org/10.1007/s12144-003-1018-2

Robinson, E.J., & Whitfield, M.J. (1985). Improving the efficiency of patients' comprehension monitoring: A way of increasing patients' participation in general practice consultations. *Social Science & Medicine*, *21*(8), 915–919. https://doi.org/10.1016/0277-9536(85)90148-0

Robinson, H., Jarrett, P., Vedhara, K., & Broadbent, E. (2017). The effects of expressive writing before or after punch biopsy on wound healing. *Brain, Behavior & Immunity*, 61, 217–227. https://doi.org/10.1016/j.jpsychores.2022.110987

Robinson, M., & Savic, A. (2019) *Creating better content for users with low health literacy. NHS Digital.* https://digital.nhs.uk/blog/transformation-blog/2019/creating-better-content-for-users-with-low-health-literacy

Rodrigues A.M., O'Brien N., French D.P., Glidewell L., & Sniehotta F.F. (2015). The question–behavior effect: Genuine effect or spurious phenomenon? A systematic review of randomized controlled trials with meta-analyses. *Health Psychology*, *34*, 61–78. https://doi.org/10.1037/hea0000104

Roediger, H. L., 3rd, & Karpicke, J. D. (2006). The power of testing memory: basic research and implications for educational practice. *Perspectives on Psychological Science*, *1*(3), 181–210. https://doi.org/10.1111/j.1745-6916.2006.00012.x

Rogers, E.M. (2003). *Diffusion of innovations* (5th ed.). Free Press

Rollo S., & Prapavessis, H. (2020). A combined health action process approach and mHealth intervention to increase non-sedentary behaviours in office-working adults–A randomised controlled trial. *Applied Psychology, Health & Well Being*, *12*(3), 660–686. https://doi.org/10.1111/aphw.12201

Rondet, C., Parizot, I., Cadwallader, J.S., Lebas, J., & Chauvin, P. (2015). Why underserved patients do not consult their general practitioner for depression: Results of a qualitative and a quantitative survey at a free outpatient clinic in Paris, France. *BMC Family Practice*, *May 8*(16), 57. doi: 10.1186/s12875-015-0273-2

Rook, K.S. (1984). The negative side of social interaction: Impact on psychological well-being. *Journal of Personality and Social Psychology*, *46*, 1097–1108. https://doi.org/10.1037//0022-3514.46.5.1097

Rosen, M.I., Rigsby, M.O., Salahi, J.T., Ryan, C.E., & Cramer, J.A. (2004). Electronic monitoring and counseling to improve medication adherence. *Behaviour Research and Therapy*, *42*(4), 409–422. https://doi.org/10.1016/S0005-7967(03)00149-9

Rosenman, R.H., Brand, R.J., Sholtz, R.I., & Friedman, M. (1976). Multivariate prediction of coronary heart disease during 8.5 year follow-up in the western collaborative group study. *American Journal of Cardiology*, *37*, 903–910. https://doi.org/10.1016/0002-9149(76)90117-x.

Rosenman, R.H., Friedman, M., Straus, R., Wurm, M., Kositchek, R., Hahn, W., & Werthessen, N.T. (1964). A predictive study of coronary heart disease. *Journal of the American Medical Association*, *189*, 15–22. https://doi.org/10.1001/jama.1964.03070010021004

Rosenstock, I.M., Strecher, V.J., & Becker, M.H. (1988). Social learning theory and the health belief model. *Health Education Quarterly*, *15*, 175–183. https://doi.org/10.1177/109019818801500203

Rosenthal, R., & Rubin, D.B. (1982). A simple, general purpose display of magnitude of experimental effect. *Journal of Educational Psychology*, *74*(2), 166–169. https://doi.org/10.1037/0022-0663.74.2.166

Roter, D.L., Hall, J.A., Merisca, R., Nordstrom, B., Cretin, D., & Svarstad, B. (1998). Effectiveness of interventions to improve patient compliance: A meta-analysis. *Medical Care*, *36*(8), 1138–1161. https://doi.org/10.1097/00005650-199808000-00004

Rothman, A.J., Salovey, P., Antone, C., Keough, K., & Martin, C.D. (1993). The influence of message framing on intentions to perform health behaviors. *Journal of Experimental Social Psychology*, *29*(5), 408–433. https://doi.org/10.1006/jesp.1993.1019

Rothman, A.J., & Sheeran, P. (2021). The operating conditions framework: Integrating mechanisms and moderators in health behavior interventions. *Health Psychology*, *40*(12), 845–857. https://doi.org/10.1037/hea0001026

Rovelli, M., Palmeri, D., Vossler, E., Bartus, S., Hull, D., & Schweizer, R. (1989). Noncompliance in organ transplant recipients. *Transplantation Proceedings*, *21*(1), 833–834.

Royal College of General Practitioners (2020). Top 10 tips for successful GP video consultations. https://www.rcgp.org.uk/blog/covid-19-video-consultations

Ruiter, R.A.C., Abraham, C., & Kok, G. (2001). Scary warnings and rational precautions: A review of the psychology of fear appeals. *Psychology & Health*, *16*(6), 613–630. https://doi.org/10.1080/08870440108405863

Ruiter, R., Crutzen, R., de Leeuw, E., & Kok, G. (2020). Changing behavior using theories at the interpersonal, organizational, community, and societal levels. In M. Hagger, L. Cameron, K. Hamilton, N. Hankonen, & T. Lintunen (Eds.), *The handbook of behavior change* (Cambridge Handbooks in Psychology, pp. 251–266). Cambridge: Cambridge University Press. https://10.1017/9781108677318.018

Rush, K.L., Howlett, L., Munro, A., & Burton, L. (2018). Videoconference compared to telephone in healthcare delivery: A systematic review. *International Journal of Medical Information*, *118*, 44–53. doi: 10.1016/j.ijmedinf.2018.07.007

Ruskin, D.A., Dentakos, S., Craig, S., Campbell, F., Isaac, L., Stinson, J., Tyreell, J., Lyon, R.E., O'Connor, K., & Brown, S.C. (2022). Don't judge a book by its cover: Exploring low self-reported distress and repressive coping in a pediatric chronic pain population. *Journal of Child Health*, in press. https://doi.org/10.1177/13674935221096925

Rutledge, T., & Hogan, B.E. (2002). A quantitative review of prospective evidence linking psychological factors with hypertension development. *Psychosomatic Medicine*, *64*, 758–766. https://doi.org/10.1097/01.psy.0000031578.42041.1c

Rymarczyk, K., Turbacz, A., Strus, W., & Cieciuch, J. (2020). Type C personality: Conceptual refinement and preliminary operationalization. *Frontiers in Psychology*, *11*, 2369. https://doi.org/10.3389/fpsyg.2020.552740

Sackett, D.L., & Snow, J.C. (1979). The magnitude of compliance and non-compliance. In R.B. Haynes, D.W. Taylor, & D.L. Sackett (Eds.), *Compliance in health care* (pp. 11–22). Johns Hopkins University Press.

Sandhu, H.K., Booth, K., Furlan, A.D., Shaw, J., Carnes, D., Taylor, S.J.C., Abraham, C., Alleyne, S., Balasubramanian, S., Betteley, L., Haywood, K.L., Iglesias-Urrutia, C.P., Krishnan, S., Lall, R., Manca, A., Mistry, D., Newton, S., Noyes, J., Nichols, V., Padfield, E., . . . Underwood, M. (2023). Reducing opioid use for chronic pain with a group-based intervention: A randomized clinical trial. *JAMA*, *329*(20), 1745–1756. https://doi.org/10.1001/jama.2023.6454

Sapolsky, R.M. (1993). Endocrinology alfresco: Psychoendocrine studies of wild baboons. *Recent Progress in Hormone Research*, *48*, 437–468. https://doi.org/10.1016/b978-0-12-571148-7.50020-8

Sara, J.D., Prasad, M., Eleid, M.F., Zhang, M., Widmer, R.J., & Lerman, A. (2018). Association between work-related stress and coronary heart disease: A review of prospective studies through the Job Strain, Effort-Reward Balance, and Organizational Justice models. *Journal of the American Heart Association*, *7*, e008073. https://doi.org/10.1161%2FJAHA.117.008073

Sarafino, E. (2008). *Health psychology: Biopsychosocial interaction*, (6th Edn.). New York: Wiley. ISBN-13: 978-0470129166.

Sargent, R.P., Shepard, R.M., & Glantz, S.A. (2004). Reduced incidence of admissions for myocardial infarction associated with public smoking ban: Before and after study. *BMJ*, *328*(7446), 977–980. https://doi.org/10.1136/bmj.38055.715683.55

Sarma, E.A., Silver, M.I., Kobrin, S., Marcus, P.M., & Ferrer, R.A. (2019). Cancer screening: Health impact, prevalence, correlates, and interventions. *Psychology & Health*, *32*, 1036–1072. https://doi.org/10.1080/08870446.2019.1584673

Savage, R., & Armstrong, D. (1990). Effect of a general practitioner's consulting style on patients' satisfaction: A controlled study. *BMJ*, *301*(6758), 968–970. https://doi.org/10.1136/bmj.301.6758.968

Scharloo, M., Kaptein, A.A., Weinman, J.A., Willems, L.N., & Rooijmans, H.G. (2000). Physical and psychological correlates of functioning in patients with chronic obstructive pulmonary disease. *The Journal of Asthma*, *37*(1), 17–29. https://doi.org/10.3109/02770900009055425

Schaufeli, W.B., Leiter, M.P., & Maslach, C. (2009). Burnout: 35 years of research and practice. *Career Development International*, *14*, 204–220. https://doi.org/10.1108/13620430910966406

Scheier, M.F., & Carver, C.S. (1987). Dispositional optimism and physical well-being: The influence of generalized outcome expectations on health. *Journal of Personality*, *55*, 169–210. https://doi.org/10.1111/j.1467-6494.1987.tb00434.x

Scheier, M.F., & Carver, C.S. (1992). Effects of optimism on psychological and physical well-being: Theoretical overview and empirical update. *Cognitive Therapy and Research*, *16*, 201–228. https://doi.org/10.1007/BF01173489

Scheier, M.F., Matthews, K.A., Owens, J., et al. (1999). Optimism and rehospitalization after coronary artery bypass graft surgery. *Archives of Internal Medicine*, *159*, 829–835. https://doi.org/10.1001/archinte.159.8.829

Scheier, M.F., Matthews, K.A., Owens, J., Magovern, G.J. Sr., Lefebvre, R.C., Abbott, R.A., & Carver, C.S. (1989). Dispositional optimism and recovery from coronary artery bypass surgery: The beneficial effects of physical and psychological well-being. *Journal of Personality and Social Psychology*, *57*, 1024–1040. https://doi.org/10.1037//0022-3514.57.6.1024

Scheier, M.F., Swanson, J.D., Barlow, M.A., Greenhouse, J.B., Wrosch, C., & Tindle, H.A. (2021). Optimism versus pessimism as predictors of physical health. A comprehensive reanalysis of dispositional optimism research. *American Psychologist*, *76*, 529–548. https://doi.org/10.1037/amp0000666

Scheier, M.F., Weintraub, J.K., & Carver, C.S. (1986). Coping with stress: Divergent strategies of optimists and pessimists. *Journal of Personality and Social Psychology*, *51*, 1257–1264. https://doi.org/10.1037/0022-3514.51.6.1257

Schinke, S.P., & Gordon, A.N. (1992). Innovative approaches to interpersonal skills training for minority adolescents. In R.J. DiClemente (Ed.), *Adolescents and AIDS: A generation in jeopardy.* (pp. 181–193). Sage Publications, Inc.

Schneider, G.M., Jacobs, D.W., Gevirtz, R.N., & O'Connor, D.T. (2003). Cardiovascular haemodynamic response to repeated mental stress in normotensive subjects at genetic risk of hypertension: Evidence of enhanced reactivity, blunted adaptation, and delayed recovery. *Journal of Human Hypertension*, *17*, 829–840. https://doi.org/10.1038/sj.jhh.1001624

Schulz, P., Schlotz, W., & Becker, P. (2011). *The Trier Inventory of Chronic Stress (TICS) – Manual* (W. Schlotz, supported by Google Translate, Trans.). Göttingen, Germany: Hogrefe. (Original work published 2004).

Schüz, B., Conner, M., Wilding, S., Alhwatan, R., Prestwich, A., & Norman, P. (2021). Do socio-structural factors moderate the effects of health cognitions on COVID-19 protection behaviours? *Social Science and Medicine*, *285*, 114261. https://doi.org/10.1016/j.socscimed.2021.114261

Schwartz, G.E. (1982). Testing the biopsychosocial model: The ultimate challenge facing behavioral medicine? *Journal of Consulting and Clinical Psychology*, *50*(6), 1040–1053. https://doi.org/10.1037//0022-006x.50.6.1040

Schwartz, J.E., Neale, J., Marco, C., Shiffman, S.S., & Stone, A.A. (1999). Does trait coping exist? A momentary assessment approach to the evaluation of traits. *Journal of Personality and Social Psychology*, *77*, 360–369. https://doi.org/10.1037//0022-3514.77.2.360

Schwartz, M.D, Rimer, B.K., Daly, M., Sands, C., & Lerman, C. (1999). A randomized trial of breast cancer risk counseling: The impact on self-reported mammography use. *American Journal of Public Health*, *89*, 924–926. https://doi.org/10.2105/AJPH.89.6.924

Schwarzer, R. (2001). Stress, resources and proactive coping. *Applied Psychology: An International Review*, *50*, 400–407.

Schwarzer, R., & Luszczynska, A. (2015). Health action process approach. In M. Conner & P. Norman (Eds.), *Predicting and changing health behaviour: Research and practice with social cognition models* (3rd Edn.; pp. 252–278). Maidenhead: Open University Press.

Sears, S.R., Stanton, A.L., & Danoff-Burg, S. (2003). The yellow brick road and the emerald city: Benefit finding, positive reappraisal coping and posttraumatic growth in women with early-stage breast cancer. *Health Psychology*, *22*, 487–497. https://doi.org/10.1037/0278-6133.22.5.487

Seelig, D., Wang, A.L., Jagannathan, K., Loughead, J.W., Blady, S.J., Childress, A.R., Romer, D., & Langleben, D.D. (2014). Low message sensation health promotion videos are better remembered and activate areas of the brain associated with memory encoding. *PloS One*, *9*(11), e113256. https://doi.org/10.1371/journal.pone.0113256

Segerstrom, S.C., & O'Connor, D.B. (2012). Stress, health and illness: Four challenges for the future. *Psychology and Health*, *27*, 128–140. https://doi.org/10.1080/08870446.2012.659516

Segerstrom, S.C., & Smith, G.T. (2019). Personality and coping: Individual differences in responses to emotion. *Annual Review of Psychology*, *70*, 651–671. https://doi.org/10.1146/annurev-psych-010418-102917

Segerstrom, S.C., Taylor, S.E., Kemeny, M.E., & Fahey, J.L. (1998). Causal attributions predict rate of immune decline in HIV-seropositive gay men. *Health Psychology*, *15*, 485–493. https://doi.org/10.1037//0278-6133.15.6.485

Seligman, M.E.P. (2019). Positive psychology: A personal history. *Annual Review of Clinical Psychology*, *15*, 1–23. https://doi.org/10.1146/annurev-clinpsy-050718-095653

Selye, H. (1950). Stress and the general adaptation syndrome. *British Medical Journal*, *1*, 1383–1392. https://doi.org/10.1136%2Fbmj.1.4667.1383

Selye, H. (1956). *The stress of life*. New York: McGraw-Hill.

Shankar, A., McMunn, A., Banks, J., & Steptoe, A. (2011). Loneliness, social isolation, and behavioral and biological health indicators in older adults. *Health Psychology*, *30*, 377–385. https://doi.org/10.1037/a0022826

Sharp, D., Lorenc, A., Morris, R., Feder, G., Little, P., Hollinghurst, S., Mercer, S.W., & MacPherson, H. (2018). Complementary medicine use, views, and experiences: A national survey in England. *BJGP Open*, *2*(4), bjgpopen18X101614. https://doi.org/10.3399/bjgpopen18X101614

Sheeran, P., & Abraham, C. (2003). Mediator of moderators: Temporal stability of intention and the intention-behavior relationship. *Personality and Social Psychology Bulletin*, *29*, 205–215. https://doi.org/10.1177/0146167202239046

Sheeran, P., Abraham, C., & Orbell, S. (1999). Psychosocial correlates of heterosexual condom use: A meta-analysis. *Psychological Bulletin*, *125*(1), 90–132. https://doi.org/10.1037/0033-2909.125.1.90

Sheeran, P., Aubrey, R., & Kellett, S. (2007). Increasing attendance for psychotherapy: Implementation intentions and the self-regulation of attendance-related negative affect. *Journal of Consulting and Clinical Psychology*, *75*(6), 853–863. https://doi.org/10.1037/0022-006X.75.6.853

Sheeran, P., Bosch, J.A., Crombez, G., Hall, P.A., Harris, J.L., Papies, E.K., & Wiers, R.W. (2016). Implicit processes in health psychology: Diversity and promise. *Health Psychology*, *35*(8), 761–766. https://doi.org/10.1037/hea0000409

Sheeran, P., Klein, W.M.P., & Rothman, A.J. (2017). Health behavior change: Moving from observation to intervention. *Annual Review of Psychology*, *68*, 573–600. https://doi.org/10.1146/annurev-psych-010416-044007

Sheeran, P., Maki, A., Montanaro, E., Avishai-Yitshak, A., Bryan, A., Klein, W.M., Miles, E., & Rothman, A.J. (2016). The impact of changing attitudes, norms, and self-efficacy on health-related intentions and behavior: A meta-analysis. *Health Psychology*, *35*(11): 1178–1188. doi: 10.1037/hea0000387

Sher, L. (2004). Daily hassles, cortisol, and the pathogenesis of depression. *Medical Hypotheses*, *62*, 198–202. https://doi.org/10.1016/s0306-9877(03)00320-7

Sherif, M. (1936). *The psychology of social norms*. Harper.

Sherman, S.J. (1980). On the self-erasing nature of errors of prediction. *Journal of Personality and Social Psychology*, *39*, 211–221. https://doi.org/10.1037/0022-3514.39.2.211

Shipley, B.A., Weiss, A., Der, G., Taylor, M.D., & Deary, I.J. (2007). Neuroticism, extraversion, and mortality in the UK health and lifestyle survey: A 21-year prospective cohort study. *Psychosomatic Medicine*, *69*, 923–931. https://doi.org/10.1097/PSY.0b013e31815abf83

Siegel, P.A., Post, C., Brockner, J., Fishman, A.Y., & Garden, C. (2005). The moderating influence of procedural fairness on the relationship between work-life conflict and organizational commitment. *Journal of Applied Psychology*, *90*, 13–24. https://doi.org/10.1037/0021-9010.90.1.13

Siegler, I.C., Feaganes, J.R., & Rimer, K. (1995). Predictors of adoption of mammography in women under age 50. *Health Psychology*, *14*, 274–278. https://doi.org/10.1037/0278-6133.14.3.274

Siegrist, J. (1996). Adverse health effects of high-effort/low-reward conditions. *Journal of Occupational Health Psychology*, *1*, 27–41. https://doi.org/10.1037//1076-8998.1.1.27

Siegrist, J. (2012). Effort reward imbalance at work – Theory evidence and measurement. Retrieved 1st July 2023. https://www.uniklinik-duesseldorf.de/fileadmin/Fuer-Patienten-und-Besucher/Kliniken-Zentren-Institute/Institute/Institut_fuer_Medizinische_Soziologie/Dateien/ERI/ERI-Website.pdf

Silverman, J., Kurtz, S., & Draper, J. (2005, 2nd Edn.). *Skills for communicating with patients*. Radcliffe Medical Press.

Simpson, M., Buckman, R., Stewart, M., Maguire, P., Lipkin, M., Novack, D., & Till, J. (1991). Doctor-patient communication: The Toronto consensus statement. *BMJ*, *303*(6814), 1385–1387. https://doi.org/10.1136/bmj.303.6814.1385

Skinner, B.F. (1974). *About behaviorism*. Knopf.

Skinner, E.A., Edge, K., Altman, J., & Sherwood, H. (2003). Searching for the structure of coping: A review and critique of category systems for classifying ways of coping. *Psychological Bulletin*, *129*, 216–269. https://doi.org/10.1037/0033-2909.129.2.216

Skinner, T.C., Hampson, S.E., & Fife-Schaw, C. (2002). Personality, personal model beliefs, and self-care in adolescents and young adults with Type 1 diabetes. *Health Psychology*, *21*(1), 61–70. https://doi.org/10.1037/0278-6133.21.1.61

Sloan, D.M., & Marx, B.P. (2004). Taking pen to hand: Evaluating theories underlying the written disclosure paradigm. *Clinical Psychology: Science and Practice*, *11*, 121–137. https://doi.org/10.1093/clipsy.bph062

Smith, J.A., & Osborn, M. (2007). Pain as an assault on the self: An interpretative phenomenological analysis of the psychological impact of chronic benign low back pain. *Psychology & Health*, *22*(5), 517–534. https://doi.org/10.1080/14768320600941756

Smith, K.E., Mason, T.B., Schaefer, L.M., Anderson, L.N., Critchley, K., Crosby, R.D., Engel, S.G., Crow, S.J., Wonderlich, S.A., & Peterson, C.B. (2021). Dynamic stress responses and real-time symptoms in binge-eating disorder. *Annals of Behavioral Medicine*, *55*, 758–768. https://doi.org/10.1093/abm/kaaa061

Smith, K.J., & Victor, C. (2022). The association of loneliness with health and social care utilisation in older adults in the general population: A systematic review. *The Gerontologist*, *62*, e578–e596. https://doi.org/10.1093/geront/gnab177

Smith, T.W. (1994). Concepts and methods in the study of anger, hostility, and health. In A.G. Seigman & T.W. Smith (Eds.), *Anger, hostility and the heart* (pp. 23–42). Hillsdale, NJ: Lawrence Erlbaum.

Smith, T.W., Glazer, K., Ruiz, J.M., & Gallo, L.C. (2004). Hostility, anger, aggressiveness, and coronary heart disease: An interpersonal perspective on personality, emotion, and health. *Journal of Personality*, *72*, 1217–1270. https://doi.org/10.1111/j.1467-6494.2004.00296.x

Sniehotta, F.F., Presseau, J., & Araujo-Soares, V. (2014). Time to retire the theory of planned behaviour. *Health Psychology Review*, 8, 1–7. https://doi.org/10.1080/17437199.2013.869710

Snow, H. (1893). *Cancer and the cancer process*. London: J. and A. Churchill.

Snyder, C.R., Sympson, S.C., Ybasco, F.C., Borders, T.F., Babyak, M.A., & Higgins, R.L. (1996). Development and evaluation of the State Hope Scale. *Journal of Personality and Social Psychology*. 70, 321–335. https://doi.org/10.1037/0022-3514.70.2.321

Solberg, M.A., Gridley, M.K., & Peters, R.M. (2021). The factor structure of the Brief Cope: A systematic review. *Western Journal of Nursing Research*, 44, 612–627. https://doi.org/10.1177/01939459211012044

Solberg Nes, L., & Segerstrom, S.C. (2006). Dispositional optimism and coping: A meta-analytic review. *Personality and Social Psychology Review*, *10*, 235–251. https://doi.org/10.1207/s15327957pspr1003_3

Somerfield, M.R. (1997). The utility of systems models of stress and coping for applied research. *Journal of Health Psychology*, *2*, 133–151. https://doi.org/10.1177/135910539700200202

Somers, M.J., & Casal, J. (2021). Patterns of coping with work-related stress: A person-centred analysis with text data. *Stress and Health*, *37*, 223–231. https://doi.org/10.1002/smi.2990

Song, Z., Foo, M-D., Uy, M.A., & Sun, S. (2011). Unraveling the daily stress crossover between unemployed individuals and their employed spouses. *Journal of Applied Psychology*, *96*, 151–168. https://doi.org/10.1037/a0021035

Sonnentag, S., Binnewies, C., & Mojza, E.J. (2008). "Did you have a nice evening?" A day-level study on recovery experiences, sleep, and affect. *Journal of Applied Psychology*, *93*, 674–684. https://doi.org/10.1037/0021-9010.93.3.674

Sonnentag, S, & Zijlstra, F.R.H. (2006). Job characteristics and off-job activities as predictors of need for recovery, well-being, and fatigue. *Journal of Applied Psychology*, *91*, 330–350. https://doi.org/10.1037/0021-9010.91.2.330

Speed, B.C., Goldstein, B.L., & Goldfried, M.R. (2018). Assertiveness training: A forgotten evidence-based treatment. *Clinical Psychology Science and Practice*, *25*, e12216. https://doi.org/10.1111/cpsp.12216

Spittal, T.Y., LaMontagne, A.D., & Milner, A.J. (2020). Psychosocial work stressors and risk of all-cause and coronary heart disease mortality: A systematic review and meta-analysis. *Scandinavian Journal of Work, Environment and Health*, *46*, 19–31. https://doi.org/10.5271/sjweh.3854

Staines, G.L. (1980). Spillover versus compensation: A review of the literature on the relationship between work and non-work. *Human Relations*, *33*, 111–129. https://doi.org/10.1177/001872678003300203

Stajkovic, A.D., & Luthans, F. (1998). Self-efficacy and work-related performance: A meta-analysis. *Psychological Bulletin*, *124*(2), 240–261. https://doi.org/10.1037/0033-2909.124.2.240

Steele, C.M. (1988). The psychology of self-affirmation: Sustaining the integrity of the self. In L. Berkowitz (Ed.), *Advances in experimental social psychology* (Vol. 21, pp. 261–302). Academic Press. https://doi.org/10.1016/S0065-2601(08)60229-4

Steele, G.P., Henderson, S., & Duncan-Jones, P. (1980). The reliability of reporting adverse experiences. *Psychological Medicine*, *10*, 301–306. https://doi.org/10.1017/s0033291700044056

Steptoe, A., Dockray, S., & Wardle, J. (2009). Positive affect and psychobiological processes relevant to health. *Journal of Personality*, *77*, 1747–1776. https://doi.org/10.1111%2Fj.1467-6494.2009.00599.x

Steptoe, A., & Kivimaki, M. (2013). Stress and cardiovascular disease: An update on current knowledge. *Annual Review of Public Health*, *34*, 337–354. https://doi.org/10.1146/annurev-publhealth-031912-114452

Steptoe, A., & Marmot, M. (2005). Impaired cardiovascular recovery following stress predicts 3-year increases in blood pressure. *Journal of Hypertension, 23*, 529–536. https://doi.org/10.1097/01.hjh.0000160208.66405.a8

Steptoe, A., Shankar, A., Demakakos, P., & Wardle, J. (2013). Social isolation, loneliness, and all-cause mortality in older men and women. *Proceedings of the National Academy of Sciences, 110*, 5797–5801. https://doi.org/10.1073/pnas.1219686110

Steptoe, A., & Wardle, J. (2005). Positive affect and biological function in everyday life. *Neurobiology of Aging, 26*, S108–S112. https://doi.org/10.1016/j.neurobiolaging.2005.08.016

Steventon, A, Bardsley, M., Billings, J., Dixon, J., Doll, H., Hirani. S., Cartwright. M., Rixon, L, Knapp, M., Henderson, C., Rogers, A., Fitzpatrick, R., Hendy, J., & Newman, S. (2012). Whole System Demonstrator Evaluation Team. Effect of telehealth on use of secondary care and mortality: Findings from the Whole System Demonstrator cluster randomised trial. *BMJ, 344*, e3874. doi: 10.1136/bmj.e3874.

Stewart, M.A. (1995). Effective physician-patient communication and health outcomes: A review. *CMAJ, 152*(9), 1423–1433

Stewart, S-J., Moon, Z., & Horne, R. (2023). Medication nonadherence: Health impact, prevalence, correlates and interventions. *Psychology & Health, 38*, 726–765. https://doi.org/10.1080/08870446.2022.2144923

Stewart-Williams, S. (2004). The placebo puzzle: Putting together the pieces. *Health Psychology, 23*(2), 198–206. https://doi.org/10.1037/0278-6133.23.2.198

Stieger, M., Flückiger, C., Rüegger, D., Kowatsch, T., Roberts, T.W., & Allemand, M. (2021). Changing personality traits with the help of a digital personality change intervention. *Proceedings of the National Academy of Sciences, 118*(8), e2017548118. https://doi.org/10.3389/fpsyg.2020.552740

Stone, J., Aronson, E., Crain, A.L., Winslow, M.P., & Fried, C.B. (1994). Inducing hypocrisy as a means of encouraging young adults to use condoms. *Personality and Social Psychology Bulletin, 20*(1), 116–128. https://doi.org/10.1177/0146167294201012

Strack, F., & Deutsch, R. (2004). Reflective and impulsive determinants of social behavior. *Personality and Social Psychology Review, 8*, 220–247. https://doi.org/10.1207/s15327957pspr0803_1

Strickhouser, J.E., Zell, E., & Krizan, Z. (2017). Does personality predict health and well-being? A metasynthesis. *Health Psychology, 36*(8), 797–810. https://doi.org/10.1037/hea0000475

Stronks, K., van de Mheen, H., Looman, C.W.N., & MacKenbach, J.P. (1998). The importance of psychosocial stressors for socioeconomic inequalities in perceived health. *Social Science and Medicine, 46*, 611–623. https://doi.org/10.1016/s0277-9536(97)00206-2

Stults-Kolehmainen, M.A., & Sinha, R. (2014). The effects of stress on physical activity and exercise. *Sports Medicine, 44*, 81–121. https://doi.org/10.1007/s40279-013-0090-5

Sturgeon, J.A. (2014). Psychological therapies for the management of chronic pain. *Psychology Research and Behavior Management, 7*, 115–124. https://doi.org/10.2147/PRBM.S44762

Sultan, S., Epel, E., Sachon, C., Vaillant, G., & Hartemann-Heurtier, A. (2008). A longitudinal study of coping, anxiety and glycemic control in adults with type 1 diabetes. *Psychology and Health, 23*, 73–89. https://doi.org/10.1080/14768320701205218

Sutton, S. (1997). Predicting and explaining intentions and behavior: How well are we doing? *Journal of Applied Social Psychology, 28*, 1317–1338. https://doi.org/10.1111/j.1559-1816.1998.tb01679.x

Sutton, S. (2000). A critical review of the transtheoretical model applied to smoking cessation. In P. Norman, C. Abraham & M. Conner (Eds.), *Understanding and changing health behaviour: From health beliefs to self-regulation* (pp. 207–225). Reading: Harwood Academic Press.

Sutton, S. (2015). Stage theories. In M. Conner & P. Norman (Eds.), *Predicting and changing health behaviour: Research and practice with social cognition models* (3rd Edn.; pp. 279–320). Maidenhead: Open University Press.

Swaithes, L., Paskins, Z., Duffy, H., Evans, N., Mallen, C., Dziedzic, K., & Finney, A. (2021). Experience of implementing and delivering group consultations in UK general practice: A qualitative study. *The British Journal of General Practice, 71*(707), e413–e422. https://doi.org/10.3399/BJGP.2020.0856

Taber, J.M., Leyva, B., & Persoskie, A. (2015). Why do people avoid medical care? A qualitative study using national data. *Journal of General Internal Medicine, 30*(3), 290–297. https://doi.org/10.1007/s11606-014-3089-1

Takahashi, Y., Edmonds, G.W., Jackson, J.J.III, & Roberts, B.W. (2012). Longitudinal correlated changes in conscientiousness, preventative health-related behaviors, and self-perceived physical health. *Journal of Personality, 81(4)*, 417–427. https://doi.org/10.1037/gpr0000065

Tannenbaum, M.B., Hepler, J., Zimmerman, R.S., Saul, L., Jacobs, S., Wilson, K., & Albarracín, D. (2015). Appealing to fear: A meta-analysis of fear appeal effectiveness and theories. *Psychological Bulletin, 141*(6), 1178–1204. https://doi.org/10.1037/a0039729

Temoshok, L., Heller, B.W., Sagabiel, R., et al. (1985). The relationship of psychosocial factors to prognostic indicators in cutaneous malignant melanoma. *Journal of Psychosomatic Research, 29*, 139–154. https://doi.org/10.1016/0022-3999(85)90035-2

Theorell, T., & Rahe, R.H. (1971). Psychosocial factors and myocardial infarction: An inpatient study in Sweden. *Journal of Psychosomatic Research, 15*, 25–31. https://doi.org/10.1016/0022-3999(71)90070-5

Thorsen, H., Witt, K., Hollnagel, H., & Malterud, K. (2001). The purpose of the general practice consultation from the patient's perspective—Theoretical aspects. *Family Practice, 18*(6), 638–643. https://doi.org/10.1093/fampra/18.6.638

Tighe, S.A, Ball, K., Kensing, F., Kayser, L., Rawstorn, J.C., & Maddison R. (2020). Toward a digital platform for the self-management of noncommunicable disease: Systematic review of platform-like interventions. *Journal of Medical Internet Research, 22*(10), e16774. doi: 10.2196/16774.

Tolman, E.C. (1948). Cognitive maps in rats and men. *Psychological Review, 55*(4), 189–208. https://doi.org/10.1037/h0061626

Tolmunen, T., Lehto, S.M., Heliste, M., Kurl, S., & Kauhanen, J. (2010). Alexithymia is associated with increased cardiovascular mortality in middle-aged Finnish men. *Psychosomatic Medicine, 72*, 187–191. https://doi.org/10.1097/psy.0b013e3181c65d00

Triplett, N. (1898). The dynamogenic factors in pacemaking and competition. *The American Journal of Psychology, 9*(4), 507–533. https://doi.org/10.2307/1412188

Troy, A.S., Willroth, E.C., Shallcross, A.J., Giuliani, N.R., Gross, J.J., & Mauss. I.B. (2023). Psychological resilience: An affect-regulation framework. *Annual Review of Psychology, 74*, 547–576. https://doi.org/10.1146/annurev-psych-020122-041854

Turk, D.C., & Burwinkle, T.M. (2005). Clinical outcomes, cost-effectiveness, and the role of psychology in treatments for chronic pain sufferers. *Professional Psychology: Research and Practice, 36*(6), 602–610. https://doi.org/10.1037/0735-7028.36.6.602

Turk, D.C., & Salovey, P. (1986). Clinical information processing: Bias inoculation. In R.E. Ingham (Ed.) *Information processing approaches to clinical psychology* (pp. 305–323). New York: Academic Press.

Turner, J.C. (1991). *Social influence*. Open University Press.

Turner-McGrievy, G., Hutto, B., Bernhart, J.A., & Wilson, MJ. (2022). Comparison of the Diet ID Platform to the Automated Self-administered 24-hour (ASA24) dietary assessment tool for assessment of dietary intake. *Journal of the American Nutrition Association, 41*(4), 360–382. doi: 10.1080/07315724.2021.1887775

Tversky, A., & Kahneman, D. (1981). The framing of decisions and the psychology of choice. *Science, 211*(4481), 453–458. https://doi.org/10.1126/science.7455683

Twisk, J.W.R., Snel, J., Kemper, H.C.G., & van Mechelen, W. (1999). Changes in daily hassles and life events and the relationship with coronary heart disease risk factors: A 2-year longitudinal study in 27–29-year-old males and females. *Journal of Psychosomatic Research, 46*, 229–240. https://doi.org/10.1016/s0022-3999(98)00088-9

Tyler, R. (2001). BSE/'mad cow disease' crisis spreads throughout Europe. www.wsws.org/articles/2001/jan2001/bse-j23.shtml

Uchino, B.N. (2009). Understanding the links between social support and physical health: A life-span perspective with emphasis on the separability of perceived and received support. *Perspectives on Psychological Science, 4*, 236–255. https://doi.org/10.1111/j.1745-6924.2009.01122.x

Uchino, B.N., Bowen, K., Kent de Grey, R., Mikel, J., & Fisher, E.B. (2018a). Social support and physical health: Models, mechanisms, and opportunities. In E.B. Fisher, L.D. Cameron, A.J. Christensen, U Ehlert, Y. Guo, B. Oldenburg, & F.J. Snoek (Eds), *Principles and concepts of behavioral medicine* (pp. 341–372). New York, NY: Springer.

Uchino, B.N., Trettevik, R., Kent de Grey, R.G., Cronan, S., Hogan, J., & Baucom, B.R.W. (2018b). Social support, social integration and inflammatory cytokines: A meta-analysis. *Health Psychology, 37*, 462–471. https://doi.org/10.1037/hea0000594

Vaananen, A., Buunk, B.P., Kivimaki, M., Pentti, J., & Vahtera, J. (2005). When it is better to give than to receive: Long-term health effects of perceived reciprocity in support exchange. *Journal of Personality and Social Psychology, 89*, 176–193. https://doi.org/10.1037/0022-3514.89.2.176

van der Doef, M., & Maes, S. (1998). The job demand-control (-support) model and physical outcomes: A review of the strain and buffer hypotheses. *Psychology and Health, 13*, 909–936. https://doi.org/10.1080/08870449808407440

van der Doef, M., & Maes, S. (1999). The job demand-control (-support) model and psychological well-being: A review of 20 years of empirical research. *Work and Stress, 13*, 87–114. https://doi.org/10.1080/026783799296084

van der Klink, J.L., Blonk, R.W.B., Schene, A.H., & van Dijk, F.J.H. (2001). The benefits of interventions for work-related stress. *American Journal of Public Health, 91*, 270–276. https://doi.org/10.2105%2Fajph. 91.2.270

van Helvoort, D., Merckelbach, H., van Nieuwenhuizen, C., & Otgaar, H. (2022). Traits and distorted symptom presentation: A scoping review. *Psychological Injury and Law, 15*(2), 151–171. https://doi.org/10.1007/s12207-022-09446-0

van Hooff, M.L.M., Guerts, S.A.E., Beckers, D.G.J., & Kompier, M.A.J. (2011). Daily recovery from work: The role of activities, effort and pleasure. *Work and Stress, 25*, 55–74. https://doi.org/10.1080/02678373.2011.570941

van Vegchel, N.V., de Jonge, J., & Landsbergis, P.A. (2005). Occupational stress in (inter)action: The interplay between job demands and job resources. *Journal of Organizational Behavior, 26*, 535–560. https://psycnet.apa.org/doi/10.1002/job.327

van Vegchel, N.V., de Jonge, J., Meijer, T., & Hamers, J.P.H. (2001). Different effort constructs and effort-reward imbalance: Effects on employee well-being in ancillary health care workers. *Journal of Advanced Nursing, 34*, 128–136. https://doi.org/10.1046/j.1365-2648.2001.3411726.x

Vartiainen, E., Paavola, M., McAlister, A., & Puska, P. (1998). Fifteen-year follow-up of smoking prevention effects in the North Karelia Youth Project. *American Journal of Public Health, 88*(1), 81–85. https://doi.org/10.2105/AJPH.88.1.81

Vas, J., Méndez, C., Perea-Milla, E., Vega, E., Panadero, M.D., León, J.M., Borge, M.A., Gaspar, O., Sánchez-Rodríguez, F., Aguilar, I., & Jurado, R. (2004). Acupuncture as a complementary therapy to the pharmacological treatment of osteoarthritis of the knee: question controlled trial. *BMJ, 329*(7476), 1216. https://doi.org/10.1136/bmj.38238.601447.3A

Verkuil, B., Brosschot, J.F., Meerman, E.E., & Thayer, J.F. (2012). Effects of momentary assessed stressful events and worry episodes on somatic health complaints. *Psychology and Health, 27*, 141–158. https://doi.org/10.1080/08870441003653470

Verma. N., Buch, B., Taralekar, R. & Acharya, S. (2023). Diagnostic concordance of telemedicine as compared with face-to-face care in primary health care clinics in rural India: Randomized crossover trial. *JMIR Form Res., 23*(7), e42775. doi: 10.2196/42775

Vickers, A., & Zollman, C. (1999). ABC of complementary medicine. The manipulative therapies: Osteopathy and chiropractic. *BMJ, 319*(7218), 1176–1179. https://doi.org/10.1136/bmj.319.7218.1176

Victor, C.R., Scambler, S.J., Bowling, A., & Bond, J. (2005). The prevalence of, and risk factors for, loneliness in later life: A survey of older people in Great Britain. *Ageing and Society, 25*, 357–375.

Victor, C.R., & Yang, K. (2012). The prevalence of loneliness among adults: A case study of the United Kingdom. *Journal of Psychology, 146*, 85–104. https://doi.org/10.1017/S0144686X04003332

Villa, G., Lanini, I., Amass, T., Bocciero, V., Scire Calabrisotto, C., Chelazzi, C., Romagnoli, S., De Gaudio, A.R., & Lauro Grotto, R. (2020). Effects of psychological interventions on anxiety and pain in patients undergoing major elective abdominal surgery: A systematic review. *Perioperative Medicine, 9*, 38. https://doi.org/10.1186/s13741-020-00169-x

Vodovotz, Y., Barnard, N., Hu, F. B., Jakicic, J., Lianov, L., Loveland, D., Buysse, D., Szigethy, E., Finkel, T., Sowa, G., Verschure, P., Williams, K., Sanchez, E., Dysinger, W., Maizes, V., Junker, C., Phillips, E., Katz, D., Drant, S., Jackson, R. J., . . . Parkinson, M. D. (2020). Prioritized research for the prevention, treatment, and reversal of chronic disease: Recommendations from the Lifestyle Medicine Research Summit. *Frontiers in Medicine, 7*, 585744. https://doi.org/10.3389/fmed.2020.585744

Vollrath, M., Knoch, D., & Cassano, L. (1999). Personality, risky behaviour and perceived susceptibility to health risks. *European Journal of Personality, 13*, 39–50. https://doi.org/10.1002/(SICI)1099-0984(199901/02)13:1<39::AID-PER328>3.0.CO;2-J

Vollrath, M.E. (Ed.) (2006). *Handbook of personality and health.* Chichester: Wiley.

Wadsworth, K.H., Archibald, T.G., Payne, A.E., Cleary, A.K., Haney, B.L., & Hoverman, A.S. (2019). Shared medical appointments and patient-centered experience: A mixed-methods systematic review. *BMC Family Practice, 20*(1), 97. https://doi.org/10.1186/s12875-019-0972-1

Wakefield, D., Bayly, J., Selman, L.E., Firth, A.M., Higginson, I.J., & Murtagh, F.E. (2018) Patient empowerment, what does it mean for adults in the advanced stages of a life-limiting illness: A systematic review using critical interpretive synthesis. *Palliative Medicine, 32*(8), 1288–1304. doi:10.1177/0269216318783919

Waldron, I. (1988). Why do women live longer than men? *Journal of Human Stress, 2*, 2–13. https://doi.org/10.1080/0097840X.1976.9936063

Waldstein, S.R., Kauhanen, J., Neumann, S.A., & Katzel, L.I. (2002). Alexithymia and cardiovascular risk in older adults: Psychosocial, psychophysiological and biomedical correlates. *Psychology and Health, 17*, 597–610. https://doi.org/10.1080/08870440290025803

Walker, M. (2017). *Why we sleep*. London: Penguin Books.

Wang., C., Lê-Scherban, F., Taylor, J., Salmoirago-Blotcher, E., Allison, M., Gefen, D., Robinson, L., & Michael, Y.L. (2021). Associations of job strain, stressful life events, and social strain with coronary heart disease in the Women's Health Initiative Observational Study. *Journal of the American Heart Association*, *10*, e017780. https://doi.org/10.1161/jaha.120.017780

Wang, F., & Wang, J. D. (2021). Investing preventive care and economic development in ageing societies: Empirical evidences from OECD countries. *Health Economics Review*, *11*(1), 18. https://doi.org/10.1186/s13561-021-00321-3

Wang, S., Repetti, R.L., & Campos, B. (2011). Job stress and family social behaviour: The moderating role of neuroticism. *Journal of Occupational Health Psychology*, *16*, 441–456. https://doi.org/10.1037/a0025100

Wanless, D. (2002). *Securing our future health: Taking a long-term view*. HMSO.

Wardle, J., & Steptoe, A. (1991). The European and behaviour survey: Rationale, methods and initial results from the United Kingdom. *Social Science & Medicine*, *33*(8), 925–936.

Ware, J., Jr, Kosinski, M., & Keller, S.D. (1996). A 12-item short-form health survey: Construction of scales and preliminary tests of reliability and validity. *Medical Care*, *34*(3), 220–233. https://doi.org/10.1097/00005650-199603000-00003

Warr, P. (1987). *Work, unemployment and mental health*. Oxford: Oxford University Press.

Watson, D. (1988). Intraindividual and interindividual analyses of positive and negative affect: Their relation to health complaints, perceived stress, and daily activities. *Journal of Personality and Social Psychology*, *54*, 1020–1030. https://doi.org/10.1037//0022-3514.54.6.1020

Watson, D., & Clark, L.A. (1984). Negative affectivity: The disposition to experience aversive emotional states. *Psychological Bulletin*, *96*, 465–490. https://doi.org/10.1037/0033-2909.96.3.465

Watson, D., & Hubbard, B. (1996). Adaptational style and dispositional structure: Coping in the context of the five factor model. *Journal of Personality*, *64*, 737–774. https://doi.org/10.1111/j.1467-6494.1996.tb00943.x

Watson, D., & Pennebaker, J.W. (1989). Health complaints, stress and distress: Exploring the central role of negative affectivity. *Psychological Review*, *96*, 234–254. https://doi.org/10.1037/0033-295X.96.2.234

Webb, T.L., Miles, E., & Sheeran, P. (2012). Dealing with feeling: A meta-analysis of the effectiveness of strategies derived from the process model of emotion regulation. *Psychological Bulletin*, *138*(4), 775–808. https://doi.org/10.1037/a0027600

Weinberger, D.A., Schwartz, G.E., & Davidson, R.J. (1979). Low-anxious, high-anxious, and repressive coping styles: Psychometric patterns and behavioral and physiological responses to stress. *Journal of Abnormal Psychology*, *88*, 369–380. https://doi.org/10.1037//0021-843x.88.4.369

Werbrouck, A., Swinnen, E., Kerckhofs, E., Buyl, R., Beckwée, D., & de Wit, L. (2018). How to empower patients? A systematic review and meta-analysis. *Translational Behavioral Medicine*, *8*(5), 660–674. https://doi.org/10.1093/tbm/iby064

West, R. (2005). Time for a change: Putting the transtheoretical (stages of change) model to rest. *Addiction*, *100*, 1036–1039. https://doi.org/10.1111/j.1360-0443.2005.01139.x.

West, R. (2017). Tobacco smoking: Health impact, prevalence, correlates and interventions. *Psychology & Health*, *32*, 1018–1036. https://doi.org/10.1080/08870446.2017.1325890

West, R., McNeill, A., & Raw, M. (2000). Smoking cessation guidelines for health professionals: An update. Health Education Authority. *Thorax*, *55*(12), 987–999. https://doi.org/10.1136/thorax.55.12.987

Whelan J. (2002). WHO calls for countries to shift from acute to chronic care. *BMJ*, *324*(7348), 1237.

White, K.P. (2000). Psychology and complementary and alternative medicine. *Professional Psychology: Research and Practice*, *31*(6), 671–681. https://doi.org/10.1037/0735-7028.31.6.671

Whitlock, J.L., Powers, J.L., & Eckenrode, J. (2006). The virtual cutting edge: The internet and adolescent self-injury. *Developmental Psychology*, *42*, 407–417. https://doi.org/10.1037/0012-1649.42.3.407

Whittaker, A.C., Ginty, A., Hughes, B., Steptoe, A., & Lovallo, W.R. (2021). Cardiovascular stress reactivity and health: Recent questions and future directions. *Psychosomatic Medicine*, *83*, 756–766. https://doi.org/10.1097/psy.0000000000000973

WHOQOL Group (1995). The World Health Organization Quality of Life Assessment (The WHOQOL): Position paper from the World Health Organization. *Social Science & Medicine*, *41*(10), 1403–1409. https://doi.org/10.1016/0277-9536(95)00112-k

Wicke, P., & Bolognesi, M.M. (2020). Framing COVID-19: How we conceptualize and discuss the pandemic on Twitter. *PloS One*, *15*(9), e0240010. https://doi.org/10.1371/journal.pone.0240010

Wiedenfeld, S.A., O'Leary, A., Bandura, A., Brown, S., Levine, S., & Raska, K. (1990). Impact of perceived self-efficacy in coping with stressors on components of the immune system. *Journal of Personality and Social Psychology*, *59*(5), 1082–1094. https://doi.org/10.1037//0022-3514.59.5.1082

Wilding, S., Conner, M., Sandberg, T., Prestwich, A., Lawton, R., Wood, C., Miles, E., Godin, G., & Sheeran, P. (2016). The question-behaviour effect: A theoretical and methodological review and meta-analysis. *European Review of Social Psychology*, *27*, 196–230. https://doi.org/10.1080/10463283.2016.1245940

Wilding, S., O'Connor, D.B., Ferguson, E., Wetherall, K., Cleare, S., O'Carroll, R.E., Robb, K.A., & O'Connor, R.C. (2022). Information seeking, mental health and loneliness: Longitudinal analyses of adults in the UK COVID-19 Mental Health & Wellbeing Study. *Psychiatry Research*, *317*, 114876. https://doi.org/10.1016%2Fj.psychres.2022.114876

Wilkinson, R.G. (1996). *Unhealthy societies: I afflictions of inequality*. Routledge.

Williams, K.J., & Alliger, G.M. (1994). Role stressors, mood spillover, and perceptions of work-family conflict in employed parents. *Academy of Management Journal*, *37*, 837–868. https://doi.org/10.2307/256602

Williams, L., O'Connor, R.C., Howard, S., et al. (2008). Type D personality mechanisms of effect: The role of health-related behaviour and social support. *Journal of Psychosomatic Research*, *64*, 63–69. https://doi.org/10.1016/j.jpsychores.2007.06.008

Williams-Piehota, P., Latimer, A.E., Katulak, N.A., Cox, A., Silvera, S.A.N., Nowad, L., & Salovey, P. (2009). Tailoring messages to individual differences in monitoring-blunting styles to increase fruit and vegetable intake. *Journal of Nutrition Education and Behavior*, *41*, 398–405. https://doi.org/10.1016/j.jneb.2008.06.006

Williams-Piehota, P., Pizarro, J., Schneider, T.R., Mowad, L., & Salovey, P. (2005). Matching health messages to monitor-blunter coping styles to motivate screening mammography. *Health Psychology*, *24*, 58–67. https://doi.org/10.1037/0278-6133.24.1.58

Willis, T.A., O'Connor, D.B., & Smith, L. (2005). The influence of morningness-eveningness on anxiety and cardiovascular responses to stress. *Physiology and Behavior*, *85*, 125–133. https://doi.org/10.1016/j.physbeh.2005.03.013

Witte, K. (1992). Putting the fear back into fear appeals: The extended parallel process model. *Communication Monographs*, *59*(4), 329–349. https://doi.org/10.1080/03637759209376276

Witte, K., & Allen, M. (2000). A meta-analysis of fear appeals: Implications for effective public health campaigns. *Health Education & Behavior*, *27*(5), 591–615. https://doi.org/10.1177/109019810002700506

Wittrock, M.C., & Alesandrini, K. (1990). Generation of summaries and analogies and analytic and holistic abilities. *American Educational Research Journal*, *27*(3), 489–502. https://doi.org/10.3102/00028312027003489

Wolferz, R., Jr, Arjani, S., Bolze, A., & Frates, E.P. (2019). Students teaching students: Bringing lifestyle medicine education to middle and high schools through student-led community outreach programs. *American Journal of Lifestyle Medicine*, *13*(4), 371–373. https://doi.org/10.1177/1559827619836970

Wood, C., Conner, M., Sandberg, T., Taylor, N., Godin, G., & Sheeran, P. (2015). The impact of asking intention or self-prediction questions on subsequent behavior: A meta-analysis. *Personality and Social Psychology Bulletin*, *20*, 245–268. https://doi.org/10.1177/1088868315592334

Wood, R., & Bandura, A. (1989). Impact of conceptions of ability on self-regulatory mechanisms and complex decision making. *Journal of Personality & Social Psychology*, *56*(3), 407–415. https://doi.org/10.1037/0022-3514.56.3.407

Wood, W., Kallgren, C. A., & Mueller Preisler, R. (1985). Access to attitude-relevant information in memory as a determinant of persuasion: The role of message attributes. *Journal of Experimental Social Psychology*, *21*(1), 73–85. https://doi.org/10.1016/0022-1031(85)90007-1

World Health Organization (1948). *Preamble to the Constitution of the World Health Organization as adopted by the International Health Conference, New York, 19–22 June, 1946; signed on 22 July 1946 by the representatives of 61 States (Official Records of the World Health Organization, 2, 100) and entered into force on 7 April 1948*. https://hero.epa.gov/hero/index.cfm/reference/details/reference_id/80385

World Health Organization (2021). *Obesity and overweight*. June 9, 2021. https://www.who.int/news-room/fact-sheets/detail/obesity-and-overweight

Wright, C.C., Barlow, J.H., Turner, A.P., & Bancroft, G.V. (2003). Self-management training for people with chronic disease: An exploratory study. *British Journal of Health Psychology*, *8*(4), 465–476. https://doi.org/10.1348/135910703770238310

Xanthopoulu, D., Bakker, A.B., Demerouti, E., & Schaufeli, W.B. (2007). The role of personal resources in the job demand-resources model. *International Journal of Stress Management*, *14*, 121–141. https://psycnet.apa.org/doi/10.1037/1072-5245.14.2.121

Yalcin, S., Hurmuz, P., McQuinn, L., & Naing, A. (2017). Prevalence of complementary medicine use in patients with cancer: A Turkish comprehensive cancer center experience. *Journal of Global Oncology*, *4*, 1–6. https://doi.org/10.1200/JGO.2016.008896

Yates, L.B., Djoussé, L., Kurth, T., Buring, J.E., & Gaziano, J.M. (2008). Exceptional longevity in men: modifiable factors associated with survival and function to age 90 years. *Archives of Internal Medicine*, *168*(3), 284–290.

Zhang, C.-Q., Zhang, R., Schwarzer, R., & Hagger, M.S. (2019). A meta-analysis of the health action process approach. *Health Psychology, 38*(7), 623–637. https://doi.org/10.1037/hea0000728.supp

Zhang, J., Luximon, Y., & Li, Q. (2022). Seeking medical advice in mobile applications: How social cue design and privacy concerns influence trust and behavioral intention in impersonal patient–physician interactions. *Computers in Human Behavior, 130*, 107178. https://doi.org/10.1016/j.chb.2021.107178.

Zajenkowski, M., Jonason, P.K., Leniarska, M., & Kozakiewicz, Z. (2020). Who complies with the restrictions to reduce the spread of COVID-19?: Personality and perceptions of the COVID-19 situation. *Personality and Individual Differences, 166*, 110199. https://doi.org/10.1016/j.paid.2020.110199

Zautra, A.J., & Reich, J.W. (2011). Resilience: The meanings, methods, and measures of a fundamental characteristic of human adaptation. In S. Folkman (Ed.), *The Oxford handbook of stress, health and coping*. Oxford: Oxford University Press.

Zhu, P., Chen, C., Liu, X. Gu, W., & Shang, X. (2022). Factors associated with benefit finding and mental health of patients with cancer: A systematic review. *Support Care Cancer, 30*, 6483–6496. https://doi.org/10.1007/s00520-022-07032-3

Zola, I.K. (1973). Pathways to the doctor – From person to patient. *Social Science & Medicine, 7*(9), 677–689. https://doi.org/10.1016/0037-7856(73)90002-4

Zolnierek, K.B., & Dimatteo, M.R. (2009). Physician communication and patient adherence to treatment: A meta-analysis. *Medical Care, 47*(8), 826–834. https://doi.org/10.1097/MLR.0b013e31819a5acc

INDEX

For Product Safety Concerns and Information please contact our EU
representative GPSR@taylorandfrancis.com Taylor & Francis Verlag GmbH,
Kaufingerstraße 24, 80331 München, Germany

Printed and bound by CPI Group (UK) Ltd, Croydon, CR0 4YY
08/06/2025
01897009-0013